Adult-Gerontology Acute Care Nurse Practitioner Q&A Review

Dawn Carpenter, DNP, ACNP-BC, CCRN, is an assistant professor at the University of Massachusetts Medical School, Graduate School of Nursing, where she coordinates the Adult-Gerontology Acute Care Nurse Practitioner (AG-ACNP) program. Dr. Carpenter possesses a passion for educating acute and critical-care nurses and nurse practitioner (NP) students and has more than 25 years of experience as a critical-care nurse, NP, and faculty member. Dr. Carpenter maintains her advanced practice clinical skills as an acute care nurse practitioner in the surgical and trauma intensive care units at UMass Memorial Medical Center, the clinical partner of the Academic Medical Center.

As a faculty, Dr. Carpenter has developed an expansive curriculum teaching critical care content to diverse levels of nurses. She has developed and teaches a specialty curriculum for both nurses and AG-ACNP students who desire to specialize in critical care.

She is actively engaged at the national level with the National Organization of Nurse Practitioner Faculties (NONPF) and the American Association of Critical-Care Nurses (AACN). She has served as both an exam-item writer and participant on the exam-development committee for AACN. She is the cochairperson of the Acute Care Special Interest Group of NONPF and is a member of the preceptor development committee.

Adult-Gerontology Acute Care Nurse Practitioner Q&A Review

Dawn Carpenter, DNP, ACNP-BC, CCRN

Editor

SPRINGER PUBLISHING COMPANY

Springer Publishing Company, LLC
11 West 42nd Street
New York, NY 10036
www.springerpub.com

Acquisitions Editor: Elizabeth Nieginski
Compositor: diacriTech

ISBN: 978-0-8261-6478-0
ebook ISBN: 978-0-8261-6482-7

19 20 21 22 23 / 5 4 3 2

The author and the publisher of this Work have made every effort to use sources believed to be reliable to provide information that is accurate and compatible with the standards generally accepted at the time of publication. Because medical science is continually advancing, our knowledge base continues to expand. Therefore, as new information becomes available, changes in procedures become necessary. We recommend that the reader always consult current research and specific institutional policies before performing any clinical procedure. The author and publisher shall not be liable for any special, consequential, or exemplary damages resulting, in whole or in part, from the readers' use of, or reliance on, the information contained in this book. The publisher has no responsibility for the persistence or accuracy of URLs for external or third-party Internet websites referred to in this publication and does not guarantee that any content on such websites is, or will remain, accurate or appropriate.

The AACN and ANCC do not endorse any AG-ACNP exam review resources or have a proprietary relationship with Springer Publishing Company.

Library of Congress Cataloging-in-Publication Data
Names: Carpenter, Dawn, editor.
Title: Adult-gerontology acute care nurse practitioner Q&A review / Dawn
    Carpenter, editor.
Description: New York, NY : Springer Publishing Company, LLC, [2019] |
    Includes bibliographical references and index.
Identifiers: LCCN 2018028864 | ISBN 9780826164780 | ISBN 9780826164827
Subjects: | MESH: Nurse Practitioners–education | Geriatric
    Nursing–education | Critical Care Nursing–education | Test Taking Skills
    | Examination Questions
Classification: LCC RC954 | NLM WY 18.2 | DDC 618.97/0231076–dc23
LC record available at https://lccn.loc.gov/2018028864

Contact us to receive discount rates on bulk purchases.
We can also customize our books to meet your needs.
For more information please contact: sales@springerpub.com

Publisher's Note: New and used products purchased from third-party sellers are not guaranteed for quality, authenticity, or access to any included digital components.

Printed in the United States of America.

This book is dedicated to my current and former students, who have honed my skills as a teacher, coach, and mentor throughout the years. You have been the nidus for this book, providing the encouragement to fill a gap in available resources for AG-ACNP students and graduates. I excitedly encourage current and future students to continue to provide additional feedback and ideas for the next edition.

Contents

SECTION I: PREPARING FOR THE EXAMINATION

SECTION II: PRACTICE QUESTIONS—CLINICAL JUDGMENT/CLINICAL PRACTICE

SECTION III: PRACTICE QUESTIONS—ROLE, PROFESSIONAL RESPONSIBILITY, AND HEALTHCARE SYSTEMS

SECTION IV: COMPREHENSIVE PRACTICE EXAM

SECTION V: AFTER THE CERTIFICATION EXAM

Contributors

Jennifer Adamski, DNP, APRN, ACNP-BC, CCRN   Adult-Gerontology Acute Care Nurse Practioner Program Director and Assistant Professor, Critical-Care Nurse Practitioner, Emory University, Atlanta, Georgia

Kathleen Ballman, DNP, APRN, ACNP-BC, CEN   Associate Professor of Clinical Nursing and Coordinator, Adult-Gero Acute Care Nurse Practitioner Program, University of Cincinnati, College of Nursing, Cincinnati, Ohio

Dawn Carpenter, DNP, ACNP-BC, CCRN   Assistant Professor and Coordinator of Adult-Gerontology Acute Care Nurse Practitioner Track, University of Massachusetts Medical School, Graduate School of Nursing, Worcester, Massachusetts

Carla Carten, PhD   Assistant Vice Chancellor, Diversity and Inclusion Office, University of Massachusetts Medical School, Worcester, Massachusetts

Victoria Creedon, MS, ACNP-BC   Instructor, Adult Gerontology-Acute Care Nurse Practitioner Track, University of Massachusetts Medical School, Graduate School of Nursing, Worcester, Massachusetts

James Fain, PhD, RN, BC-ADM, FAAN   Associate Dean for Academic Affairs, University of Massachusetts Medical School, Graduate School of Nursing, Worcester, Massachusetts

Leanne H. Fowler, DNP, MBA, AG-ACNP-BC, CNE   Assistant Professor of Clinical Nursing and Director of Nurse Practitioner Programs, Coordinator of Adult-Gerontology Acute Care Nurse Practitioner Concentration, Louisiana State University–Health, New Orleans School of Nursing, New Orleans, Louisiana

Donna Gullette, PhD, APRN, AG-ACNP-BC, ACNP-BC   Associate Dean for Practice, College of Nursing, University of Arkansas for Medical Sciences, Little Rock, Arkansas

Carol Hartigan, MA, RN   Certification and Policy Strategist, American Association of Critical-Care Nurses, AACN Certification Corporation, Aliso Viejo, California

Joan E. King, PhD, ACNP-BC, ANP-BC, FAANP   Professor of Nursing, Vanderbilt University School of Nursing, Nashville, Tennessee

Stefanie La Manna, PhD, MPH, ARNP, AG-ACNP, FNP-C Associate Professor and Coordinator of Clinical Services, Advance Practice Registered Nursing Program, College of Nursing, Health Professions Division, Nova Southeastern University, Palm Beach Gardens, Florida

Kimberly Langer, DNP, APRN, CNP Assistant Professor, Adult-Gerontology Acute Care Nurse Practitioner Program Coordinator, Winona State University–Rochester, Rochester, Minnesota

Gail Lis, DNP, ACNP, BC Nurse Practitioner Program Director, Madonna University, Livonia, Michigan

Donna Lynch-Smith, DNP, ACNP-BC, APN, NE-BC, CNL Assistant Professor and Concentration Coordinator, Adult-Gerontology Acute Care Nurse Practitioner Program, University of Tennessee Health Science Center College of Nursing, Advanced Practice and Doctoral Studies Program, Memphis, Tennessee

Mary Anne McCoy, RN, PhD, ACNS, BC, ACNP-BC Assistant Professor (Clinical) and Graduate Specialty Coordinator, Adult-Gerontology Acute Care Nurse Practitioner Specialty, Wayne State University, College of Nursing, Detroit, Michigan

Anthony McGuire, PhD, CCRN-K, ACNP-BC, FAHA Professor and Chair, Nursing Department, and Nurse Practitioner Program Director, Saint Joseph's College of Maine, Standish, Maine

Beth McLear, RN, DNP, FNP-C, ACNP-BC Adult-Gerontology Acute Care Nurse Practitioner Track Coordinator, Augusta University, Athens, Georgia

Alexander Menard, MS, AG-ACNP Instructor, Adult-Gerontology Acute Care Nurse Practitioner Track, University of Massachusetts Medical School, Graduate School of Nursing, Worcester, Massachusetts

Helen Miley, RN, PhD, CCRN, AG-ACNP Specialty Director, Adult-Gerontology Acute Care Nurse Practitioner DNP Program, Rutgers School of Nursing, Newark, New Jersey

Dana Mitchell, DNP, ACNP-BC, CHFN Instructor, School of Nursing, Department of Acute, Chronic, and Continuing Care, Nurse Practitioner, Heart Failure Clinic, University of Alabama–Birmingham School of Medicine/UAB School of Nursing, Birmingham, Alabama

Hope Moser, DNP, RN, AG-ACNP, BC, ANP, BC, WHNP, BC, SCRN, CNRN, ANVP, BC Assistant Professor, Clinical Nursing, Kaplan University, Fort Lauderdale, Florida

Traci M. Motes, MNSc, APRN, AG-ACNP-BC Clinical Instructor, University of Arkansas for Medical Sciences, Little Rock, Arkansas

Nancy Munro, RN, MN, CCRN, ACNP   Faculty Associate, Georgetown University Graduate School of Nursing, Senior Acute Care Nurse Practitioner, Critical Care Medicine Department and Pulmonary Consult Service, National Institutes of Health, Bethesda, Maryland

Kenneth Peterson, PhD, FNP-BC   Assistant Professor, University of Massachusetts Medical School, Graduate School of Nursing, Worcester, Massachusetts

Stephanie Blackwell Pruitt, MSN, ACNP-BC, CCRN, BSN   Acute Care Nurse Practitioner Track Adjunct Faculty, University of Alabama–Birmingham School of Nursing, Birmingham, Alabama

Nikhil Raswant, MS, ACNP   Critical Care Nurse Practitioner, UMass Memorial Medical Center, Worcester, Massachusetts

Kristine Anne Scordo, PhD, RN, ACNP-BC, FAANP   Professor and Director, Adult-Gerontology Acute Care Nurse Practitioner Program, Wright State University, Dayton, Ohio

Audrey Snyder, PhD, RN, ACNP, FAANP, FAEN   Coordinator, Adult-Gerontology Acute Care Nurse Practioner Program, University of Northern Colorado, Greeley, Colorado

Mary Sullivan, DNP, ANP, ACNP   Assistant Professor and Coordinator, Adult-Gerontology Primary Care Track, University of Massachusetts Medical School, Graduate School of Nursing, Worcester, Massachusetts

Diane Fuller Switzer, DNP, ARNP, RN, FNP-BC, ENP-BC, ENP-C, CCRN, CEN, FAEN   Assistant Clinical Professor, Emergency Nurse Practitioner Harborview Medical Center, University of Washington, Seattle, Washington

Diane Thompkins, MS, RN   Manager, Accreditation Certification Department, American Nurses Credentialing Center, Silver Spring, Maryland

Major Damon Toczylowski, RN, MSN, CCRN, ACNP-C, CCNS, APNP   Acute Care Nurse Practitioner, Cardiothoracic/Pulmonary/Critical Care Services, David Grant Medical Center Travis Air Force Base, Fairfield, California

Carla C. Turner, DNP, CRNP, ACNP-BC   Instructor, School of Nursing, Department of Adult/Acute Health, Chronic Care and Foundations, University of Alabama–Birmingham, School of Nursing, Birmingham, Alabama

Christine Merman Woolf, PhD, EdS, MA   Assistant Professor, Department of Medicine, Director, Academic Enrichment Programs and Center for Academic Achievement, University of Massachusetts Medical School, Worcester, Massachusetts

Content Reviewers

Kathleen Ballman, DNP, APRN, ACNP-BC, CEN   Associate Professor of Clinical Nursing and Coordinator, Adult-Gero Acute Care Nurse Practitioner Program, University of Cincinnati, College of Nursing, Cincinnati, Ohio

Dawn Carpenter, DNP, ACNP-BC, CCRN   Assistant Professor and Coordinator, Adult-Gerontology Acute Care Nurse Practitioner Track, University of Massachusetts Medical School, Graduate School of Nursing, Worcester, Massachusetts

Janet Fraser Hale, PhD, RN, FNP   Professor and Associate Dean for Interprofessional and Community Partnerships, University of Massachusetts Medical School, Graduate School of Nursing, Worcester, Massachusetts

Stefanie La Manna, PhD, MPH, ARNP, AG-ACNP, FNP-C   Associate Professor and Coordinator of Clinical Services, Advance Practice Registered Nursing Program, College of Nursing, Health Professions Division, Nova Southeastern University, Palm Beach Gardens, Florida

Mary Anne McCoy, RN, PhD, ACNS-BC, ACNP-BC   Assistant Professor (Clinical) and Graduate Specialty Coordinator, Adult-Gerontology Acute Care Nurse Practitioner Specialty, Wayne State University, College of Nursing, Detroit, Michigan

Kristine Anne Scordo, PhD, RN, ACNP-BC, FAANP   Professor and Director, Adult Gerontology-Acute Care Nurse Practitioner Program, Wright State University, Dayton, Ohio

Foreword

Malcomb Knowles (1988) noted that the mission of education is to produce people who can apply their knowledge to changing conditions shaped by an explosion of information and a revolution in technology. He also observed that a fundamental competency relevant to people in all areas of knowledge is the need to engage in lifelong learning.

Educational psychologist Ausubel (1968) discussed the processes of scaffolding, or the acquiring of new knowledge by relating it to what is already known and developing a new and deeper understanding. *Scaffolding* refers to structural processes educators use to guide learners. Learning outcomes that integrate theoretical and clinical competencies have been especially meaningful when the volume and complexity of knowledge to be acquired are formidable.

Learning outcomes can be further refined using Bloom's taxonomy (Anderson & Kratwohl, 2001). Elaboration, and the later stages of Bloom's taxonomy, require an increasing depth of understanding. There are complicating factors, since many learners are strategic in choosing surface learning styles before they enter university courses. Even at the graduate level, students who know they will be tested on their acquisition of facts rather than their understanding of concepts will naturally choose a surface learning style. If the educator is aiming for a deeper level of understanding, it will be necessary to make sure that the assessment process does not derail these efforts (Newble & Entwistle, 1986).

What strategies and tools will help students learn to think, and not merely acquire information for a specific task or goal? *Adult-Gerontology Acute Care Nurse Practitioner Q&A Review* serves multiple important purposes for the adult-gerontology nurse practitioner (AG-ACNP) student, or for those AG-ACNPs preparing to take the initial certification exam or who need recertification. The essential areas addressed are exam preparedness, identification of knowledge gaps, practice questions that address diagnosing and treatment of conditions, recognition of complications, and clinical judgment. Practice questions follow the national certification template and include all areas of the exam: health promotion, cardiology, gerontology, pulmonary, neurology, renal, renal genitourinary, gastrointestinal, hematology, infectious disease, endocrine, musculoskeletal, integumentary, psychosocial, and multisystem.

Steps to achieve licensure, transition into practice and resources for employment searches, interview coaching, and negotiation strategies when an offer is made are discussed. Collaborative agreements, institutional credentialing, information on recertification, and transition into practice are also addressed.

One of the most significant contributions of this book is to allow educators to be facilitators for students as they go beyond their course of study, prepare for their standardized exam, and enter into their new practice roles. This book links learners to the critical resources needed for success.

Sheila Drake Melander, PhD, APRN, ACNP-BC, FCCM, FAANP, FAAN, MSN, DNP
Professor and Associate Dean
Graduate Programming and Faculty Practice
College of Nursing
University of Kentucky
Lexington, Kentucky

■ REFERENCES

Anderson, L. W., & Kratwohl, D. R. (2001). *A taxonomy for learning, teaching and assessing: A revision of Bloom's taxonomy of educational objectives.* New York, NY: Longman.

Ausubel, D. (1968). *Educational psychology: A cognitive view.* New York, NY: Holt, Rinehart and Winston.

Knowles, M. (1988). *The adult learner: A neglected species.* Houston, TX: Gulf.

Newble, D. I., & Entwistle, N. J. (1986). Learning styles and approaches: Implications for medical education. *Medical Educator, 20,* 162–175.

Preface

Welcome to the first edition of *Adult-Gerontology Acute Care Nurse Practitioner Q&A Review*. This book was created specifically for new AG-ACNP graduates to prepare for successful passage of the national certification examinations. It presents question styles and content material from both the American Association of Critical-Care Nurses (AACN) and American Nurses Credentialing Center (ANCC) exams. The questions in this book are written solely by faculty, many of whom have written questions for the certification exams. This book also provides detailed information to smooth the transition and successful entry into practice as a freshly board-certified AG-ACNP.

This book can also be used to support student education during the nurse practitioner educational program. Students can use this book to enhance study habits, hone test-taking skills, prepare for programmatic exams, reinforce knowledge, and avoid test-taking errors. Faculty can use these questions throughout their curriculum by integrating them into polling technology, classroom discussion, and pre- and posttest lecture to evaluate assimilation of knowledge.

The book is unique in that it provides an overview of the certification exams written specifically by representatives of the certification organizations themselves. These writers discuss key information relevant to the respective exams.

Distinctive to this book is a detailed, step-by-step process outlining the journey from classroom to exam room. Section I is written by an education specialist who is exceptional at coaching students to improve their study and test-taking habits. She outlines how best to prepare and study for the exam.

The largest section of the book contains practice questions that are tested on the exams. To reinforce your knowledge, each answer to the question includes a rationale explaining why it is correct. A practice exam that is representative in length, variety, and complexity of the board exam questions is provided, and can be taken in a timed format to assess your abilities under pressure.

The final section provides critical information in a step-by-step format to efficiently transition from a newly certified to gainfully employed AG-ACNP. Key information outlining the steps to obtain licensing, Federal Drug Enforcement Agency registration, and credentialing is detailed.

These questions will soon be integrated into a mobile device application for ease of access.

I am eager to receive feedback on this book and its questions and rationales, as well as suggestions for additions that can be incorporated into a future edition. Please send any comments, suggestions, feedback, or criticisms to Dawn Carpenter at Dawn.Carpenter@umassmed.edu.

Dawn Carpenter

Acknowledgments

This book could not have been possible without the networking opportunity provided by the National Organization of Nurse Practitioner Faculties (NONPF). NONPF provided access to magnificent faculty colleagues whose tremendous contributions are represented here. Everyone enthusiastically shared their expertise and diligently worked to meet deadlines.

I want to extend my sincerest gratitude to my colleagues who have supported this book. Specific recognition and appreciation go to Dr. Janet Fraser Hale, who provided me expert advice, never-ending encouragement, and tireless editing. You were my sounding board and constant cheerleader. You continually reinforced the vital need to fill a void in available materials and provided essential feedback and resources. Additionally, Ricardo Poza developed diagrams and formatted pictures for the book, and Victoria Rosetti provided assistance and education on endnotes. Thank you, Janet, Ricardo, and Victoria; I could not have done this without you!

The following students have contributed, reviewed, or pilot-tested materials in this book: Mary Chrabaszcz, Jacklyn Feeley, Elizabeth Ferguson, Ryan Flynn, Tyler Ingham, Nick Keeler, Megan Kennelly, Steven LoVerso, Susan Ludwig, Megan Miller, Kathryn Swider, Beatie Ultimo, and Caroline Yu. Thank you for being great students and for your patience and encouragement!

I want to specifically acknowledge Dr. Kristine Anne Scordo, who avidly and efficiently reviewed materials, quickly becoming the primary reviewer of the book. You tirelessly and expeditiously edited materials, willingly shared your expertise, and provided vital coaching and mentoring. Thank you, Kris; I learned so much from you!

Thanks to Elizabeth Nieginski and Rachel Landes at Springer Publishing Company for providing the opportunity to publish this book, and for patiently answering my many questions. You have made this project come to fruition. It has been a pleasure to work with you.

Most importantly, I am eternally grateful to my loving husband, Andy, who has unwaveringly supported my career. You have provided infinite love, patience, and sustenance to help make this book a reality—I love you!

Preparing for the Examination

1

Introduction to National Certification Examinations

DAWN CARPENTER, CAROL HARTIGAN, AND DIANE THOMPKINS

Congratulations on your successful completion of an adult-gerontology acute care nurse practitioner (AG-ACNP) program. Your program included content and experiences designed to prepare you for certification as an AG-ACNP. To obtain AG-ACNP certification, you must complete an accredited graduate program, have your application for certification testing approved, and successfully pass the certification examination. To ensure you pass the AG-ACNP certification exam on the first attempt, it is important to prepare thoroughly, honing not only your knowledge base, but also your test-taking skills. While your program provided a solid foundation, a breadth and depth of knowledge is needed to successfully pass the exam. We recommend that you use multiple modalities to prepare for the AG-ACNP exam, including a review of materials from your graduate courses, a comprehensive certification exam review course, and this book.

ABOUT THIS BOOK

This book is intended for AG-ACNP program students/graduates

- As preparation for quizzes and exams during their AG-ACNP programs
- To review and reinforce knowledge
- To prepare for the AG-ACNP certification exams
- As preparation for recertification by examination
- To provide knowledge for practice
- To identify knowledge gaps

Faculty can utilize the content

- For in-class review
- For pre- and posttest assessments

- To gather ideas for questions for programmatic exams
- For new faculty to learn how board exam questions are formatted

This book is NOT intended to:

- Replace comprehensive and detailed reading, in-depth studying, or mastery of content. In other words, this book is NOT the "Cliff Notes" for certifying exams.
- Be a diagnostic readiness exam, although there is a practice exam of similar length and complexity at the end of the book.
- Guarantee passing the certification exam. Mastery of these questions will help you prepare, but will not be the only material you will need to know or review to pass the exams.

The book format is structured into five major sections. Section I reviews how to prepare for the exams. Section II presents practice questions on clinical content, including diagnosing and treating conditions, as well as recognition of complications. This section tests your clinical judgment and is organized by physiologic systems. Section III presents practice questions focused on the AG-ACNP role, professional responsibilities, and healthcare systems. Section IV is a practice exam that mimics the national certification exams in length, difficulty, and variety of questions. Section V discusses next steps to achieve licensure and transition into practice once certified. This section provides resources on employment search, interview coaching, and negotiations once an offer is made. Last, Section V provides information on recertification and some words of wisdom as your progress into practice.

■ ROLE AND SCOPE OF PRACTICE OF THE AG-ACNP

To set the stage for certification exam preparation, it is critical to review the role, scope, and standards of practice for nurse practitioners (NPs) and specifics for the AG-ACNP. The *AACN Scope and Standards of Acute Care Nurse Practitioner Practice* (2017) and AG-ACNP *Competencies* (2016) define the practice for the AG-ACNPs.

Professional Role of the NP

The American Association of Nurse Practitioners (AANP) defines the professional role of NPs as follows:

> Nurse practitioners (NPs) are licensed, independent practitioners who practice in ambulatory, acute and long-term care as primary and/or specialty care providers. Nurse practitioners assess, diagnose, treat, and manage acute episodic and chronic illnesses. NPs are experts in health promotion and disease prevention. They order, conduct, supervise, and interpret diagnostic and laboratory tests, prescribe pharmacological agents and nonpharmacologic therapies, as well as teach and counsel patients, among other services. As licensed, independent clinicians, NPs practice autonomously and in coordination with healthcare professionals and other individuals. They may serve as healthcare researchers, interdisciplinary consultants, and patient advocates. NPs provide a wide-range of healthcare services to individuals, families, groups, and communities. (AANP, 2015)

Adult-Gerontology Acute Care Nurse Practitioner

The role, scope, and standards for practice for the AG-ACNP are clearly delineated by the American Association of Critical-Care Nurses (AACN) in the *AACN Scope and Standards of Acute Care Nurse Practitioner Practice* (2017) and the AG-ACNP *Competencies* (2016). The AG-ACNP is an APRN, educated at the graduate level to provide advanced nursing care to independently meet the specialized needs of adult-gerontology patients. The adult-gerontology population includes late adolescents, young adults, adults, and older adults.

AG-ACNP practice focuses on caring for patients who are:

- Physiologically unstable
- Technologically dependent
- Highly vulnerable to complications (AACN, 2017)

AG-ACNPs manage patients with:

- Acute health conditions
- Complex chronic health conditions
- Critical health conditions (AACN, 2017)

Patients may be experiencing:

- Episodic critical illness
- Stable chronic illness
- Acute exacerbation of chronic illness
- Acute injury and/or terminal illness (AACN, 2017)

AG-ACNPs provide a range of services to:

- Stabilize patient conditions
- Prevent complications
- Strive to restore an improved health state
- Transition the focus toward palliation and comfort (AACN, 2017)

This care is continuous and comprehensive across the variety of healthcare settings (AACN, 2018). It is important to recognize that the scope of practice (SOP) of the AG-ACNP is based upon patient acuity and needs, not a physical location or setting where the patient is seen. This is elaborated upon further in Section V.

Competencies

The National Organization of Nurse Practitioner Faculties (NONPF) and American Association of Colleges of Nursing (AACN) define the core and population-focused competencies that delineate the minimum standard for entry into practice. The population-focused competencies build upon the core competencies. Core and population competencies are divided into several categories, including: scientific foundations, leadership, quality, practice inquiry, technology and information literacy, policy, healthcare delivery systems, ethics, and independent practice. These competencies are the basis for the educational programs and national certification exams used to determine whether an individual meets the minimum criteria for entry into practice.

Scope of Practice

It is crucial to understand the legal SOP for NPs, which may vary greatly between states.

The term SOP identifies activities a NP is legally authorized to perform and delineates the boundaries of a NP's practice. The NP SOP is based on educational preparation and certification (AACN, 2017). State statutes and regulations define the range of responsibilities legally authorized in each state (Markowitz, Adams, Lewitt, & Dunlop, 2017). In each state, the legislature establishes the nurse practice act, which governs the practice of the profession within that state (Hartigan, 2016). State practice acts are intentionally written broadly so that they will not require frequent changes through legislative processes. Administrative rules and regulations provide more detailed and specific provisions to operationalize the practice act (Hartigan, 2016).

The nurse practice act or resultant regulations specify the degree of practice independence, which ranges from full autonomous practice to collaborative or consultative arrangements with physicians and supervisory relationships. State laws also specify the prescriptive authority for a NP, delineating whether physician involvement is required and sometimes the types of medications the NP may prescribe. The regulatory environment for NPs varies by state. Restrictive practice requirements create barriers to practice, reduce patient access to care, delay patient care, and disrupt continuity of care (Markowitz et al., 2017).

Collaborative Practice Agreements

Among the 50 states and District of Columbia, NPs practice with varying levels of legal autonomy. These practice requirements may allow full autonomous practice upon certification, a transition to practice period after certification prior to full practice authority, or permanent formal collaborative practice agreements or supervision by physicians in order to practice. The AANP tracks licensure and practice requirements and levels of independence in each state. As of this writing, NPs in 23 states (including the District of Columbia) have full autonomous practice authority, while NPs in 16 states have reduced practice autonomy and NPs in 12 states have restricted practice (AANP, 2018).

The federal definition of "collaboration" identifies it as "a process by which an NP works with a physician to provide healthcare within the providers' SOP and expertise, whereby the physician provides medical direction and supervision as provided by jointly developed guidelines that are in congruence with the state laws where the services are provided" (42 U.S.C.S. § 1395x(aa)(6) in Buppert, 2018). This definition does not imply that direct or on-site supervision is required. Rather, the respective state statute or board of nursing and/or medicine regulations define the type of supervision or collaboration that is required. Check with the specific statute and regulations in the state where you are applying for licensure to obtain the most up-to-date information.

Institutional Credentialing

Before beginning practice, an AG-ACNP must complete the credentialing process and be granted practice privileges by the hospital. The credentialing process includes a primary review and verification of the AG-ACNP's educational preparation, licensure, certification, and experience references, and a background check.

Clinical privileges are delineated based on state SOP, institutional medical staff bylaws, the patient population to be cared for, the primary duties, and any procedures to be performed within the specific institution. Examples of clinical privileges include performing history and physicals, ordering and interpreting diagnostic testing, prescribing, procedures that may be performed, and so on. Ongoing and renewal of credentialing occurs at prespecified time periods by the institution and requires maintenance of licensure, board certification, and clinical skills to maintain and renew credentialing and, thus, employment.

■ OVERVIEW OF CERTIFICATION EXAMS

The purpose of national certification exams is to ensure the NP meets a minimal competency level for safe entry into practice. There are two exam options for national board certification as an AG-ACNP. The two organizations offering the AG-ACNP national certification examination are the AACN and the American Nurses Credentialing Center (ANCC). AACN uses the acronym ACNPC-AG® for "acute care nurse practitioner certified in adult-gerontology," whereas ANCC uses the acronym AG-ACNP for "adult-gerontology acute care nurse practitioner." Both certifications are recognized by all 50 state boards of nursing (SBON). Employers accept both certification exams. For the purposes of this book, we will use AG-ACNP to refer to adult-gerontology acute care nurse practitioners regardless of which certification is held, not in deference to ANCC, but rather to align with the AG-ACNP competencies written by the AACN and the NONPF (AACN, 2017).

Certification exams and the questions within them are written by actively practicing ACNPs, who are clinicians and/or from faculty healthcare systems, colleges, and universities. The item writers possess diverse clinical experience and are experienced and seasoned NPs. In addition to scope and standards and competency documents, exam content is based on current surveys of NPs working with acutely and critically ill patients. Exams test both medical and nursing knowledge and integrate foundational material such as advanced pathophysiology, advanced pharmacology, evidence-based practice, and advanced health assessment concepts. Both exams test your ability to:

- Diagnose and treat conditions
- Identify and manage complications and side effects
- Recognize indications, contraindications, and complications of procedures
- Effectively communicate
- Recognize and respond to medical legal issues
- Work within the SOP
- Apply evidence-based practice concepts
- Manage healthcare systems and policy challenges

Exam blueprints are readily available on the respective certification websites. We recommend you become familiar with the exam blueprints before deciding which exam to take.

Which Exam to Take

This is a very personal decision that warrants thoughtful consideration. An informed decision can be made by exploring and understanding the two exams, and by discussing this with your faculty. Start by reviewing the following two sections, which provide an overview and are written by each of the certifying organizations. Thoroughly explore each of their websites, exam blueprints, and styles of practice questions. The practice questions found in this book contain the type and style of questions found on each exam.

You need to pass only one examination to be certified. Thus, there is no need or benefit to take both examinations. That being said, some students who are concerned about passing an exam may choose to sign up for both in hopes of passing at least one of them on the first attempt.

About the Content and Questions

Content on the certifying exams is based on well-established standards of care. Exams are routinely updated every few years. As such, there is lag time, sometimes up to 2 to 3 years, between when new evidence or updated clinical practice guidelines are published and when the content is integrated into the exams. We recommended you review the resources listed for each exam and keep this lag time in mind when you respond to questions.

The exams consist of multiple-choice questions with four possible answers. All the answers options are written to be plausible, but only one answer is correct.

Exam questions are written at high levels of difficulty. Rather than simply testing your ability to recall facts or understand content, the questions will test knowledge at the application or evaluation level. This requires analysis and synthesis of the information provided. In other words, you will need to understand facts and be able to apply them to a clinical scenario to make a diagnosis or a treatment decision. Many questions require you to make a diagnosis, then prioritize an intervention and/or treat a complication. Remember: if a question asks for an intervention, answer with an intervention and not an assessment. In addition, items may evaluate multiple elements in one question. Many professional role, SOP, communication skills, patient education, advocacy, ethical, legal, and quality metrics may be integrated into clinical scenarios, rather than as stand-alone questions.

Questions are straightforward and contain only essential elements of data to answer the question. They do not contain extraneous information or information to confuse the examinee. Some questions are more difficult than others, but unlike the NCLEX® exam, variation in question difficulty does not change in response to examinees' answers.

What is NOT on the exam? There will be no fill-in-the-blank, matching, or true/false questions. You are not likely to find exam questions with "All of the above" or "None of the above" as answers. Nor should you find questions with negatively worded stems, such as "Which of the following is NOT . . . " or "All of the following EXCEPT . . . "

With these tenets in mind, the questions in this book are written to be representative of the style of questions found on both exams, including content that could be on the exam. The questions are written in the same format and at the same level of difficulty, and cover similar content areas.

The following two sections are written by the respective national board certification exam organizations, AACN and ANCC. They highlight key information you need to know. Please note that website links can change over time. The best way to access the most current information for what you are seeking is to go to the AACN and ANCC websites.

■ AACN CERTIFICATION CORPORATION

About the AACN Certification Corporation

The mission of the AACN Certification Corporation (AACN CertCorp) is to drive patient health and safety through comprehensive credentialing of acute and critical care nurses ensuring practice consistent with standards of excellence. A sister organization to the AACN, the largest nursing specialty organization in the world, the AACN CertCorp began certifying RNs in critical care in 1975. The ACNPC-AG certification program aligns with AACN's extensive expertise as the specialty organization that understands the practice of ACNPs. In 1995, AACN CertCorp partnered with the ANCC to offer the first ACNP certification exam program. From 1995 through 2001, Adult ACNPs were jointly credentialed by both organizations. In 2001, AACN CertCorp sold its share of the program to ANCC. In 2007, AACN CertCorp relaunched its Adult ACNP program, and subsequently integrated the gerontology components to become the AG-ACNP board certification.

AG-ACNP Board Certification

AACN CertCorp is a separately incorporated 501(c)(6) organization governed by the AACN CertCorp Board of Directors, which confers board certification for all of its examination programs. The ACNPC-AG examination is nationally accredited by the National Commission for Certifying Agencies (NCCA), meets the National Council of State Boards of Nursing (NCSBN®) criteria for APRN certification exams and is compliant with the Consensus Model for APRN Regulation: Licensure, Accreditation, Certification, and Education. The exam meets regulatory sufficiency for all SBON as a proxy NP licensure exam. The certification credential is approved by the Veterans Health Administration, the Centers for Medicare and Medicaid Services (CMS), and insurance providers for reimbursement purposes.

Determining Exam Content

The first step in exam development is to determine the content. To be used for regulatory (licensure) purposes, an examination must be targeted to entry level practice; measure only job-related knowledge, skills, and abilities; assess competence at the minimum level required for safe and effective practice; and be psychometrically sound (Zara, 2000). To assure job relatedness, certification organizations conduct studies variously referred to as studies of practice, job analysis studies, role delineation studies (RDS), and so on, in order to learn the critical abilities required for the target practitioner to perform safely and effectively in practice. At this point in the exam development process, we often see some divergence in the focus of the educational community/professional associations and the certification/regulatory community. The role of the education/professional community is to advance the profession and to set standards for excellence in clinical practice. The role of the certification/regulatory community in conducting a job analysis is to provide for patient safety by documenting the key components of the actual practice of competent practitioners as it currently exists, not to analyze practice as we wish it would be delivered and then to develop an examination based on that ideal scenario (Hartigan, 2007).

To develop the study of practice survey instrument, AACN CertCorp convenes an expert panel comprised of geographically and demographically representative current practitioners in the role, which may include faculty from AG-ACNP programs, from a variety of practice settings, including large and small facilities, rural and urban sites, and teaching and community hospitals. All examination development panels are oriented to their roles and assisted in their activities by the test service psychometrician and AACN CertCorp staff nurses. Because AG-ACNPs practice in a variety of different environments, it is essential that the panel be diverse. The panel consults the current literature, as well as resources such as hospital admission and discharge statistics and morbidity and mortality data, to determine current disease and acuity trends in constructing the survey. After a pilot test, the survey is sent to current practitioners to gather demographic information about their practice settings and conditions, as well as the types of patients they care for on a regular basis.

All of AACN CertCorp's certification examinations include the AACN Synergy Model for Patient Care (Synergy Model) as one of the major content domains, or organizing structures. The Synergy Model was developed to link nursing clinical practice with patient outcomes. The Synergy Model APRN competencies have been incorporated into the national competencies used to develop the AG-ACNP exam.

The purpose of the exam program is to help ensure public protection. New graduate NPs are required to pass a legally defensible and psychometrically sound exam that measures the advanced practice competencies needed to perform safely and effectively as a newly licensed, entry-level AG-ACNP. NCSBN criteria and SBON requirements for regulatory sufficiency state that APRN exams must test both core role and population-focus competencies as validated by the most recent job analysis survey or study of practice, and must cover the entire test plan.

The final job analysis survey consists of the NP core competencies, the AG competencies, patient care problems, and nursing interventions or procedures, as well as a series of demographic questions. The job analysis survey is sent to current practitioners, and they are asked to rate each item on the importance to their practice. When the survey results are received, the panel members are assisted by the psychometric expert from the test service to interpret the data and determine, based on the responses, what content must be included on the exam and what percentage of the total exam should be devoted to particular content areas. Because the exam is national, a variety of subgroup analyses are conducted to be certain that it is not biased toward a particular region of the country or toward urban areas or only toward community hospitals. All candidates must have an equal opportunity to pass the exam. The content panel forwards its recommendations to the Board of Directors, which makes the final decision on the test plan. Job analysis studies are conducted every 5 years for all AACN CertCorp examination programs.

Exam Development Process

A second group of volunteers, or subject-matter experts (SMEs), make up the Item Writer Committee (IWC). These IWC members must be experts on the knowledge and practice competencies that are required for the newly licensed AG-ACNP to practice safely and effectively at entry level, and are often ACNP faculty and ACNPs who regularly work with new graduate ACNPs. With assistance from the test service psychometrician and AACN CertCorp staff, IWC members compose items at the application and analysis level whenever possible. Items must be written to cover the entire test plan, including the patient care problems and the core and population competencies. The exam is made up of multiple-choice items and the candidate must select the best response. In the stem, or question, only the information needed to respond to the item is provided; no extraneous data is given, to avoid excess scrolling or reading. There are no "trick" questions or negative stems (e.g., "all of the following *except*"; "which of the following would *not* be"); drugs are provided with both generic and trade name (e.g., dopamine [Intropin]); and normal laboratory values are provided. Item writers are encouraged to draw from their own clinical experiences in developing items. New items are pre-tested before they may be used for scored testing. The ACNPC-AG exam is 3½ hours and consists of 175 multiple-choice items. Of the 175 items, 150 are scored. The remaining 25 items are pre-test items, but are indistinguishable from scored items.

Exam Development Committee (EDC) volunteer SMEs, who are familiar with the required competencies of newly licensed AG-ACNPs, review the statistical data on the items written by the that have been administered as unscored pre-test items; evaluate the items for currency, bias, and consistency, and either unanimously approve them for use on future exams or send them back for revision; review items in the current item pool for continued use; and work with the test service and staff to put together new versions of the examination to replace versions currently in use. As versions are rotated in and out of use, they must undergo an equating process to be sure that each candidate takes an exam of equal difficulty. All versions must completely cover the test plan. Based on the statistical characteristics of the items, a new passing standard is established for the new version.

Exam Eligibility

Completion of a graduate-level advanced practice education program that meets the following requirements:

1. The program is through a college or university that offers a Commission on Collegiate Nursing Education (CCNE) or Accreditation Commission for Education in Nursing (ACEN) accredited master's or higher degree in nursing with a concentration as an AG-ACNP. The program must include in-depth competencies to care for the entire adult population (young adults, older adults, and frail elderly).

2. The program has demonstrated compliance with the National Task Force Criteria for Evaluation of Nurse Practitioner Programs (NTF Criteria).

3. Both direct and indirect clinical supervision must be congruent with current AACN and nursing accreditation guidelines.

4. The curriculum includes but is not limited to

   a. Biological, behavioral, medical, and nursing sciences relevant to practice as an AG-ACNP, including advanced pathophysiology, pharmacology, and physical assessment

   b. Legal, ethical, and professional responsibilities of the ACNP

   c. Supervised clinical practice relevant to the specialty of acute care

5. The curriculum meets the following criteria:

   a. The curriculum is consistent with competencies of AG-ACNP practice.

   b. The instructional track/major has a minimum of 500 supervised clinical hours overall.

    c. All clinical hours are focused on the direct care of acutely ill adult-gerontology patients and completed within the United States.

    d. The supervised clinical experience is directly related to the knowledge and all role components of the AG-ACNP.

Didactic coursework with content specific to care of acutely ill adult-gerontology patients is required.

The program director of the education program must complete an Educational Eligibility Form that verifies completion of the required courses. You must submit originals of all graduate-level educational transcripts showing degree(s) conferred. A secure, electronic transcript may be provided by your school directly to APRNcert@aacn.org.

Current, unencumbered U.S. RN or APRN licensure is required. An unencumbered license is not currently being subjected to formal discipline by any SBON and has no provisions or conditions that limit the nurse's practice in any way. This applies to all RN or APRN licenses you currently hold. Candidates and ACNPC-AG-certified nurses must notify AACN CertCorp within 30 days if any restriction is placed on their RN or APRN license(s). Nurses who hold an encumbered license may be eligible for conditional certification; email APRNcert@aacn.org to inquire.

Applying for the Exam

To support you as you transition into your new APRN role, AACN is pleased to provide you with a free year of AACN e-membership in the senior year of your AG-ACNP program. Benefits of e-membership include a discount on certification exams, and discounts on education resources and conferences including the National Teaching Institute/Advanced Practice Institute conference and digital versions of AACN's publications, *American Journal of Critical Care, Critical Care Nurse, and AACN Bold Voices*. Check with your program director on how to take advantage of this offer so that you can access AACN's multitude of clinical educational resources during the final year of your program.

AACN CertCorp is committed to a certification process that addresses your needs, offering a quick turnaround of exam applications, online applications for faster processing; and exams competitively priced with students and working professional nurses in mind.

You may submit your exam application any time prior to or after graduation. At the time you apply, you will receive links to free review products, including:

- Practice questions with items and rationale presented in the same style as the actual exam

- Comprehensive, self-paced review course that aligns with our detailed test plans (online and CD-ROM)

- Consultation with a nurse specialist on exam preparation strategies available upon request

Have your original, final transcript showing date degree/certificate was awarded sent to AACN. Send official transcripts of any graduate-level coursework from other schools. You will receive an email confirming that your application has been received and forwarded to a certification nurse specialist for evaluation; this certification nurse specialist will be partnered with you to answer questions and provide updates. Your eligibility will be evaluated within 2 to 3 business days of required documents being received. You will receive an email notifying you that your application has been approved and providing instructions for scheduling your exam.

After You Test

Upon completion of computer-based exams, results with a score breakdown will be presented on-site. For purposes of evaluating educational programs, exam pass/fail status and a breakdown of exam scores by content area will be reported to the candidate's program director. The SBON in the state(s) in which you have applied or intend to apply for licensure will also be notified of your pass/fail status. Within 1 week of certification, certificants, employers, SBON, and others can verify certification status free of charge at www.aacn.org/verifycert.

Your certification is valid for 5 years. Renewal requirements include 1,000 clinical practice hours and 150 continuing education (CE) points; 25 must be in pharmacology. The annual AACN membership entitles you to take advantage of free CE offerings and discounted attendance at the annual conference. To learn more, go to www.aacn.org.

■ AMERICAN NURSES CREDENTIALING CENTER

About the American Nurses Credentialing Center

The ANCC's mission is to promote excellence in nursing and healthcare globally through credentialing programs. ANCC's internationally renowned credentialing programs board certify NPs, clinical nurse specialists (CNS), and RNs in specialty areas of practice. ANCC also recognizes healthcare organizations that promote nursing excellence and quality patient outcomes while providing safe, positive work environments. In addition, ANCC accredits healthcare organizations that provide and approve continuing nursing education, interprofessional CE, residency/fellowship programs, and skills-based competency programs.

ANCC AG-ACNP Board Certification

The ANCC AG-ACNP board certification examination is a competency-based entry-level examination that provides a valid and reliable assessment of the entry-level clinical knowledge and skills of the AG-ACNP. The AG-ACNP certification exam aligns with the Consensus Model for APRN Regulation: Licensure, Accreditation, Certification, and Education (Consensus Model) (APRN Consensus Work Group, 2008). The AG-ACNP certification is accredited by the Accreditation Board for Specialty Nursing Certification (ABSNC) and the NCCA.

The ANCC AG-ACNP certification examination is accepted by the NCSBN and SBON for licensure. The U.S. Department of Veterans Affairs, CMS, and health insurance companies recognize ANCC AG-ACNP certification.

The ANCC AG-ACNP certification examination is computer based and in a multiple-choice format. The certification examination is available year round. You may apply at any time. Once you meet eligibility criteria to take the examination, you are provided a 90-day window to schedule the exam at any of the Prometric testing centers in the United States or internationally.

You are provided 4 hours to answer 175 scored and 25 pilot (unscored) multiple-choice questions. You will receive a copy of your exam results before you leave the exam center.

After successfully passing the examination, you are awarded the AG-ACNP-BC credential. This credential is valid for 5 years. You can continue to use this credential by maintaining your license to practice and meeting the renewal requirements of the certifying body that are in place at the time you are seeking renewal of the AG-ACNP certification.

Overview of the AG-ACNP Examination Content

The AG-ACNP certification exam includes clinical knowledge of young adults, including late adolescents, through the elderly and frail elderly. You are expected to apply knowledge from the APRN core content (advanced pharmacology, advanced health assessment, and advanced pathophysiology) as well as to demonstrate understanding of the NP role and healthcare systems.

Overview of the AG-ACNP Exam Development Process

The AG-ACNP examination is developed by ANCC in cooperation with a content expert panel (CEP) composed of carefully selected AG-ACNP SMEs. CEPs analyze the professional skills and abilities from RDS, which provide the evidence for the exam content outline or the exam blueprint.

Exam questions, or "items," are written by AG-ACNP certified SMEs who have received training by ANCC staff in writing exam questions. The items are then reviewed by the CEP with the ANCC staff and pilot tested to ensure validity and psychometric quality before being used as scored items on the actual examinations. ANCC adheres to exam development standards to ensure that the items are appropriate. This includes editing and coding items, referencing items to the approved exam content outlines and reference books, and screening items for bias and stereotypes. The validity and reliability of the examination is monitored by ANCC staff. Certification examinations are updated approximately every 3 to 5 years.

Eligibility for the AG-ACNP Certification Examination

AG-ACNP eligibility criteria aligns with the Consensus Model requirements for graduate preparation for APRNs. Because eligibility criteria are regularly reviewed, consult the ANCC website for the most current version. When you apply for certification, you will need to meet the criteria as stated on the ANCC website. A general overview of the AG-ACNP eligibility criteria is provided as follows:

- Hold a current, active RN license in a state or territory of the United States or hold the professional, legally recognized equivalent in another country.

- Hold a master's, postgraduate, or doctoral degree from an AG-ACNP program accredited by the CCNE or the ACEN (formerly NLNAC I National League for Nursing Accrediting Commission). The degree-granting graduate AG-ACNP program must be able to demonstrate the following:

  ■ A minimum of 500 faculty-supervised clinical hours are in the AG-ACNP role and population

◼ Three separate, comprehensive graduate-level courses in:

- Advanced physiology/pathophysiology, including general principles that apply across the life span

- Advanced health assessment, which includes assessment of all human systems, advanced assessment techniques, concepts, and approaches

- Advanced pharmacology, which includes pharmacodynamics, pharmacokinetics, and pharmacotherapeutics of all broad categories of agents

◼ Content covering health promotion and/or maintenance and differential diagnosis and disease management

Note: Candidates may be authorized to take the AG-ACNP examination after all coursework and faculty-supervised clinical practice hours for the degree are complete, prior to degree conferral and graduation, provided that all other eligibility requirements are met. For more information, contact ANCC directly via email at certification@ana.org or telephone 1.800.284.2378 if you have questions about testing after completing all AG-ACNP courses and clinical requirements, prior to the conferral of your degree.

Preparing for the Certification Examination

ANCC provides the current AG-ACNP exam-content outline, sample questions with answers, and reference list at the ANCC website for free. ANCC does not endorse any review materials, books or courses, or companies. Completing any review materials, including a review course, does not guarantee you will pass the exam.

Create Your ANCC Online Account

At any time, create your ANCC certification online account. You will be able to complete your application to take the exam via this account. In addition, this site offers the opportunity to store all your professional development activities throughout the certification period. This provides an efficient means to complete the application or renewal.

Study Plan

Approximately 6 months before taking the exam, develop a study plan. This could include self-study, finding a study buddy or group, taking a review course, reviewing current textbooks and articles, or other methods. The key is to have a study plan and follow through with it. It is also important to focus on known areas of weakness.

Exam Content Outline

The AG-ACNP exam-content outline, also known as the exam blueprint, identifies the content areas covered on the examination. In addition, it provides the number and percentage of items in each major category.

Sample Questions

For practice, there are sample questions that are similar to those on the actual examination but do not represent the full range of content or levels of difficulty. There is no time limit associated with reviewing the sample questions, and you can review them as many times as you wish, for free.

Reference List

For additional reading, a review of authoritative texts is recommended. While the list is not all-inclusive, it may act as a guide for preparation. Your school materials and resources are also excellent resources.

Primary Source Verification of Certification

After you have tested, you can request a primary source verification of your certification to be sent to individuals, SBON, or employers you designate. ANCC does not automatically send a verification of certification. Verification of AG-ACNP certification can be requested via the ANCC certification website (https://www.nursingworld.org/certification/).

Maintaining AG-ACNP Certification, Also Referred to as Certification Renewal

After you successfully pass the examination, you are awarded the AG-ACNP-BC credential. This credential and certification is valid for 5 years. You can maintain your certification and continue to use the AG-ACNP credential by maintaining your license to practice and meeting the mandatory 75 CE hours, 25 of which must be in pharmacology and at least one of the eight renewal categories in place at the time you renew AG-ACNP certification.

You can find more information on the ANCC Certification website.

Review the renewal requirements, create a plan to complete the professional development activities to renew the certification, and maintain the ability to continue to use the AG-ACNP-BC credential.

ANCC AG-ACNP Resources and Latest Information

Visit the ANCC Certification website for the latest information including these AG-ACNP resources:

- Exam-content outline
- Sample exam questions and answers
- Reference list
- Prometric testing centers
- Create your ANCC certification account
- Certification general testing and renewal handbook
- Verification of certification

For any questions, you can send an email to certification@ana.org or call 1.800.284.2378.

■ THE JOURNEY FROM CLASSROOM TO CERTIFICATION

Once you have completed coursework, there is a stepwise, logical sequence to follow to ensure timely and successful transition from school to employment. The first and most important step is to become nationally board certified as an AG-ACNP. The following steps are a guide to help you in this sometimes confusing, complex, and evolving process.

Certifying bodies may allow you to take the exam before you actually have officially graduated, or "walked across the stage." This is the date the school will confer or grant your official degree. Thus, based on when you want to take the exam, some of the following steps are flexible.

1. First, you must finish all coursework for your AG-ACNP program, including assignments and clinical hours. This determines your program completion date.

2. Develop a study plan and strategies, including an in-depth review of this book's introduction section, reviewing each certification organization's exam and the chapter on study planning.

3. Decide on which exam to take.

4. Notify your program director of which exam you plan to take and request the required certifying organization's form.
   - AACN requires the Educational Eligibility Form: ACNPC-AG Certification for Adult-Gerontology Acute Care Nurse Practitioners form to be filled out by your program director. The form is found on page 27 of the ACNPC-AG exam handbook at www.aacn.org/~/media/aacn-website/certification/get-certified/handbooks/acnpcagexamhandbook.pdf
   - ANCC requires a Validation of Advanced Practice Nursing Education Form be filled out by your program director. The form can be found at nursecredentialing.org/APRN-Validation-Form

5. Submit your application for the certification examination. Be certain you have supplied all the required information.

6. Study while you wait for the organization to verify your application. You will then receive notification to schedule your exam, often referred to as "authorization to test."

7. Submit your final transcript with your master's or doctoral degree conferred on it. Be sure to read the directions of AACN and ANCC to see if either or both require an "official" transcript.

8. Prepare for the exam. Be sure to review Section I of this book. Review course content, notes, and coursework from previous classes. Consider taking a review course. Most importantly, be sure to practice answering questions, such as the ones in this book.

9. Schedule your exam. This can be done prior to your degree being conferred if you are ready for the exam and are confident in your knowledge base and test-taking abilities.

10. Take the exam.

11. Results are immediately available to you at the completion of your exam. However, official notification from the organization may take 2 weeks or longer to arrive in the mail.

12. Lastly, be sure to let your program coordinator and/or program director know your results. Schools are required to track student outcomes and pass rates.

■ FREQUENTLY ASKED QUESTIONS

1. Does it matter which exam I take?
   No, they are both nationally recognized exams accepted by all 50 states and the District of Columbia. Thoroughly review each website, exam handbook, practice questions, and exam blueprint, and then decide which examination to take.

2. When can I apply for the certification exam?
   You can begin the application process prior to graduation. The additional lead time for processing paperwork can streamline the process and turnaround time. The certifying organizations' policies and practices have been evolving over time, so it is important to carefully review their respective websites and exam handbooks because changes may have been made since the publication of this book.

3. Can I take the exam at any time of the year?
   Yes, you can apply for the computer-based testing throughout the year and test within the 90-day period after you receive authorization to test.

4. Can I get a discount on the exams?
   Yes, both organizations offer discounts. Check their respective websites for details.

   • AACN offers discounts if you are a member of AACN, and offers group discounts for groups of 10 or more applicants.

   • ANCC offers varying levels of discounts with the American Nurses Association (ANA), AANP, Gerontological Advanced Practice Nurses Association (GAPNA), and the National Gerontological Nursing Association (NGNA).

5. What is an "official transcript"?
   The official transcript is a legal document that contains (a) the signature and title of the certifying official, (b) the institutional seal and date of issue, and (c) a statement forbidding the release of information from the transcript to a third party, as required by the FERPA of 1974. Official transcripts are sealed and directly sent to the certification body. You will request a copy of your transcript through the registrar's office at your school. It may be done electronically through the website or in writing, and there may or may not be a nominal fee. Check your schools registrar's website for specifics to your institution.

6. How long does it take to process applications?
   Processing of applications can take up to 2 to 4 weeks, depending on how long it takes to receive all required documentation. Once all the required paperwork is received, it is usually quite an efficient turnaround. Please check the websites to explore offers for expedited reviews. An additional fee is customarily associated with this service, and it is a personal choice whether or not to use it.

7. How will I know if I'm cleared to schedule the exam?
   You will receive an email notifying you of your "approval to test" or "authorization to test." You will have 90 days in which to schedule and take your exam.

8. When should I schedule my exam?
   You should schedule your exam once you have worked out your study plan (discussed in Section I of this book) and allowed sufficient time for review and practice questions.
   That being said, there are other scheduling considerations. You want to also consider scheduling your exam early to secure your preferred date and time. Early scheduling provides you flexibility to schedule your examination based on religious, personal, or other needs. Waiting until the end of the 90-day period may limit appointment availability.
   Another important consideration is that you'll have the greatest success if the exam is taken in close proximity to your clinical and didactic coursework, when the content is freshest in your mind. Most faculty recommend taking the exam in the first few months after graduation.

9. What if my targeted testing date/time is not available?

Depending on how eager you are to take the exam and how flexible you are, you could investigate other testing-site locations for availability. This may require additional travel time or travel to another state, but it allows for you to attempt to secure the date and time of your preference.

10. What normal values must I know?

You will need to know normal and abnormal vital signs; hemodynamic profiles; and basic laboratory values, including but not limited to complete blood count, basic metabolic profile, and troponin. Candidates for the AACN exam do not need to know the following values:

Phosphate	BUN	Serum ammonia level
Calcium	Creatinine	Serum magnesium
Amylase	Urine specific gravity	Serum osmolality

BUN, blood urea nitrogen.

For these values, there will be an indicator if these values are "high" or "low."

11. How will data be provided?

Data may either be presented in table format or written into the stem of the question. AACN presents data in table format; the following are examples of what to expect.

BP	138/75
HR	110
RR	22
Temperature	99°F (37.2°C)
SpO_2	92%
$EtCO_2$	38

BP, blood pressure; HR, heart rate; RR, respiration rate.

pH	7.36
$PaCO_2$	36
PaO_2	86
HCO_3^-	19
BE	2 mEq/L
SaO_2	91%

BE, base excess.

Mode	Assist control
FiO_2	0.50
Rate	12
Tidal volume	500
PEEP	5 cm H_2O

PEEP, positive end expiratory pressure.

MAP	50 mmHg
CVP	22 mmHg
PAP	38/18 mmHg
PAOP	5 mmHg
CO	9.6 L/min
CI	7.0 L/min/m^2
SVR	1,300 dynes/sec/cm^5
PVR	22 dynes/sec/cm^5

CI, cardiac index; CO, carbon monoxide; CVP, central venous pressure; MAP, mean arterial pressure; PAOP, pulmonary artery occlusion pressure; PAP, pulmonary artery pressure; PVR, pulmonary vascular resistance; SVR, systemic vascular resistance.

Whereas ANCC presents data integrated into the stem of the question, such as

- The patient's laboratory values are blood urea nitrogen of 12 mg/dL, creatinine of 0.8 mg/dL, PaCO$_2$ of 37 mmHg.
- The patient weighs 132 lb (59.9 kg). The serum osmolality is 320 mOsm/L kg H$_2$O.

12. What medication names do I need to know?
Drug names will be presented with both trade and generic names.

13. What other data will be on the exams?
You should expect telemetry rhythms, 12-lead ECGs and chest x-rays, and possibly other x-rays or diagnostic tests—all of which require interpretation—to be on the exams.

14. What abbreviations must I know?
The certification bodies follow The Joint Commission and Institute for Safe Medication Practices (ISMP) recommendations regarding abbreviations. Most diagnoses will be written out (e.g., hypertension, not "HTN"). The idea is to test your knowledge about the content area and not your familiarity with abbreviations, which may vary across the United States.

15. When will I receive results of the exam?
For computer-based testing, you will be given the results of your exam by the testing center staff prior to leaving the testing center. For paper-and-pencil exam, candidates will receive results within 3 to 4 weeks.

16. What happens if I fail the exam?
You will receive a score report upon completing the exam. This will provide you information on overall performance and assessment of the various areas of the exam. This report is helpful to develop a new plan. Please refer to Chapter 29 of Section V of this book for additional information and next steps.

17. What if I need to reschedule my exam?
Please check the PSI/AMP and Prometrics websites for their specific policies on rescheduling. You can reschedule exams with advance notice, but rescheduling within 48 to 72 hours is more complicated and will incur a fee as the testing site likely will not be able to fill your time slot. For extreme extenuating circumstances, call both the testing site and your certifying body for additional guidance.

18. If there is a major storm, now what?

If a testing center is closed due to severe weather or other problems, the testing center will make every attempt to contact each scheduled candidate by email and phone. You can also contact the test center candidate support center; check the website for the phone number.

It's important to note that exams are usually not rescheduled if testing site personnel can reach and operate the site. They make every attempt to administer exams as scheduled. Should an exam be canceled, all scheduled candidates will receive follow-up notification regarding a rescheduled exam date or reapplication procedures.

19. After I take the exam, can I share content from the exam with my classmates or faculty?

No! You have signed a confidentiality agreement with the certifying body. Nurses are the number one most trusted profession (Gallop Poll, 2017). As such, we are accountable for honoring this confidentiality agreement, which protects the integrity of the certification exam which in turn protects patient safety.

It is especially inappropriate for candidates to post information on listserv and chats. It's well known that you can't take notes out of the exam with you, but once your friends find out that you have tested, they will start asking you for information. You can have an answer ready and should practice this in anticipation. Simply say, "I'm sorry, I can't share content; I signed a confidentiality agreement."

In addition, newer faculty do not realize it is inappropriate to quiz graduates about what was on the exam. This happens simply because nobody has ever told them not to ask. As a candidate, it is important you recognize that this is an element of the honor statement you sign as part of your application.

20. How does my state board of nursing know I passed the examination?

You will need to request that the certification body send verification to the desired SBON. Alternatively, the SBON can verify your certification through the certification bodies' respective websites. Please check your SBON for specifics for your respective state.

21. What else do I have to do to be able to practice?

Please review Section V of this book for additional steps. The next steps will vary from state to state, but typically applying for state licensure is the very next step. You'll need to contact the relevant SBON to find the appropriate application.

22. How do I display my credentials?

The preferred order of displaying credentials is as follows:

a. Academic degrees before clinical degree (e.g., PhD, APRN or DNP, APRN)

b. Highest earned degree (e.g., MS, MSN, DNP)

c. Licensure (e.g., RN)

d. State designations or requirements (e.g., APRN, NPC)

e. National certifications

   i. For ANCC, your credentials will be AG-ACNP-BC

   ii. For AACN, your credentials will be ACNPC-AG

f. Awards and honors (e.g., FAAN)

g. Other recognitions (EMT)

h. Example: Jane Doe, DNP, NPC, AG-ACNP-BC, FAAN, CCRN, (ANCC, 2013)

■ REFERENCES

Adult-Gerontology NP Competencies Work Group. (2016). *Adult-gerontology acute care and primary care NP competencies.* Retrieved from http://c.ymcdn.com/sites/www.nonpf.org/resource/resmgr/competencies/NP_Adult_Geri_competencies_4.pdf

American Association of Critical Care Nurses. (2017). *AACN scope and standards for acute care nurse practitioner practice 2017* (L. Bell, Ed.). Aliso Viejo, CA: American Association of Critical Care Nurses.

American Association of Critical Care Nurses. (2018). *Certification Corporation ACNPC-AG certification handbook*. Aliso Viejo, CA: AACA. Retrieved from https://www.aacn.org/~/media/aacn-website/certification/get-certified/handbooks/acnpcagexamhandbook.pdf?la=en

American Association of Nurse Practitioners. (2015). *Scope of practice for nurse practitioners*. Retrieved from https://aanp.org/images/documents/publications/scopeofpractice.pdf

American Association of Nurse Practitioners. (2018). *States categorized by type*. Retrieved from https://www.aanp.org/66-legislation-regulation/state-practice-environment/1380-state-practice-by-type

American Nurses Credentialing Center. (2013). *How to display your credentials: Common questions and answers about displaying your credentials in the proper order*. Retrieved from http://www.nursecredentialing.org/DisplayCredentials-Brochure.pdf

APRN Consensus Work Group & National Council of State Boards of Nurses APRN Advisory Committee. (2008). *Consensus model for APRN regulation: Licensure, accreditation, certification and education*. Retrieved from https://www.ncsbn.org/Consensus_Model_for_APRN_Regulation_July_2008.pdf

Buppert, C. (2018). *Nurse practitioner's business practice and legal guide* (6th ed.). Boulder, Co: Jones & Bartlett.

Gallup Poll. (2017). *Nurses ranked #1 most ethical profession by 2017 Gallup poll*. Retrieved from https://nurse.org/articles/gallup-ethical-standards-poll-nurses-rank-highest/

Hartigan, C. (2007). Certification and the synergy model. In M. A. Q. Curley. (Ed.), *Synergy: The unique relationship between nurses and patients*. Indianapolis, IN: Sigma Theta Tau International.

Hartigan, C. (2016). Scope of practice. *Critical Care Nurse, 36*(5), 70–72. doi:10.4037/ccn2016325

Markowitz, S., Adams, E. K., Lewitt, M. J., & Dunlop, A. L. (2017). Competitive effects of scope of practice restrictions: Public health or public harm? *Journal of Health Economics, 55*, 201–218. doi:10.1016/j.jhealeco.2017.07.004

Zara, A. (2000). The mission of the National Council of State Boards of Nursing. In C. G. Schoon & I. L. Smith (Eds.), *The licensure and certification mission: Legal social and political foundations* (pp. 189–193). New York, NY: Professional Examination Services.

2

Study Planning

CHRISTINE MERMAN WOOLF AND
DAWN CARPENTER

REVIEW EXAM BLUEPRINTS

For each exam, carefully review the exam outlines, known as exam blueprints.

- The American Association of Critical-Care Nurses (AACN, 2017) publishes the *ACNPC-AG Exam Handboo*k http://www.aacn.org/~/media/aacn-website/certification/get-certified/handbooks/acnpcagexamhandbook.pdf

- The American Nurses Credentialing Center (ANCC, 2017a,b) produces a test-content outline: https://www.nursingworld.org/our-certifications/adult-gerontology-acute-care-nurse-practitioner/

You will determine your study system based on which exam you are going to take. Ask your faculty, preceptors, and alumni about the exams. Faculty may share historical data and alumni success rates for each exam. Plan to study with peers who anticipate taking the same exam. Both exams are fair assessments of your beginning skills as an adult-gerontology acute care nurse practitioner (AG-ACNP). By graduating from an accredited program, feel confident you have the knowledge needed to succeed on your certification exam.

STUDY MATERIALS

Once you have determined which exam you will take, use that exam's blueprint as your study guide. The test blueprint provides an outline of content contained on the exam along with the percentage of which each topic is tested within the exam.

Assemble resources to study. Use your notes, textbooks, articles, and presentations from your AG-ACNP program. In addition, each certification organization has a list of references it used to create exam items. Utilize these resources as you prepare for the exam. Use clinical practice guidelines that are at least 2 years old, as newer guidelines may not have yet been incorporated into the exam.

Use this book to gain detailed knowledge about how to work through exam questions. Practice questions train you on how to reason through questions and apply your knowledge. Your performance on the questions throughout this book will highlight areas where you'll need to do additional reading.

■ DEVELOP A STUDY PLAN

The first issue to consider is how much time you have to prepare for the exam. If you performed very well throughout your program and had compressive exams at various times in your program, you may be ready to take the exam relatively soon after graduation. Try a few of the questions in each area of this book. If you perform very well on the practice questions, then consider taking the practice exam. The sooner you take the exam, the better—knowledge will be fresh. Be certain to read this chapter first.

Study Planning

Formulate a study plan. Decide how many days and number of hours each day you can devote to studying. Be realistic and note if you need time for work, family events, appointments, and so on. Build these dates and times into your plan to avoid stress later on. Here is one example:

Monday	Tuesday	Wednesday	Thursday	Friday	Saturday	Sunday
1	2	3	4	5	6	7
4 hr	4 hr	0 hr	5 hr	5 hr	3 hr	6 hr
8	9	10	11	12	13	14
4 hr	4 hr	0 hr	5 hr	5 hr Catch-up	3 hr	6 hr
15	16	17	18	19	20	21
4 hr	4 hr	0 hr	5 hr	5 hr	3 hr	6 hr
22	23	24	25	26	27	28
4 hr	4 hr	0 hr	5 hr	5 hr Catch-up	3 hr	6 hr
29	30	31	1	2	3	4
4 hr	4 hr	0 hr	5 hr	5 hr	3 hr Practice exam	6 hr Catch-up/off
5	6	7	8	9	10	11
4 hr	4 hr	0 hr	5 hr	0 hr	Exam	Celebrate!

■ PRIORITIZE CONTENT

The exam includes both clinical content and, for lack of better words, nonclinical material. Nonclinical material focuses on role, scope of practice, healthcare systems, research and evidence-based practice, nurse practitioner/patient relationship, communication, patient education, ethics and patient advocacy, and so on. It is important to study all materials.

Clinical Content

Review the clinical content in the exam blueprints. For the ANCC (2017b) exam, clinical practice comprises 46% of the exam and the APRN *Core Competencies* is 16% of the exam, whereas for the AACN (2017), clinical judgment comprises 73% of the exam.

ANCC	AACN
• Head, eyes, ears, nose, and throat • Respiratory • Cardiovascular • Gastrointestinal • Genitourinary • Musculoskeletal • Neurological (including psychiatric) • Endocrine • Hematopoietic • Immune • Integumentary	• Cardiovascular • Pulmonary • Endocrine • Musculoskeletal • Hematology/immunology/oncology • Neurology • Gastrointestinal • Renal • Genitourinary • Integumentary • Multisystem • Psychosocial/behavioral/cognitive health

AACN, American Association of Colleges of Nursing; ANCC, American Nurses Credentialing Center.

Both exams assess your knowledge in an integrated manner; thus it is important to review content in all systems. Look at the list previously given for the exam you are taking and note next to each your level of comfort with the material in that system. Rate them as:

- 1 (very challenging—top priority)
- 2 (somewhat challenging—middle priority)
- 3 (feel fine with content, but still need to review)

As you rate each area, consider the following:

- How did you score on your academic exams for each of these systems?
- How much clinical experience or exposure did you get related to the systems?
- Consider how long ago you studied or clinically experienced these systems.

Read the details of the test blueprint; note specifics within each system and decide if you want to change your previously noted level of priority. For the AACN exam, you have an extra step—add the percentage of exam content next to each system. Rank order priorities with content areas by its percentage of the exam. Here is an example:

Priority 1 (Very Challenging—Top Priority)
- Neurology (7%)
- Hematology/immunology/oncology (4%)

- Musculoskeletal (3%)
- Psychosocial/behavioral/cognitive health (3%)

Priority 2 (Somewhat Challenging—Middle Priority)
- Cardiovascular (21%)
- Pulmonary (12%)
- Multisystem (9%)
- Integumentary (2%)

Priority 3 (Feel Fine With Content, but Still Need to Review)
- Gastrointestinal (5%)
- Renal/genitourinary (4%)
- Endocrine (3%)

Nonclinical Content

While physiological organ systems comprise the majority of both exams, the other, nonclinical content is essential to review. On the ANCC (2017b) exam, 38% of the content tests role, professional responsibility, and healthcare systems. On the AACN (2017), professional caring and ethical practice account for 26% of the assessment. For the ANCC (2017b), be sure to focus on the advanced pharmacology content of anti-infective and antineoplastic medications, as well as the other pharmacology-related issues listed. These medications are also essential for the AACN (2017).

Review the topics in the blueprint and determine how many hours you need to review this content. If you are unsure, complete some of the questions in this book from those sections. Determine if these topics are a priority level 1, 2, or 3.

■ CREATE A STUDY SCHEDULE

Start with the end in mind. Enter review time into the schedule for the week before the exam. These days are helpful to allow you to address unexpected challenges. During this review week, you will do the comprehensive practice exam in this book.

Then go to the first day of the calendar and add your top-priority topics into the calendar (an example follows). Once you have decided how many study hours you have in each day, decide how many days you want/need to study each topic. If you feel significantly concerned about a particular topic, consider if you should stop after 3 days on the topic. Oftentimes, after 3 days it is hard to stay as focused on one topic. For example, you may be worried about your level of knowledge of endocrinology and would like to spend weeks on endocrinology. However, after 2 or 3 days on the topic, you might be ready to focus on something else. You can always go back to a topic if necessary. You know yourself best. If you can focus on a topic intensely beyond 3 days, that is fine, as long as you have the time to do so. When you are studying for only a few hours each day, then more than 3 days may not be concerning.

Monday	Tuesday	Wednesday	Thursday	Friday	Saturday	Sunday
1	2	3	4	5	6	7
4 hr Cardio-vascular—1	4 hr Cardio-vascular—1	0 hr	5 hr Pul-monary—1	5 hr Role—1	3 hr Ethics—1	6 hr Multi-systems—1
8	9	10	11	12	13	14
4 hr Endocrine—2	4 hr MSK—2	0 hr	5 hr EBP—2	5 hr Catch-up	3 hr Geriatric—2	6 hr Renal—1
15	16	17	18	19	20	21
4 hr Hemato-poietic/ oncology—1	4 hr	0 hr	5 hr ID—2	5 hr ID—2	3 hr HP&DP—3	6 hr Policy—2
22	23	24	25	26	27	28
4 hr Psychol-ogy—2	4 hr Palliative care—2	0 hr	5 hr Quality—2	5 hr Catch-up	3 hr Integu-mentary—3	6 hr Coding—2
29	30	31	1	2	3	4
4 hr Patient Education—3	4 hr Caring—3	0 hr	5 hr Review	5 hr Review	3 hr Practice exam	6 hr Catch-up
5	6	7	8	9	10	11
4 hr Review	4 hr Review	0 hr	5 hr Review	0 hr	Exam	Celebrate!

EBP, evidence-based practice; HP&DP, health promotion and disease prevention; ID, infectious disease; MSK, musculoskeletal.

After you list your priority topics in order and for as many days/hours as you would prefer, see if you need to make adjustments. If everything does not fit, consider the following:

- Do you have any hours you can add to the calendar for studying?
- Can you get out of some obligations during your weeks of study?
- Are there friends/family that can help you with tasks so that you have more time to study?
- Are you overestimating how long you need to study topics?

■ REORDER SCHEDULE

If you work through your top priorities and feel frustrated or overwhelmed, it is acceptable to reorder topics as done in the following chart. However, do not move a high-priority topic to the end of the calendar. On the next page is another example:

1	2	3	4	5	6	7
4 hr Level 1 priority—Neurology	4 hr Level 1 priority—Neurology	0 hr	5 hr Level 1 priority—Neurology	5 hr Level 1 priority—Hematopoietic/Oncology/Immune	3 hr Level 1 priority—Hematopoietic/Oncology/Immune	6 hr Level 1 priority—Hematopoietic/Oncology/Immune
8	**9**	**10**	**11**	**12**	**13**	**14**
4 hr Was Musculoskeletal (Level 1 priority), for 2 days but due to fatigue will now study gastrointestinal (Level 3) that was planned for later this week	4 hr Was Musculoskeletal (was to be Level 1) switched to renal/genitourinary (Level 3) that was planned for later this week	0 hr	5 hr Musculoskeletal (Level 1)	5 hr Catch-up/off	3 hr Musculoskeletal (Level 1)	6 hr Musculoskeletal (Level 1)

Once you have adjusted the schedule to fit everything into the calendar and reprioritized the schedule based on the percentage the content is worth on the exam, if you are still feeling concerned, consider if you need to reschedule your exam. Check the certifying organization and testing center websites for information regarding moving exam dates. Do not change your exam date unless absolutely necessary. Make the decision to change your exam date after you have engaged in some studying.

◼ WHAT TO DO DURING STUDY TIME

For each content area, it is essential to plan time to
- Read and review content material on the topic of the day
- Complete practice questions and rationales on the topic of the day
- Complete practice questions on content previously reviewed
- Go back and review information for topics already studied
- Repeat practice questions

Start to study by working through your highest priorities first. These days may be draining, but they are preparing you for the exam and, by studying them, you will feel more confident. Realize the topics at the end of your calendar should be more familiar, and thus less demanding, and go more smoothly. Breaking up materials and tasks during the day helps to keep you engaged.

Review Content

Spend time actively reviewing content for part of the day. Reread your textbooks, review notes, and PowerPoint slides on the materials scheduled for that particular day. Some students prefer to
- Read the content aloud
- Listen to recordings
- Draw out concepts like anatomy or physiology
- Make electronic cards
- Handwrite index cards
- Write in a notebook
- Annotate a resource book
- Make tables comparing similar diseases to differentiate among them

Create a system that allows you to capture essential information and is easily accessed. Avoid having to hunt for where you wrote information during your review time. Tables and images may already be available in your resources; if so, mark them so that they can easily be found again. Drawing can help you to recall information.

Review the most essential content for the topic, without neglecting aspects that you know best. Be mindful of how you are dedicating your time to the subtopics within the topic. Spend the most time on areas of concern while still reviewing the entire topic.

Identify the level of knowledge needed to become proficient with that material. For example, if you got a question about leukemia incorrect, did you forget the name of the medication to treat that type of leukemia, or did you forget how to distinguish among the types of leukemia? Be sure to understand the entirety of the disease of concern as identified through your performance on the questions. Questions in this book or other resources are examples of potential questions that could be asked.

Take Practice Questions

During part of each day, you will take practice questions in this book for the respective content area for the day. It is best to do some studying and then step away from the topic by doing other content review, and then take questions on the topic you studied earlier in the day. By doing this, you will test your ability to recall information.

There will be questions you do not know the answer to right away. Reason through them, reflect on what you do know, and apply it to the question. Practice reasoning through all the questions when you are studying and you will be more efficient on exam day. Refer to the "Read the Questions" section at the beginning of Chapter 3.

If you feel very confident about your knowledge of a topic and only have 1 day to review the material or if it is a priority level 3, then you may want to start with questions on the topic before studying resources. By starting with the questions, you will know which areas need more review and then you can use your time more wisely by going to specific subtopics within your resources.

During part of each day, take practice questions on topics you have already studied. When you do these questions, draw from multiple topic areas. By mixing questions you will switch your thinking from one system to another system rapidly, and as such it will mimic the national board exam.

Track where in the exam you get more questions incorrect (i.e., in the first third, second third, or last third of a test). If you find that you miss more questions later in the exam, it may be due to fatigue. Take longer practice question sessions to condition you for this longer testing period of 3 to 4 hours.

Review Question Rationale/Feedback

Review the rationales on questions you got correct to reinforce material on the content. The question rationales assume you have a foundation of knowledge. If you do not have a deep enough understanding, to enhance your learning you will need additional content that can be obtained from the reference material. Take time to learn/relearn the material. When you answer a question incorrectly, take time to analyze the information related to the correct answer. It may be that you just forgot a detail about the content, or maybe you realize that you were incorrectly reasoning through the physiology of the organ system. If you did not know the material, go back to your study materials and reread and update your notes.

Review Previously Studied Materials

Every study day, to keep content fresh in your mind, allocate time to review previous material and questions. Review notes, flash cards, and so on that were made for areas of concern identified through doing questions. Repeated exposure to material reinforces and commits it to memory.

Repeat Questions

To assess if you learned and retained the information, it is fine to repeat or "redo" questions. Be sure you can reason through the content and are not just picking an answer because you recall it. Try to give the answer after reading the question, but before reading the answer options. Also, do not use questions you are seeing a second time as the best indicator of your readiness. New questions should be used to assess your knowledge close to exam day, hence the reason to save the practice exam toward the final week of your study calendar.

In summary, a day of studying may look something like this:

6 hours total time to study:

- 3 hours reading resources on cardiovascular
- 1 hour reviewing areas of concern from topics already studied
- 1 hour doing cardiovascular questions and reviewing the feedback
- 1 hour doing mixed questions on topics already studied and reviewing the feedback

■ PACING

If your pacing has been fine in classroom exams, then doing the practice questions in an untimed mode is fine, meaning you can do a question and immediately review the answer feedback.

If you are someone who had pacing issues throughout your training, then consider doing all your questions in a timed mode. This means going from one question to the next without checking your answers until you've completed all the questions you had planned.

When you do the mixed review questions, try doing them in a timed mode as well. It may be more challenging, since you are paging through this book to find the questions, so pause the timer as you move from one section of the book to another. Consider tabbing the pages from which you are drawing questions so you can find them more easily.

Pacing Challenges

It can be challenging to move on from one question when you believe the answer will come to you if you just spend a little more time on it. The concern is that a little time can end up being 2 or more minutes spent on one question. Some questions will be a little easier for you and require less time, allowing a few extra seconds to devote to more challenging questions. The concern can become a real issue when 2 or more minutes is spent on multiple questions, leading to a lack of time for other questions that you could have answered correctly. If you spend significantly more time on some questions and end up finishing the questions within the time limit, then there is no problem. The issue needs to be addressed if you:

- Spend a lot of time on some questions and have to rush at the end to finish questions
- Finish questions just by completely guessing answers without reading the questions thoroughly, to make up for lost time
- Leave questions blank because you ran out of time

Consequences

A consequence of spending too much time on certain items is that it can increase your anxiety or create a negative feedback loop—thoughts like, "you should know this one," "you are not going to do well on this exam if you do not know this question, because you studied it," and so on. Negative messages like these are counterproductive. It is much better to mark the item, move on, and tell yourself, "I can come back to it." Perhaps another question will trigger your recollection of additional information.

Assess Data

Mark questions you are unsure of when you take practice questions and the practice exam. Keep a list of the questions that took too much time so that you can easily identify them. See how many of the ones on which you dwelled you got correct. Then count how many items you rushed through, skipped, or completely guessed. Assessing this data should convince you to move on and not spend too much time on individual items.

Review the items which you rushed through, skipped, or completely guessed. Did you know the answers to all, most, or some of these questions? If so, then it was most likely not worth spending too much time on other questions. Not only did you potentially lose points due to not being able to put forth your best work on those questions, you also caused unnecessary stress for yourself during the exam.

Reduce Time on Questions

To reduce extended time on individual questions, review the content identified previously that needs additional review. You spent time on these questions because you thought the answers were within your reach. Therefore, take time to learn the content so it is retrievable the next time you see a similar question.

To make sure you are progressing through the exam at the pace needed, periodically check the clock. This system is especially helpful to those who are unaware they are spending too much time on individual questions. If you are someone who checks the time toward the end of the exam and then realizes she or he is very far behind and has to quickly rush and guess, then this system might be helpful.

Alternatively, employ regular time checks after a specific number of questions. For example, you have 1 hour to finish 50 questions. Teach yourself to check the time on every 10th item. Write yourself a grid on your scratch paper:

- Item 10, want 50 minutes remaining
- Item 20, want 40 minutes remaining
- Item 30, want 30 minutes remaining
- Item 40, want 20 minutes remaining
- Item 50, want 10 minutes remaining

Then after all items are finished, you will still have 10 minutes to review.

The goal is to keep you from spending too much time on one item. Use the system for short sets of questions. Try to do 10 questions in 10 minutes, and then have 2 minutes to review marked items. Remember to mark ones on which you were spending too much time or were unsure of the answer.

If you find checking the time every 10 minutes is too overwhelming, or if pacing is not a significant concern, then you can check at item 25 or another pattern that best meets your needs. At a minimum, use this system for the practice exam.

■ PRACTICE EXAM

There is a sample practice exam in Section IV of this book. Save this exam until you have completed studying materials. This should be about a week or so before your exam date. Use this test to evaluate overall performance. Results will determine where additional studying is required prior to taking the national examination.

Take your practice as a timed exam, without checking answers until you have finished all the questions on the exam. This will mirror your exam day experience. Be sure to take this practice exam in a quiet, distraction-free environment. Take it when you are able to focus. If possible, start it at the same time your actual exam is scheduled.

Before starting the questions, set your timer for these limits:

- The AACN exam is 175 questions in 3.5 hours, meaning you will have 72 seconds per question.

- The ANCC exam is 200 questions in 4 hours, meaning you will have 80 seconds for each question.

■ CHANGING ANSWERS

When you are first working through questions, it is fine to change answers. These questions are new to you. As your studying progresses, practice not changing answers.

When you are taking practice questions, keep data on why you changed answers. Develop a data-tracking sheet to assess reasons. The simple form that follows can be filled out quickly while you are taking practice questions or the practice exam.

Question Number That Was Changed	Changed From (You do not need to log the one you changed to because you have that information)	Reason Changed N (new information) M (misread first time) C (considered info for first time) D (doubted self) O (other)
9	B	M
17	A	N

At the end of the practice questions, analyze the data. Do you always change to incorrect? If so, stop changing answers. Does it work for you when you logged N, M, and C, but not when you logged the reason as D? If so, then do not change when the only reason was D.

▪ CHALLENGES ADHERING TO STUDY PLANS

There are many reasons that you may not be able to adhere to your study plan.

- Were you were unrealistic about the time you had available to study? If that is the case, adjust your calendar and see if you can still get through all the studying you planned.

- Do you not have enough hours to get through the content because it is more challenging than you expected to recall the information?

- Free up more time to study. Ask others for assistance in managing your nonstudy tasks. Take advantage of these options:

  - Can a friend pick up your children from school?
  - Can your spouse pick up a few more chores?
  - Can your boss limit your shifts?
  - Can your neighbor walk your dog?

- Remind family and friends that you are almost finished and need their support as you complete your final step toward your goal. They may see that you are not in class and be happy to have time with you. That is wonderful, but, if you can, ask them to wait until after the exam: and let those who are helping you know they are appreciated.

If you maximized the catch-up time, will you be able to finish by your current exam date? If so, maintain your exam date. If not, consider if you are so far behind that you need to change your exam date. Then when you change your date, allow yourself sufficient time to prepare. Update your calendar.

▪ DIFFICULTY STUDYING

Studying for certification exams can be overwhelming. You have finished classes and are excited about working as an AG-ACNP, but something may be stopping you from focusing. Remember that the certification exam is simply designed to demonstrate your proficiency as a beginning safe practitioner.

Although study habits vary, and you may have difficulty focusing on the task, consider the following: Although many graduates stay focused, others find studying intimidating, frustrating, tedious, and perhaps, scary. Do you

- Avoid studying?
- Only engage in the study activities you like?
- Have difficulty concentrating on study materials?
- Have insomnia?

If you are experiencing any of these difficulties, you may want to obtain academic support services and work with professionals trained to develop study systems. Your nursing program may offer these services, or there may be individuals in private practice to assist with these concerns. If you seek a service outside of the school, ensuring they are familiar with your national certification exam is immensely beneficial.

You may also need additional support. Consider seeking the advice of your primary care providers or psychologists, psychiatrists, counselors, or other mental health professionals that are trained to offer support for anxiety, depression, attention deficit, and other mental health concerns. Check to see if your employer offers these services for free or at a reduced rate.

ACADEMIC ACCOMMODATIONS

Both national board certification examinations are compliant with the Americans with Disabilities Act (ADA). As such, students who have a history of learning, mental health, or medical conditions requiring accommodations are encouraged to request reasonable accommodations during their application process. The process and format for supporting documentation differs with eachcertifying body. While not explicitly stated on the websites, it is helpful and adds strength to your request to have had formal academic accommodations granted while in your educational program and to be able to provide documentation of such. Whether or not you have had accommodations in your program, it is wise to seek the assistance of your school's disability office when filling out forms or submitting your request and supporting documentation. Alternatively, an education specialist who works in an academic achievement department can provide similar support.

Although not specifically stated on the websites, it is helpful if your documentation includes *ICD-10* or *DSM-5* codes, and any significant educational history that supports your need for accommodations (i.e., individualized education program [IEP], Section 504 Plan, Educational Program Placement).

Specific requirements included on each organization's website are found at the following web links:

- ANCC: https://www.nursingworld.org/~4ac3ba/globalassets/certification/renewals/GeneralTestingandRenewalHandbook

- AACN: www.aacn.org/~/media/aacn-website/certification/get-certified/handbooks/certpolicyhndbk.pdf?la=en. See pages 10 and 22 to 23 in the January 2018 publication. Review the form requirements and the AACN test administration process. That allows you to have a comprehensive discussion with your provider resulting in the accurate completion of the form.

Certifying bodies may request additional documentation or clarifications. Thus, it is important that you do NOT schedule your exam date until you have an answer to your request for accommodations and have ensured the testing center can facilitate your approved accommodations. Once accommodations have been approved, then you can schedule your exam date and time. Should you receive a denial letter, you will want to seek assistance of your school's disability office or student ADA coordinator for guidance.

ADVICE

First and foremost, if you were granted and utilized accommodations during your academic career, we highly recommend you seek accommodations for your national board certification exam. This certification exam can lead to a much more stressful situation and you want to create optimal conditions for success. We advise AGAINST trying to take the exam without accommodations. The risk of failing the exam without accommodations goes up exponentially. In addition, failing the exam creates a significant negative impact on your confidence level, making the second exam encounter even more intimidating.

Second, it is important that your request matches the recommendations the provider submits. Submit a copy of your request or form to the provider so he or she sees what has been requested.

Third, it is helpful to include all application paperwork, such as request and supporting letters for accommodations, in one envelope for ease and efficiency of processing. Single or additional pieces of paperwork mailed separately can get lost or take longer to collate within the organization. Make sure your name is included and easily located on each page submitted.

Fourth, processing paperwork may take time. Submit the accommodations and application paperwork as soon as your program indicates that you are eligible to sit for the exam. If needed, plan in advance to meet with your provider to discuss your current needs, previous history, and/or update testing.

Last, if you have any questions regarding the process, please be sure to ask your student ADA coordinator and contact the accrediting or certifying agency if needed.

■ REFERENCES

American Association of Critical-Care Nurses. (2017). *Certification corporation ACNPC-AG certification handbook*. Retrieved from https://www.aacn.org/~/media/aacn-website/certification/get-certified/handbooks/certpolicyhndbk.pdf?la=en

American Nurses Credentialing Center. (2017a). *Adult-gerontology acute care nurse practitioner*. Retrieved from https://www.nursingworld.org/~4accca/globalassets/certification/certification-specialty-pages/resources/test-content-outlines/adultgerontologyacutecarenp-tco.pdf

American Nurses Credentialing Center. (2017b). *Test content outline*. Retrieved from http://nursecredentialing.org/Exam62-AdultGeroAcuteCareNP-TCO-Jan2017

Nolting, P. D. (1997). *Winning at math*. Bradenton, FL: Academic Success Press.

3

Test-Taking Strategies and Succeeding on Exam Day

CHRISTINE MERMAN WOOLF AND
DAWN CARPENTER

READ THE QUESTIONS

Carefully read each question. A major mistake is to skim the questions. Read the question, also known as the *stem*, for key words such as "assess," "teach," "diagnose," or "treat" (Thompson, 2016). These words direct you to what action is expected by the adult-gerontology acute care nurse practitioner (AG-ACNP) for the scenario. Identify what the question is asking and use your diagnostic reasoning skills and logic to problem solve and think critically. Highlight important words or phrases, or write them on the paper or whiteboard provided by the testing center. Pay particular attention to details in the scenario, including age group of the patient, gender, and past medical history (Thompson, 2016). These details are specifically included to help you identify the correct answer. Avoid reading into the stem—stay with the information given.

EVALUATE THE ANSWERS

Formulate an answer before you look at the possible answers. Then look to see if the answer is among the possible answers or if one of them closely approximates your thoughts. Read each distractor carefully. There may be more than one correct answer; thus, answer with the best option. If a question asks for an intervention, then answer with an intervention. Eliminate options that you know to be incorrect. If any part of an answer is wrong, the entire option is wrong.

REPHRASE THE QUESTION

Turn the question around. That is, take the distractor and turn that into a statement. For instance, "Which of the following medications may increase liver enzymes?" If an answer is vancomycin, then simply think: Does vancomycin increase liver enzymes? No? Then look for another answer. That being said, avoid rewriting the question in your head as you think it "should" be worded. Simply read the question at face value, choosing a response that simply answers the question.

■ USE EVIDENCE

Use evidence-based practice knowledge to answer the question. Avoid the tendency to apply your personal anecdotal experience to determine the correct answer. Do not think of what they do in your hospital. Consider the best evidence to make a diagnosis or treatment decision. When doing practice questions, review material on questions you get incorrect or do not know. Add notes to study materials.

■ PROBLEM SOLVING

There will be questions for whose content area you are unaware. If the question is about a patient on asthma medication and you think to yourself, I do not remember asthma medication information, do not guess. Instead, relax and think about breaking down the parts and elements you do know. Reason through it. For example:

> *"Okay I know patients can be on long-term control or quick-relief medications. For long-term the patient may be on corticosteroids. How do those work? I remember that corticosteroids can be inhaled to reduce inflammation in the lungs. However, reducing inflammation takes time and may not help this patient fast enough because this patient is waking up at night, complaining of chest tightness, and has stopped playing sports. Okay so I do not think the answer is related to long-term control. That leaves the quick-relief offered by SABAs. I think that medication relaxes the airway muscles, but I am not confident. However, I know it works quickly. So I ruled out the long-term medication, I think it might be a SABA, and the other two options do not address the significant lung concerns since one is basically related to just resting and the other is related to educating the patient about asthma, they will not provide the relief needed to address the airway issue. I'll pick the SABA."* (National Institutes of Health [NIH], 2012)

■ CHANGING ANSWERS

There are only four reasons to change your answer to an item. It is acceptable to change your answers only if:

- You misread the question or did not read the entire item and all the answer options. You may have been anxious when you read it, or rushed because you were worried about the time.

- You did not consider all the information when you read it. Did you see an option, presumed it to be correct, and did not fully read the other options or fully consider the information?

- You have new information to consider when you read the item again. This may happen if a question later in the exam prompts you to remember something about a disease that you had forgotten when you first read the question.

- You misclicked on the computer and discovered an error upon reviewing the exam.

Keep data as noted in Chapter 2. Identify when changing works for you, and only in those instances change the answer. If changing answers typically negatively impacts your score, then you can write yourself a note: "Don't change answers!" (Nolting, 1997). Consider deciding not to do a second pass at the items if it is too challenging for you not to change answers.

TESTING ON A COMPUTER

If you are worried about the computer format of the exam, then be sure to do many practice questions on the computer. Even if you have to redo the questions multiple times, it is worth immersing yourself in the experience. Go to a library or somewhere that has computers set up for public use. Try to work through questions on those computers. Taking questions near other people and on a computer that is not yours is good practice for exam day. Also, solving practice questions when others are moving around is helpful, because on exam day people will be getting up and leaving the exam room when you are taking your exam.

SUCCEEDING ON EXAM DAY

What to Expect the Day of the Exam

Be aware of what to expect on exam day. Review all the relevant information at the relevant exam website. For American Nurses Credentialing Center (ANCC, 2017), you will take the exam at a Prometric center. For American Association of Critical-Care Nurses (AACN, 2017), you will take the exam at a PSI/AMP center. Procedures change over time, so be certain you read the current exam policies. Do not rely on statements from peers and coworkers about these issues. You do not want to have an unexpected outcome on exam day.

These are questions you should be able to answer:

- What forms of identification do I need to bring?
- What proof is needed to show I am taking the exam on the certification exam day?
- Do I need to bring documentation showing I am to receive accommodations?
- What are the security procedures?
- How do I take breaks and how do they impact my exam time?
- What can I bring to the exam center?

Visit the Exam Center

Prior to taking the exam, drive to the site. This helps you plan your drive time and lessen anxiety. Note traffic patterns, and plan your drive around the same day of the week and time that you will take your exam. Observe for school buses, city buses, construction, and so on. Developing a driving plan will decrease stress on exam day. Be sure to give yourself sufficient time for any unexpected delays. Arrive early to allow time for check-in procedures.

Attire

Check the website for information regarding proper attire. Wear comfortable clothes and shoes. Remember you will be sitting for a few hours. Exam rooms may be cool, so dress accordingly.

Insomnia Before the Exam

AVOID alcohol the night before the exam. If you wake up due to not being able to sleep, that does not mean you will have a terrible exam day. You may have had trouble sleeping before other exams. If you have a history of poor sleep before exams, then try to get a good night's sleep for multiple days before your exam day. That way, one night of poor sleep will not have as much of an impact. Try your best to get to sleep by doing your usual routines to sleep. If you are up early and you know that you will not be able to get back to sleep, then try to relax and eat a good breakfast. Avoid studying, but if you must study, review content you know well to remind yourself that you are ready for the exam.

On Exam Day

Remember—you have the knowledge you need to succeed. You have been exposed to many exams, so you have experience taking exams. The questions you worked through on a regular basis are likely to be similar to the ones you will see on the exam.

At the Start of the Exam

Read the directions. Do not skip or skim directions. Take the practice or sample questions to ensure you are answering correctly (Nolting, 1997).

Pacing on Exam Day

At times examinees are nervous on the day of their exam; this can throw off your usual system. Once you notice you are not following your system, pause, take a deep breath, and try your best to relax and remind yourself that your system works.

Going Too Fast

If you notice you are going too fast, consider if you are just skimming items or not reading the entire item or all the options. Slow down, and read carefully and critically.

Going Too Slowly

If you are going slowly, then remember the way you handled dwelling on items when you were practicing and set time limits on answering questions. Mark only questions you are uncertain of and go back to them. Use the skills you practiced, including tracking your time and marking questions to come back to once you have answered the majority of the questions.

Changing Answers

DO NOT GO BACK and change your answers. Your first answer is most often the correct one. If you are changing answers more than usual, then use your system on your exam day and track reasons for changing answers. Tell yourself your system worked at home/library/school and will work at the center. Take a few moments for a deep breath and a calming thought to help you refocus. Only flag or mark questions you have no idea about. You should not flag more than three to five questions.

Use the Tools Provided on Exam Day

Use the laminate board or scratch paper you receive at the exam center to help you keep track of key words, your reasoning or questions you want to review, and reasons for changing answers. You most likely used paper to do those tasks when working with practice questions, so use the tools at the center the same way. Do not start a new system on the day of your exam.

When you are using the computer to answer items, be sure you are not accidentally clicking. If you pick an answer and then move your cursor around within the page, be sure you do not inadvertently change your chosen answer.

Manage Anxiety

Do not exaggerate the importance or significance of the exam. Avoid negative feedback, as it will increase your anxiety. Take 30 to 60 seconds to sit back and relax. Use some mindfulness and relaxation techniques, such as deep breathing.

Computer Issues/Unexpected Events on Exam Day

Sometimes unexpected events occur. There may be a computer hardware or software issue. There may be a power issue or a number of other challenges. Know these events are rare and that the center staff members know how to address them. If something happens to your computer and it takes time to fix, the best reaction is to stay calm, remain professional, and request assistance. If the staff instruct you to follow up by contacting the association either through email or phone, then be professional in those communications as well. And if there is a massive snowstorm or hurricane, double-check with the testing center to be certain it is open.

■ REFERENCES

American Association of Critical-Care Nurses. (2017). *Certification corporation ACNPC-AG certification handbook*. Retrieved from https://www.aacn.org/~/media/aacn-website/certification/get-certified/handbooks/certpolicyhndbk.pdf?la=en

American Nurses Credentialing Center. (2017). *Adult-gerontology acute care nurse practitioner*. Retrieved from http://nursecredentialing.org/AdultGeroAcuteCareNP

National Institutes of Health. (2012). *Asthma care quick reference: Diagnosing and managing asthma*. Retrieved from https://www.nhlbi.nih.gov/files/docs/guidelines/asthma_qrg.pdf

Nolting, P. D. (1997). *Winning at math*. Bradenton, FL: Academic Success Press.

Thompson, D. L. (2016). Useful test-taking strategies when preparing for the WOCNCB continence examination. *Journal of Wound, Ostomy and Continence Nursing, 43*(4), 425–426. doi:10.1097/WON.0000000000000246

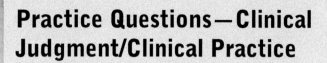

Practice Questions—Clinical Judgment/Clinical Practice

4

Health Promotion, Disease Prevention, and Factors Influencing Health Status

BETH McLEAR, STEFANIE LA MANNA, AND GAIL LIS

HEALTH PROMOTION, DISEASE PREVENTION, AND FACTORS INFLUENCING HEALTH STATUS QUESTIONS

1. Healthcare disparities among African American, Hispanic, and Caucasian Americans of all age groups have been decreasing since 2014. This is largely due to:

   a. Access to health insurance
   b. Genetic modifications
   c. Better patient education
   d. Enhanced diet

2. A 64-year-old male patient has undergone a prostectomy to remove and control localized prostate cancer. This is an example of:

   a. Primary prevention
   b. Secondary prevention
   c. Tertiary prevention
   d. Definitive prevention

3. The AG-ACNP performs a hepatitis screening panel and the results are as follows: negative HBsAg, positive anti-HBs, negative anti-HBc. The correct interpretation of these results is:

   a. The patient has an active hepatitis B infection and is contagious
   b. The patient has an active hepatitis B infection and is not contagious
   c. The patient has had a hepatitis B infection in the past and has natural immunity
   d. The patient has had a hepatitis B vaccine in the past and has passive immunity

4. A 55-year-old patient is seen by the AG-ACNP in the cardiology office for follow up of his congestive heart failure. He has a 35-pack-year history of smoking and is a current smoker. He inquired about the possibility his shortness of breath is due to lung cancer. The AG-ACNP orders:

   a. Chest x-ray
   b. Low-dose computed tomography of the chest
   c. Pulmonary function test
   d. Six-minute walk test

5. A 54-year-old female patient presents to the thoracic surgery clinic for follow-up of her lung cancer. Her medical history is significant for asthma which is well controlled with a low dose corticosteroid inhaler. She is a nonsmoker and has two glasses of wine weekly. She has no other personal or family history of cancer. She inquires when her mammogram is due. The AG-ACNP informs her she should be receiving:

    a. Biennial mammogram

    b. Annual mammogram

    c. Biannual mammogram

    d. Mammogram not indicated

6. The AG-ACNP is evaluating a 62-year-old male patient who had a colonoscopy 5 years ago. The colonoscopy was normal and he has no personal or family history that puts him at higher risk for colon cancer. The evidence-based recommendation for repeat colonoscopy in this patient is:

    a. Repeat colonoscopy this year

    b. Flex sigmoidoscopy this year

    c. No further testing is recommended

    d. Repeat colonoscopy in 5 years

7. The AG-ACNP is discharging a 74-year-old male who has been hospitalized for pneumonia. During this admission it was noted he had difficulty ambulating due to severe osteoarthritis in his left knee. Physical therapy has recommended use of a cane. The discharge planning should include a home visit for fall risk assessment, review of medications, and instructions:

    a. To use cane on right side

    b. To use cane when he feels unsteady

    c. To use cane on left side

    d. Use cane when outside of home environment only

8. The AG-ACNP is admitting a 47-year-old male with a diagnosis of an acute upper gastrointestinal hemorrhage. The venous thromboembolism (VTE) prophylaxis that is indicated at this time is:

    a. None is indicated

    b. Low molecular weight heparin

    c. Vitamin K antagonist

    d. Intermittent pneumatic compression device

9. A 22-year-old college student is being discharged after a motor vehicle crash. His surgical care included a splenectomy and right femur rodding. Which of the following vaccines are needed upon discharge?

    a. Diptheria-tetanus and human papillomavirus (HPV)

    b. Influenza and poliomyelitis

    c. PNEUMOVAX®23 (Pneumococcal Vaccine Polyvalent) (PPSV23) and quadrivalent meningiococcal vaccine

    d. Hepatitis A and B

10. Which of the following patients requires stress ulcer prophylaxis?

    a. A 54-year-old female admitted for elective right knee replacement

    b. A 67-year-old male patient admitted for evaluation of chest pain

    c. A 21-year-old female admitted for cesarean delivery

    d. A 76-year-old male patient on mechanical ventilation due to acute respiratory failure

11. The AG-ACNP is evaluating a 35-year-old female patient with a body mass index (BMI) of 28. Her medical history is negative except for allergic rhinitis which is well controlled. She expresses an interest in losing weight. The initial plan should include:

    a. Education regarding exercise and caloric intake
    b. Referral for gastric sleeve for rapid weight loss
    c. Pharmacotherapy for rapid weight loss
    d. Referral to psychiatry for behavior modification training

12. The AG-ACNP is caring for a patient who is on mechanical ventilation. Which of the following is a strategy prevents ventilator-associated pneumonia (VAP)?

    a. Change the ventilator circuit every 24 hours
    b. Perform spontaneous breathing trials every 24 hours
    c. Interrupt sedation once every 72 hours
    d. Perform spontaneous breathing trials every 48 hours

13. A 33-year-old HIV-positive patient presents to the HIV clinic for a follow-up and asks the AG-ACNP about receiving the pneumococcal vaccine. The current recommendation is vaccination with the:

    a. PCV13 (Pneumococcal Conjugate Vaccine) now and revaccination with PPSV23 (PNEUMOVAX®23 [Pneumococcal Vaccine Polyvalent]) in 1 year
    b. PCV13 now and revaccination with PPSV23 in 8 weeks
    c. PPSV23 now and revaccination with PCV13 in 8 weeks
    d. PPSV23 now and revaccination with PCV13 in 1 year

14. An AG-ACNP is educating a patient with chronic obstructive pulmonary disease (COPD) about tobacco cessation. According to the U.S. Department of Health and Human Services Treating Tobacco Use and Dependence Guideline, the components of an intervention for treating tobacco use include:

    a. Ask, advise, assess, assist, arrange
    b. Ask, advise, assess, assist, teach
    c. Ask, advise, arrange, manage, teach
    d. Ask, assess, advise, treat, manage

15. A contraindication for the herpes zoster vaccine is:

    a. Allergy to penicillin
    b. History of zoster infection
    c. Current chemotherapy treatment
    d. Current treatment for chronic obstructive pulmonary disease

16. The AG-ACNP is providing a client who is ready to quit using tobacco with an evidence-based treatment plan for treating tobacco use and dependence. The client's medical history is significant for a history of seizures 10 years ago. He is not on any medications at this time. The treatment plan should include which of the following?

    a. A tricyclic antidepressant and counseling
    b. A nicotine patch and bupropion XR
    c. A nicotine lozenge and counseling
    d. Bupropion XR and varenicline (Chantix)

17. Our national health promotion framework, Healthy People 2020, has two overarching goals for all people. These goals are:

    a. To increase the quality and years of a healthy life and eliminate health disparities
    b. To increase the number of patients covered by health insurance and decrease health disparities
    c. To decrease the number of uninsured patients and increase years of productive life
    d. To decrease emergency room visits and increase the number of patients with health insurance

18. AG-ACNPs discuss code status with all patients admitted to the hospital. This is an example of:

    a. Primary prevention
    b. Secondary prevention
    c. Tertiary prevention
    d. Quaternary prevention

19. A 76-year-old patient with progressive Parkinson's disease has had multiple admissions for aspiration pneumonia. The patient's functional capacity is also declining and his wife has indicated that she would like to continue his care. The AG-ACNP caring for this patient would like to integrate palliative care in the overall care management. Which of the following questions should be asked initially to assist the patient and family in establishing goals of care?

    a. Are you afraid you are going to die?
    b. Do you practice a particular faith?
    c. Would you like me to tell you about your prognosis?
    d. What do you currently understand about your Parkinson's disease?

20. An 82-year-old female with a history of metastatic colon cancer, and enrolled on the palliative care service, is receiving medical treatment for a bowel obstruction. The patient reports that she feels short of breath and this is making her quite anxious. Upon exam, an ill-appearing, anxious female is evaluated, sitting upright in bed and breathing 28 breaths per minute. Her oxygen saturation is 96% on room air. The initial goal of management for this patient is to:

    a. Determine the underlying cause
    b. Enroll the patient into hospice care
    c. Provide symptom management to decrease the respiratory rate
    d. Provide symptom management to attain a subjective improvement in breathlessness

21. A 69-year-old male with stage IV lung cancer indicates to the staff that he would like to discontinue his treatment and move to hospice care. The patient is concerned that his family will not support his wishes and wants to know how to make sure his end of life wishes are honored. In order to assist with this request, the AG-ACNP should do which of the following first?

    a. Ask the patient if he has identified a durable power of attorney
    b. Ask the patient if he has an advance directive
    c. Ask the patient if he has discussed this with his family
    d. Ask the patient if he would like to speak with a chaplain

■ HEALTH PROMOTION, DISEASE PREVENTION, AND OTHER FACTORS INFLUENCING HEALTH STATUS ANSWERS AND RATIONALES

1. **a) Access to health insurance.** The Affordable Care Act provided increased health insurance options for young adults, early retirees, and Americans with pre-existing conditions. These were implemented in October 2013 with coverage beginning in January 2014. Expanded access to Medicaid in many states began in January 2014. This resulted in a reduction of health access disparities for Americans.

2. **c) Tertiary prevention.** Categories of prevention include primary, secondary, or tertiary prevention. Primary prevention aims to remove or reduce risk factors for disease (e.g., immunizations), secondary prevention strategies promote early detection of disease (e.g., Pap smear screening to detect carcinoma or dysplasia of the cervix), and tertiary prevention measures are aimed at limiting the impact of an established disease (e.g., mastectomy for breast cancer).

3. **d) The patient has had a hepatitis B vaccine in the past and has passive immunity.** A positive HBsAg result indicates acute or chronic infection. Testing for antibodies to HBsAg (anti-HBs) and anti-HBc is also done as part of a screening panel to help distinguish between infection and immunity. Acute hepatitis B infection is characterized by the appearance of HBsAg and followed by the appearance of anti-HBc. The disappearance of HBsAg and the presence of anti-HBs and anti-HBc indicate the resolution of HBV infection and natural immunity. Anti-HBc, which persists for life, is present only after HBV infection and does not develop in persons whose immunity to HBV is due to vaccination.

4. **b) Low-dose computed tomography of the chest.** The U.S. Preventive Services Task Force recommends annual screening for lung cancer with LDCT in adults 55 to 80 years of age who have a 30-pack-year smoking history and currently smoke or have quit within the past 15 years. Chest x-ray is not as sensitive or specific as LDCT and is not recommended as screening. Pulmonary function test and 6-minute walk tests are tests to evaluate lung function and are not sensitive or specific to detection of lung cancer.

5. **a) Biennial mammogram.** The U.S. Preventive Services Task Force recommends biennial screening mammography for women aged 50 to 74 years. This recommendations applies to asymptomatic women aged 40 years or older who do not have pre-existing breast cancer or a previously diagnosed high-risk breast lesion and who are not at high risk for breast cancer because of a known underlying genetic mutation (such as a *BRCA1* or *BRCA2* gene mutation or other familial breast cancer syndrome) or a history of chest radiation at a young age.

6. **d) Repeat colonoscopy in 5 years.** The United States Preventive Services Task Force recommends screening for colorectal cancer starting at age 50 years and continuing until age 75 years. Screening with colonoscopy every 10 years, annual fecal immunochemical test (FIT), annual high-sensitivity fecal occult blood test (FOBT), or flexible sigmoidoscopy every 5 years combined with high-sensitivity FOBT every 3 years are the recommended modalities of screening. This recommendation applies to asymptomatic adults 50 years and older who are at average risk of colorectal cancer and who do not have a family history of known genetic disorders that predispose them to a high lifetime risk of colorectal cancer (such as Lynch syndrome or familial adenomatous polyposis), a personal history of inflammatory bowel disease, a previous adenomatous polyp, or previous colorectal cancer.

7. **a) To use cane on right side.** Balance and ambulation require a complex coordination of cognitive, neuromuscular, and cardiovascular function. Falls in older people are rarely due to a single cause, and effective intervention entails a comprehensive assessment of the patient's intrinsic deficits (e.g., diseases and medications) and environmental obstacles. Assistive devices, such as canes and walkers, are useful for many older adults but are often used incorrectly. Canes should be used on the "good" side. The height of walkers and canes should generally be about the level of the wrist.

8. **d) Intermittent pneumatic compression device.** For acutely ill hospitalized patients with increased risk of thrombosis who are bleeding or at high risk for major bleeding, the optimal use of mechanical thromboprophylaxis with GCS or IPC rather than no mechanical thrombo-prophylaxis is recommended. When bleeding risk decreases, and if VTE risk persists, pharmacologic thromboprophylaxis can be added to mechanical thromboprophylaxis.

9. **c) PPSV23 and quadrivalent meningiococcal vaccine.** Asplenic patients are at great risk for pneumococcal and Neisseria meningitidis infections. Meningitis vaccines are especially warranted in the college-age student. The flu and DT are both recommended; the HPV, polio, and hepatitis vaccines are not indicated. Of note, DT is indicated at the time of admission to the hospital as prophylaxis, not at the time of discharge.

10. **d) A 76-year-old male patient on mechanical ventilation due to acute respiratory failure.** Two of the most important risk factors for gastrointestinal bleeding from stress ulcers are coagulopathy and respiratory failure with the need for mechanical ventilation for over 48 hours. When these two risk factors are absent, the risk of significant bleeding is only 0.1%. Other risk factors include traumatic brain injury, severe burns, sepsis, vasopressor therapy, corticosteroid therapy, and prior history of peptic ulcer disease and gastrointestinal bleeding. Prophylaxis should be routinely administered upon admission to critically ill patients with risk factors for significant bleeding.

11. **a) Education regarding exercise and caloric intake.** Initial weight-loss plans should be focused on developing habits that will help maintain weight loss, such as dietary and activity changes. The National Institutes of Health clinical obesity guidelines state that obesity drugs may be used as a comprehensive weight-loss program for patients with a body mass index (BMI) greater than 30 or with a BMI over 27 if obesity-related risk factors are present. Gastric surgery is considered only if BMI is over 40 or over 35 with obesity-related risk factors. Although behavior modification programs exist, many of these techniques can be taught by general clinicians.

12. **b) Perform spontaneous breathing trials every 24 hours.** Daily spontaneous breathing trials are associated with extubation 1 to 2 days earlier than usual care and are a level 1 recommendation for prevention of VAP. Interruption of sedation daily is also a level 1 recommendation and should be paired with spontaneous breathing trials. There is no evidence to support that changing ventilator circuits on a regular basis decreased VAP rates and is costly, therefore changing only when visibly soiled or when there is a malfunction is the current recommendation.

13. **b) PCV13 now and revaccination with PPSV23 in 8 weeks.** According to the CDC guidelines, vaccination with the PCV13 and the PPSV23 vaccination should be given 8 weeks later for immunocompromised patients such as HIV.

14. **a) Ask, advise, assess, assist, arrange.** On every hospital or office visit, the practitioner must ask, advise, assess, assist, and arrange about tobacco use and guide the patient about tobacco cessation. This is a Medicare guideline and quality effective care.

15. **c) Current chemotherapy treatment.** A person who has ever had a life-threatening or severe allergic reaction to gelatin, the antibiotic neomycin, or any other component of shingles vaccine should not be vaccinated with the zoster vaccine. Zoster vaccine should be given with or without of a history of zoster. Zoster recurs, and there is no evidence to indicate that persons are at reduced risk for zoster for any period of time following a prior occurrence of the disease and there are no recognized safety concerns in giving the vaccine to people with prior history of zoster. The general guideline for any vaccine is to wait until the acute stage of the illness is over and symptoms resolve. The zoster vaccine is contraindicated in patients who have weakened immune systems because of HIV/AIDS or another disease that affects the immune system, treatment with drugs that affect the immune system, cancer treatment such as radiation or chemotherapy, or a cancer affecting the bone marrow or lymphatic system.

16. **c) A nicotine lozenge and counseling**. Combining counseling and medication increases abstinence rates. The first-line medications for treatment of tobacco use include bupropion SR, nicotine gum, nicotine inhaler, nicotine lozenge, nicotine nasal spray, nicotine patch, and varenicline. Certain combinations of cessation medications are effective. Bupropion is contraindicated in patients with a history of seizures. Bupropion may increase long-term cessation rates in smokers who have a past medical history of depression, but there was not sufficient evidence found for the use of bupropion in smokers with current depression.

17. **a) To increase the quality and years of a healthy life and eliminate health disparities**. The Healthy People 2020 campaign, which has been adopted by the World Health Organization, outlines two overarching goals for all people. These goals are to increase the quality and years of a healthy life and eliminate health disparities.

18. **d) Quaternary prevention**. Prevention of overmedicalization is defined as quaternary care. Primary prevention aims to remove or reduce risk factors for disease (e.g., immunizations), secondary prevention strategies promote early detection of disease (e.g., Pap smear screening to detect carcinoma or dysplasia of the cervix), and tertiary prevention measures are aimed at limiting the impact of an established disease (e.g., mastectomy for breast cancer).

19. **d) What do you currently understand about your Parkinson's disease?** It is important to initially understand what the patient and family currently know about the disease process and ask open-ended questions to facilitate the overall conversation. Once the practitioner comprehends what the patient understands, a conversation related to the prognosis will follow. Questions should be queried in an open-ended format, allowing the patient to expand upon what he is truly thinking. Questions related to faith and death are also relevant, but may not be appropriate at the onset of the conversation.

20. **d) Provide symptom management to attain a subjective improvement in breathlessness**. The symptom of breathlessness is quite distressing for most individuals, and self-reporting by the patient is considered a reliable measure because respiratory rate, pulmonary congestion, hypoxia, and hypercapnia do not correlate. The goal of treatment should be the subjective improvement in breathlessness as opposed to lowering the respiratory rate to normal. Because breathlessness is a complex pathophysiologic process, determining the underlying cause may not be timely and therefore initial symptom management is recommended. Further investigation should follow the initial symptom management. It may be time to consider hospice care, but the priority goal should initially focus on symptom management.

21. **b) Ask the patient if he has an advance directive**. Advance directives are medical documents that identify a patient's preference for future medical care. This patient is currently competent and therefore able to explicitly determine his healthcare wishes. If the patient does not have an advance directive, then one should be developed and become part of the patient's medical record. It is also important for the patient to have a discussion with his family; however, this often evolves from completion of an advance directive or living will. The durable power of attorney should have a specific designation for healthcare and would be designated within the advance directive. Spiritual support would be beneficial to consider as the patient is developing the advance directive and even having discussions with his family.

■ BIBLIOGRAPHY

Agency for Healthcare Research and Quality. (2015). *2015 National Healthcare Quality and Disparities Report and 5th anniversary update on the National Quality Strategy*. Rockville, MD: U.S. Department of Health and Human Services. Retrieved from https://www.ahrq.gov/sites/default/files/wysiwyg/research/findings/nhqrdr/nhqdr15/2015nhqdr.pdf

AIDSinfo, A. (2017). Guidelines for the prevention and treatment of opportunistic infections in HIV-infected adults and adolescents. *Progressive*. Retrieved from https://aidsinfo.nih.gov/contentfiles/lvguidelines/adult_oi.pdf

Benjamin, I. J., Griggs, R. C., Wing, E. J., & Fitz, J. G. (2010). *Andreoli and Carpenter's Cecil essentials of medicine* (8th ed.). Philadelphia, PA: Elsevier Saunders.

Braveman, P. A., Egerter, S. A., & Mockenhaupt, R. E. (2011). Broadening the focus: The need to address the social determinants of health. *American Journal of Preventive Medicine, 40*(1 Suppl. 1), S4–S18. doi:10.1016/j.amepre.2010.10.002

Centers for Disease Control and Prevention. (2009). *Shingles/herpes zoster vaccine recommendations.* Retrieved from https://www.cdc.gov/vaccines/vpd/shingles/hcp/recommendations.html

Centers for Disease Control and Prevention. (2015). *Pneumococcal vaccination: Summary of who and when to vaccinate.* Retrieved from https://www.cdc.gov/vaccines/vpd/pneumo/hcp/who-when-to-vaccinate.html

DeNisco, S. M. (2018). *Role development for the nurse practitioner.* Burlington, MA: Jones & Bartlett Learning.

Flaherty, E. R., & Resnick, B. (2014). *Geriatric nursing review syllabus: A core curriculum in advanced practice geriatric nursing.* New York, NY: American Geriatrics Society.

Guyatt, G. H., Akl, E. A., Crowther, M., Gutterman, D. D., & Schuünemann, H. J. (2012). Executive summary: Antithrombotic therapy and prevention of thrombosis (9th ed.) American College of Chest Physicians evidence-based clinical practice guidelines. *Chest, 141*(2), 7S–47S. doi:10.1378/chest.1412S3

Kasper, D., Hauser, S., Jameson, J., Fauci, A., Longo, D., & Loscalzo, J. (2015). *Harrison's principles of internal medicine* (19th ed.). New York, NY: McGraw-Hill Education.

Klompas, M., Branson, R., Eichenwald, E., Greene, L., Howell, M., Lee, G., & Berenholtz, S. (2014). Strategies to prevent ventilator-associated pneumonia in acute care hospitals: 2014 update. *Infection Control and Hospital Epidemiology, 35*(8), 915–936. doi:10.1086/677144

Pandve, H. T. (2014). Quaternary prevention: Need of the hour. *Journal of Family Medicine and Primary Care, 3*(4), 309–310.

Papadakis, M. A., McPhee, S. J., & Rabow, M. W. (2017). *Current medical diagnosis & treatment 2017.* New York, NY: McGraw-Hill Education.

Tatum, P., Talebreza, S., Ross, J. S., & Widera, E. (2017). Palliative care and special management issues. In J. B. Halter, J. G. Ouslander, S. Studenski, K. P. High, S. Asthana, M. A. Supiano, & C. Ritchie (Eds.), *Hazzard's geriatric medicine* (7th ed.). New York, NY: McGraw-Hill Education.

U.S. Department of Health and Human Services Tobacco Use and Dependence Guideline Panel. (2008). *Treating tobacco use and dependence 2008 update.* Retrieved from https://www.ncbi.nlm.nih.gov/books/NBK63952/

U.S. Department of Health and Human Services. Office of Disease Prevention and Health Promotion. (2020). *Healthy people 2020.* Retrieved from https://www.healthypeople.gov

U.S. Preventive Services Task Force. (2016). *Final update summary: Breast cancer: Screening.* Retrieved from https://www.uspreventiveservicestaskforce.org/Page/Document/UpdateSummaryFinal/breast-cancer-screening1

United States Preventive Service Task Force. (2014). *Final recommendation statement hepatitis B virus infection: Screening.* Retrieved from https://www.uspreventiveservicetaskforce.org/Page/Document/RecommendationStatementFinal/hepatitis-b-virus-infection-screening-2014#Pod1

United States Preventive Services Task Force. (2016). *Final recommendation statement: Lung cancer: Screening.* Retrieved from https://www.uspreventiveservicestaskforce.org/Page/Document/RecommendationStatementFinal/lung-cancer-screening

United States Preventive Services Task Force. (2017). *Final recommendation statement: Colorectal cancer: Screening.* Retrieved from https://www.uspreventiveservicestaskforce.org/Page/Document/RecommendationStatementFinal/colorectal-cancer-screening2

van der Meer, R. M., Willemsen, M. C., Smit, F., & Cuijpers, P. (2013). *Smoking cessation interventions for smokers with current or past depression* (CD006102). Retrieved from https://www.ncbi.nlm.nih.gov/pubmed/23963776

Wiegand, D., & Russo, M. M. (2013). *Ethical considerations* (2nd ed., Vol. 1). Pittsburgh, PA: Hospice and Palliative Nurses Association.

5 Geriatric

GAIL LIS, ANTHONY McGUIRE, AND
VICTORIA CREEDON

GERIATRIC QUESTIONS

1. An 85-year-old female admitted to the ICU with four unilateral rib fractures from a mechanical fall reports occasional short-term memory loss (forgetfulness). Her family is concerned that she sometimes has trouble hearing, especially with phone conversations. She lives independently and does not require assistance with her activities of daily living. Which condition is most consistent with the stated history?

   a. Early signs of Alzheimer's dementia
   b. Early signs of vascular dementia
   c. Normal aging process
   d. Benign paroxysmal positional vertigo

2. Normal changes associated with aging that may alter the absorption, distribution, or metabolism of drugs include which of the following?

   a. Increased fat as a percentage of body mass
   b. Increased body water
   c. Reduced number of hepatocytes
   d. Increased serum albumin

3. An AG-ACNP who works on an acute care unit for elders understands that falls can readily impact the independence of older adults. Which of the following is the most modifiable risk factor associated with falls in older adults?

   a. Medication use
   b. Diet
   c. Osteoarthritis
   d. Neuropathy

4. An AG-ACNP is caring for a 72-year-old female patient with acute exacerbation of COPD. Upon review of systems, the patient verbalizes to the nurse practitioner that she continues to smoke but has decreased the amount of cigarettes per day. The best response to this patient would be:

   a. "Since you have decreased the amount you smoke, you will likely experience no further lung damage."
   b. "It is important that you quit smoking altogether; please have your family throw away all of your cigarettes at home so you won't be tempted to smoke again."
   c. "It seems like you are trying to quit smoking; let me discuss with you some possible strategies."
   d. "Patients older than the age of 65 do not need to quit smoking, as the lung damage has already occurred."

5. An 84-year-old female patient is admitted to the orthopedic unit status post fall and hip fracture. The patient indicates that she got up to go to the bathroom during the night, became dizzy, and fell. On admission to the emergency room the patient's vital signs were as follows: blood pressure 170/82, heart rate 76, and respiration rate 18. In reviewing her medications, which one of the following medications would most likely have contributed to her fall?

   a. Diltiazem
   b. Atorvastatin
   c. Levothyroxine
   d. Tylenol PM

6. A 75-year-old patient is admitted to your unit for abdominal pain. She is found to have cholecystitis. The surgeons would like to wait a few days for the acute inflammatory process to subside. The patient has a history of HFrEF and hypertension. On exam the patient is noted to have bilateral crackles and 2+ edema of the lower extremities. The chest x-ray identifies pulmonary vascular congestion. Blood pressure 160/92, heart rate 82, and respiration rate 24. What is the best plan of action in the preoperative setting?

   a. Prescribe diuretics.
   b. Administer fluids at 50 cc/hour.
   c. Hold home medications until after surgery.
   d. Attain baseline dry weight prior to surgery.

7. The AG-ACNP is caring for an 85-year-old female who was admitted for weakness secondary to anemia. She has a history of myelodysplastic syndrome and her bone marrow is becoming less responsive. The nurse tells the AG-ACNP that the patient sleeps a lot and has a limited appetite. Upon exam, the AG-ACNP notes the patient is awake and answers all questions with minimal response. She denies pain and indicates she is tired and just wants to sleep. Physical and laboratory assessment is benign. Based on this information, identify the best intervention at this time:

   a. Prescribe a tricyclic antidepressant.
   b. Have family encourage her to interact.
   c. Administer the PHQ-9.
   d. Administer the C-SSRS.

8. An 86-year-old female is admitted to the hospital for exacerbation of COPD. Her daughter tells the AG-ACNP that her mother seems to be having a hard time hearing and wonders if her mom has wax buildup. The patient denies dizziness, gait imbalance, pain, and tinnitus. The AG-ACNP assesses the ear canal to be without wax. Based upon the AG-ACNP's understanding of the physiologic changes that occur with aging, the AG-ACNP expects the hearing loss to be:

   a. An abnormal finding, the patient likely has a perforated tympanic membrane
   b. A normal finding, the patient has developed increased elasticity and efficiency of ossicular articulation
   c. A normal finding, the patient likely has increased thickening of the tympanic membrane
   d. An abnormal finding, the patient likely has an acoustic neuroma

9. The AG-ACNP is caring for a 94-year-old female who is admitted to the hospital with mental status changes secondary to dehydration. The patient's daughter indicates that this is her third admission in a 6-month time period for dehydration. The NP understands that older adults are at risk for dehydration secondary to:

   a. Increased perception of thirst
   b. Impaired response to serum osmolality
   c. Increased ability to concentrate urine
   d. Impaired creatinine clearance

10. A 70-year-old male has undergone an open cholecystectomy. Aggressive pulmonary toileting is necessary in the post-operative period because older adults have:

    a. Decreased residual capacity
    b. Decreased forced vital capacity
    c. Increased surface area
    d. Increased chest wall compliance

11. The AG-ACNP is caring for a 66-year-old female who is diagnosed with Alzheimer's dementia. The patient's husband indicates that she was most recently started on a medication to help with her memory, but cannot recall the name. The AG-ACNP suspects this medication to belong to which of the following drug classes:

    a. Select serotonin-reuptake inhibitors
    b. Cholinesterase inhibitors
    c. Dopamine agonists
    d. Monoamine oxidase inhibitors

12. The AG-ACNP is caring for an 89-year-old female who was admitted for exacerbation of CHF. Of the following, which finding would be considered a part of normal aging?

    a. The patient's daughter indicates to you that her mother becomes angry at times and this is out of character for her.
    b. The patient's daughter indicates to you that her mother does not answer questions as quickly as she used to.
    c. The patient tells you that she has forgotten how to knit.
    d. The patient tells you that she cannot remember what year she was born.

13. The AG-ACNP is caring for a 69-year-old retired accountant whose wife is concerned that he may have Alzheimer's dementia. Of the following, which finding would be supportive of this diagnosis?

   a. The patient is able to accurately draw intersecting geometrical shapes.
   b. The patient has gait disturbances.
   c. The patient is able to count backward from 100 by sevens.
   d. The patient is unable to balance his checking account.

14. An 85-year-old frail-appearing female is admitted to the hospital for acute exacerbation of CHF (New York Heart Association Class II). The patient has a history of type 2 DM that has been diet controlled. The patient reports that her blood sugars at home have been ranging 180 to 200 and the AG-ACNP notes that the blood sugars have been the same during the patient's hospitalization. Her last hemoglobin A1C is 8. The AG-ACNP's best response is to:

   a. Prescribe glyburide
   b. Prescribe glipizide
   c. Recognize hypoglycemia is risk for elderly
   d. Start low dose insulin sliding scale at discharge

15. An 88-year-old male with a history of Alzheimer's dementia is admitted to the hospital status post fall resulting in a femur fracture. The medical record indicates that the patient has severe cognitive impairment. The family is concerned that the patient may be in pain and inquires how pain is assessed in patients with dementia. The AG-ACNP understands that patients with cognitive impairment will manifest pain by:

   a. Increase in appetite
   b. Decreased confusion
   c. Verbal abusiveness
   d. Hypotension

16. A 74-year-old female is admitted to the short-stay unit for mental status changes secondary to a UTI. Upon review of systems the patient verbalizes generalized joint pain especially in her hips and knees and inquired about pain medication. At the time of the assessment, the patient rates her pain at a level 4 out of 10. Upon physical exam the AG-ACNP notes a well-developed female who appears comfortable. Full range of motion is assessed to all joints with no swelling, warmth, or erythema noted. The patient verbalizes some pain, however, when the knees are put through range of motion. The patient has a history of hypertension and hyperlipidemia. The best recommendation for pain management would be:

   a. Acetaminophen
   b. Nonsteroidal anti-inflammatory drugs
   c. Low-dose opioids
   d. Gabapentin

■ GERIATRIC ANSWERS AND RATIONALES

1. **c) Normal aging process.** Short-term memory loss and hearing loss are normal signs of aging in an octogenarian. Short-term memory loss is a part of a constellation of symptoms often described in dementia; however, it is only one of the diagnostic criteria for major or mild neurocognitive disorder which must be present to diagnose Alzheimer's or vascular dementia. BPPV is a disorder of the inner ear, often described as a sensation of spinning, and if present could explain the fall. However, given no history of dizziness coupled with hearing loss not being associated with benign paroxysmal positional vertigo, this diagnosis is unlikely.

2. **a) Increased fat as a percentage of body mass.** Once drugs enter tissues, drug distribution to the interstitial fluid is determined primarily by perfusion. For poorly perfused tissues (i.e., muscle, fat), distribution is very slow, especially if the tissue has a high affinity for the drug.

3. **a) Medication use.** All choices place the older adult patient at risk for falls; however, both neuropathy and osteoarthritis are not modifiable risk factors. Diet in itself does not place the older adult at higher risk for fall unless the patient has hypovitaminosis, especially vitamin D. Medication use, especially polypharmacy with psychotropic use, is suggested to increase falls. Medication review with de-prescribing, if appropriate, is recommended as a means to prevent falls.

4. **c) "It seems like you are trying to quit smoking, let me discuss with you some possible strategies."** Tobacco dependence is a chronic disease that often requires multiple attempts to quit. Smoking cessation at any age will slow the decline in lung function even in the older adult. Continuous encouragement with effective strategies should be introduced to patients with any healthcare encounter. The nurse practitioner in the hospital should discuss with patients evidence-based strategies that the patient may be open to considering. The Agency for Health Care Policy and Research identifies the five A's of smoking cessation (ask, assess, advise, assist, arrange). The patient indicates readiness to quit and it is up to the nurse practitioner in the hospital setting to advise and assist the patient with treatment options and continued follow up from the primary care provider.

5. **d) Tylenol PM.** Tylenol PM contains diphenhydramine, which is an antihistamine and highly anticholinergic. Older adults typically have decreased clearance. Diphenhydramine is listed on the Beers Criteria as a potentially inappropriate medication to be used in older adults. Diltiazem is an antihypertensive that can also contribute to falls, but in a patient who is hypotensive. Diltiazem is on the Beers Criteria as a possible inappropriate medication to be used in patients with heart failure as it is noted to promote fluid retention; this patient does not have heart failure and is currently hypertensive with an appropriate heart rate. Atorvastatin and Levothyroxine typically do not cause dizziness.

6. **d) Attain baseline dry weight prior to surgery.** The process of anesthesia and overall stress of surgery places the older adult patient at increased risk for hemodynamic instability both intra- and postoperatively. The assessment data supports the fact that the patient may have fluid overload and the recommendations for older adult patients undergoing anesthesia is to achieve baseline dry weight prior to surgery, therefore, diuretics should be administered. In this patient fluids would be contraindicated as they could possibly potentiate further exacerbation of congestive heart failure. Cardiac and antihypertensive medications should be continued pre-operatively.

7. **c) Administer the PHQ-9.** Older adults often do not exhibit overt symptoms of depression. As such, these symptoms are often overlooked by practitioners. The patient in this case verbalizes ongoing fatigue despite sleeping. Healthcare providers should have a high index of suspicion for depression and document this finding with the use of appropriate screening tools. The PHQ-9 is the most common screening tool to identify depression. The patient has symptoms suggestive of depression and should not be left alone. The best single question to ask is, "Do you feel sad or depressed?" If the response is affirmative, then a standardized depression screening tool for depression should be utilized. Treatment for depression should not be instituted until some type of formal screening is carried out. First-line treatment for

depression in older adults is the use of SSRIs or SNRIs and not tricyclic antidepressants. The Columbia-Suicide Severity Rating Scale (C-SSRS) is used to screen for suicide and should be applied once depression is identified, but not as a first-line screening tool.

8. **c) A normal finding, the patient likely has increased thickening of the tympanic membrane.** Changes that occur with aging include thickening of the tympanic membrane that causes conductive hearing loss and affects low-frequency sounds. High-frequency hearing loss is associated with decreased elasticity and efficiency of ossicular articulation. Patients with acoustic neuroma could develop hearing loss, but balance disturbances typically develop first. Patients with a perforated tympanic membrane may also develop hearing loss, but will have additional symptoms of sharp pain in affected ear, "buzzing sensation," and ear drainage.

9. **b) Impaired response to serum osmolality.** Dehydration is the most common cause of fluid and electrolyte imbalance in older adults secondary to decreased perception of thirst, impaired response to serum osmolality, and reduced ability to concentrate urine. Creatinine clearance may affect urine production, but not dehydration or thirst.

10. **b) Decreased forced vital capacity.** Pulmonary function changes that occur with aging are often related to decreased chest wall compliance. Decreased chest wall compliance can lead to reduced intrathoracic negative pressure that can cause airway collapse. With this, the surface area of the lung decreases, leading to decreased forced vital capacity and increased residual capacity.

11. **b) Cholinesterase inhibitors.** The class of pharmacologic agents used to stabilize cognitive function in Alzheimer's dementia is cholinesterase inhibitors. These medications work to decrease the breakdown of neurotransmitter acetylcholine, which is thought to facilitate memory function. In addition to managing compulsive behaviors, SSRIs are antidepressants that may be used if the patient has associated depressive symptoms. Caution must be taken with SSRIs in that they may contribute to falls. Dopamine agonists are used in the treatment of Parkinson's disease for movement control. Monoamine oxidase inhibitors are used in the treatment of depression and generalized anxiety disorder and inhibit the neurotransmitters of norepinephrine, serotonin, and dopamine.

12. **b) The patient's daughter indicates to you that her mother does not answer questions as quickly as she used to.** Personality traits typically remain stable over time. Changes in personality are often associated with depression and/or dementia. Short-term memory may decline with aging, but long-term memory declines less; thus patient should remember how to knit or know her birthdate. The speed at which information is encoded, stored, and retrieved does slow with aging and it may take longer for an older adult to respond to a question.

13. **d) The patient is unable to balance his checking account.** Patients with dementia exhibit a decline in cognitive function and not typically gait disturbances until late in the disease. This particular patient is exhibiting signs and symptoms associated with moderate cognitive decline or mild to early-stage Alzheimer's disease. Patients at this stage have decreased ability to carry out complex tasks; one would be managing finances. The inability to manage finances should be quite easy for this patient as he is a retired accountant who likely has an advanced degree. Balancing a checkbook should be a very easy function for this patient. The ability to draw intersecting geometrical shapes and counting backward from 100 by sevens is measured on the Folstein Mini-Mental State Examination and reflects deficiencies in attention, calculation, and language.

14. **c) Recognize hypoglycemia is risk for elderly.** Elders with diabetes have a greater risk for hypoglycemia from altered physiologic response to low glucose levels. Many frail elders also have other comorbidities, such as cognitive and functional losses, that interfere with recognition and treatment of hypoglycemia. Hypoglycemia increases their risk for falls, fall-related fractures, seizures, and even coma, as well as exacerbation of other chronic conditions, including cognitive dysfunction and cardiac events. A hemoglobin A1c level of 8 to 8.5 is acceptable

in the elderly population. Sulfonylureas are noted to be efficacious and safe in the treatment of type 2 DM. While glyburide and glipizide are both sulfonylureas, glipizide is recommended for older adults because it is short acting with less-likely adverse reaction of hypoglycemia. However, given the patient's life expectancy, liberalizing the goal glucose level and HbgA1c is the most appropriate intervention. Metformin would not be an acceptable option, as it can impair renal function and must be closely monitored. Because the patient has a history of CHF, there is an increased risk for renal insufficiency as the CHF progresses. Starting insulin at time of discharge is not the best action, as the patient would have no monitoring to assess for hypoglycemia.

15. **c) Verbal abusiveness.** Patient with severe cognitive impairment may not be able to express pain or the degree of pain appropriately. Pain occurring from a fracture is nociceptive and will likely cause constant, gnawing pain to the affected area. Understanding that this patient is likely to experience pain will guide the nurse practitioner to assess for pain related behaviors and could include appetite changes (likely decreased), increased confusion, and verbal abusiveness. Patients in pain typically present with hypertension, not hypotension.

16. **a) Acetaminophen.** This patient did not have exposure to pain medication. Based on her age, signs, and symptoms, the pain to her hips and knees is likely related to osteoarthritis. The World Health Organization pain ladder recommends nonopioids as a place to start. In this case acetaminophen would be the best recommendation, as it provides analgesia for mild to moderate pain syndromes and patients can take up to 4 g per 24 hours in patients with normal hepatic and renal function. NSAIDs are noted to be highly effective for chronic inflammatory pain but pose additional risk to older adults, especially those with hypertension. Opioids can be used for moderate to severe pain but only after nonopioids have been trialed. Gabapentin is typically used for neuropathic pain or as adjunctive therapy.

■ BIBLIOGRAPHY

American Geriatrics Society Beers Criteria Update Expert Panel. (2015). American Geriatrics Society 2015 updated Beers criteria for potentially inappropriate medication use in older adults. *Journal of the American Geriatrics Society*, 63(11), 2227–2246. doi:10.1111/jgs.13702

American Psychiatric Association. (2013). *Diagnostic and statistical manual of mental disorders* (5th ed.). Washington, DC: Author.

American Psychological Association. (2017). *Older adult.* Retrieved from http://www.apa.org/pi/aging/resources/guides/older.aspx

Flaherty, E. R. B. (2014). *Geriatric nursing review syllabus: A core curriculum in advanced practice geriatric nursing.* New York, NY: American Geriatrics Society.

Kennedy-Malone, L., Fletcher, L. R., & Martin-Plank, L. (2014). *Advance practice nursing in the care of older adults.* Philadelphia, PA: F. A. Davis.

National Institute of Neurological Disorders and Stroke. (2017). *Dementia information page.* Retrieved from https://www.ninds.nih.gov/Disorders/All-Disorders/Dementia-Information-Page

Rosenthal, L. B. J. (2018). *Lehne's pharmacotherapeutics for advanced practice providers.* St. Louis, MO: Elsevier.

Sircar, M., Bhatia, A., & Munshi, M. (2016). Review of hypoglycemia in the older adult: Clinical implications and management. *Canadian Journal of Diabetes*, 40(1), 66–72. doi:10.1016/j.jcjd.2015.10.004

Substance Abuse and Mental Health Services Administration. (2018). *Screening tools.* Retrieved from https://www.integration.samhsa.gov/clinical-practice/screening-tools

6

Cardiovascular

KRISTINE ANNE SCORDO, JOAN E. KING,
DANA MITCHELL, AND KATHLEEN BALLMAN

■ CARDIOVASCULAR QUESTIONS

1. A 50-year-old White male with a history of hypertension, smoking (60 pack-years), angina, and chronic bronchitis (COPD) presents with 3 hours of substernal chest pain with diaphoresis. He is anxious, diaphoretic, and nauseous. His blood pressure is 90/70 mm, pulse 50 per minute, respirations 24 per minute. His lungs are clear, heart is bradycardic with no murmurs, and there is ~10 cm of jugular venous distension (estimated jugular venous pressure 15 cm). His ECG is shown in the following figure.

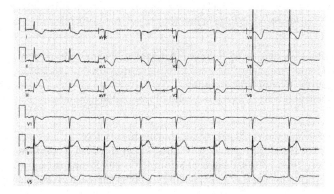

Based on these findings, which of the following diagnoses is most likely?

a. Inferior myocardial infarction with evidence of right ventricular involvement
b. Anterior myocardial infarction with lateral extension
c. Anterior myocardial infarction with aneurysm formation
d. Posterior myocardial infarction with lateral extensio

2. A patient with known CAD, post-MI, and preserved LV function presents to the office with the rhythm shown in the following ECG. His only complaint is palpitations. Vital signs are stable and he has not taken any medications for over a year because he cannot afford them. Which of the following medications should initially be prescribed?

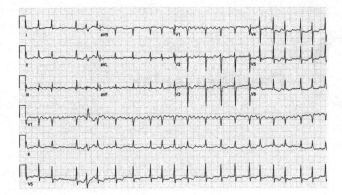

a. Amiodarone (Cordarone)
b. Metoprolol (Toprol/Lopressor)
c. Procainamide (Pronestyl)
d. Dofetilide (Tikosyn)

3. A 65-year-old male presents to the ED with new-onset chest pain. During the examination, a grade II/VI systolic murmur is auscultated, best heard at the second ICS, right sternal border. The differential diagnosis is:

a. Mitral stenosis
b. Pulmonic insufficiency
c. Aortic stenosis
d. Mitral insufficiency

4. A 67-year-old male presents with a history of aphasia and right-sided hemiparesis which has now resolved. He has 80% blockage of both carotids. The AG-ACNP understands the treatment for this patient will be:

a. Right carotid endarterectomy followed by a left cardioid endarterectomy
b. Left carotid endarterectomy followed by a right carotid endarterectomy
c. Maintenance with antiplatelet therapy
d. No treatment at this time, a repeat carotid ultrasound in 6 months

5. A 45-year-old female with a 20-pack-year smoking history recently returned from Europe with her husband. She developed pain and swelling in her right calf 8 hours into the return flight. She denies fever, chest pain, shortness of breath, abdominal pain, nausea, or vomiting. She has no bleeding conditions. She has no drug allergies but is allergic to seafood and certain types of nuts. The most appropriate next step is:

a. Administration of warfarin (Coumadin) with a target INR of 2 to 3
b. Lower extremity Doppler ultrasound study
c. Obtain ABGs and ventilation-perfusion scan
d. Administration of enoxaparin sodium (Lovenox)

6. A 24-year-old male presents to the ED with a cocaine overdose. He is awake, with tachycardia, anxiety, diaphoresis, headache, confusion, and a blood pressure of 230/120. Which of the following is the most appropriate medication to treat his hypertension?

a. Isoproterenol (Isuprel)
b. Esmolol (Brevibloc)
c. N-Acetlylcysteine (Mucomyst)
d. Phentolamine (OraVerse)

7. A 62-year-old male is 1 day postoperative cardiac bypass surgery. He suddenly develops hypotension with pulsus paradoxus and has no urinary output for the past 2 hours. Point of care two-dimensional echocardiogram demonstrates right systolic collapse. The AG-ACNP's diagnosis is which of the following?

   a. Cardiac tamponade
   b. Dissecting thoracic aortic aneurysm
   c. Hemorrhage
   d. Barotrauma

8. A patient is transferred to the ICU with a blood pressure of 90/60 mmHg, oxygen saturation of 85%, oliguria, and diffuse crackles. Pulmonary artery catheter readings reveal a cardiac output of 1.9 L/min. and a wedge pressure of 24 mmHg. Which IV medication does the AG-ACNP prescribe?

   a. Nesiritide (Natrecor)
   b. Nitroglycerin
   c. Dopamine
   d. Nitroprusside (Nipride)

9. A 32-year-old female 3 months pregnant presents to the ED with worsening dyspnea, bilateral ankle edema, and bibasilar crackles. A two-dimensional echocardiogram demonstrates a reduced ejection fraction. Which of the following medications are initially appropriate to prescribe?

   a. Lisinopril (Prinivil)
   b. Diltiazem (Cardizem)
   c. Metoprolol (Lopressor)
   d. Methyldopa (Aldomet)

10. The AG-ACNP is asked to see a patient in the postanesthesia care unit who is postop thoracotomy for coronary artery bypass surgery. The patient becomes hypotensive with a blood pressure of 90/70, pulse 120/regular, with cool clammy skin. The AG-ACNP initially prescribes:

   a. Dopamine
   b. IV fluids
   c. Digoxin (Lanoxin)
   d. Norepinephrine (Levophed)

11. A 68-year-old female cigarette smoker complains of fatigue and dyspnea. The most specific evidence for CHF in this patient would be

   a. Ankle edema
   b. Wheezes
   c. S3 gallop
   d. Weight gain

12. The AG-ACNP is making rounds in the ICU, when suddenly a postcardiac transplant patient develops symptomatic bradycardia. The AG-ACNP orders which of the following medications?

   a. Atropine
   b. Epinephrine (adrenaline)
   c. Isoproterenol (Isuprel)
   d. Aminophylline

13. A 56-year-old male presents to the ED with substernal chest pain, pain with inspiration, systolic apical murmur, and fever. His ECG demonstrates ST segment elevation in all leads. The AG-ACNP recognizes this as:

   a. Endocarditis
   b. Acute myocardial infarction
   c. Pleurisy
   d. Pericarditis

14. A 38-year-old female patient presents to the ED with fever 100.4 and sharp left chest pain. The pain is exacerbated when she lies flat, and lessened with sitting upright and leaning forward. Her heart rate is 106 beats per minute at rest and blood pressure is 116/72. An ECG shows diffuse ST elevation without troponin elevation. The most likely diagnosis is?

   a. Acute myocardial infarction
   b. Acutely decompensated heart failure
   c. Acute mitral chordae rupture
   d. Acute pericarditis

15. A 48-year-old female patient presents to the ED with complaints of palpitations and dyspnea for the past 6 hours. Upon triage, her pulse is found to be irregular with a rate of 146 beats per minute. Her blood pressure is 114/68. She is alert and oriented and denies chest pain. ECG demonstrates an irregular, narrow complex tachycardia. Which intervention is most appropriate for the AG-ACNP to order first?

   a. Order STAT transthoracic echocardiogram.
   b. Perform synchronized cardioversion immediately.
   c. Order metoprolol (Lopressor) 5 mg to be given slow IV push now.
   d. Administer adenosine (Adenocard) 6 mg rapid IV push now.

16. The AG-ACNP is providing discharge education for a 56-year-old male client with a new diagnosis of systolic heart failure related to dilated cardiomyopathy. The patient has history of heavy alcohol consumption daily for the past 8 years. Which topic is most important in the pre-discharge counselling for the client and his family?

   a. Aerobic exercise may worsen his heart function.
   b. Sexual activity is contraindicated due to his heart function.
   c. Cessation of alcohol may improve his heart function.
   d. Following a low-sodium diet will improve his heart function.

17. A 57-year-old male with a history of smoking presents to the ED with complaints of sudden, severe chest pain radiating down his back and associated dizziness. His blood pressure is 208/116. An ECG demonstrates LV hypertrophy without ischemic changes. Which initial intervention is appropriate?

   a. Chest CT with IV contrast
   b. Urgent surgical consultation
   c. Aggressive blood pressure control
   d. Transesophageal echocardiogram

18. The NP is caring for a 38-year-old African American male patient who has no known medical history, was admitted to the hospital for management of newly diagnosed type II DM and renal dysfunction with proteinuria. Throughout the hospitalization, the patient has been noted to be persistently hypertensive, with blood pressure readings in the general range of 160/90. The most appropriate first-line medication for this client would include:

    a. Metoprolol succinate (Toprol XL) 25 mg orally twice per day
    b. Amlodipine (Norvasc) 10 mg orally once per day
    c. Hydrochlorothiazide (Microzide) 25 mg orally once per day
    d. Lisinopril (Prinivil) 20 mg orally once per day

19. The AG-ACNP is caring for a 58-year-old male patient who was recently diagnosed with CAD after having an ST-segment myocardial infarction. Based on the 2013 ACC/AHA Guideline on the Treatment of Blood Cholesterol, which option for statin therapy would be most appropriate for this client when planning for hospital discharge?

    a. Atorvastatin (Lipitor) 40 mg orally once per day
    b. Lovastatin (Mevacor) 40 mg orally once per day
    c. Pravastatin (Pravachol) 40 mg orally once per day
    d. Simvastatin (Zocor) 40 mg orally once per day

20. A 48-year-old patient underwent PCI with a DES. Which antiplatelet regimen would be most appropriate for the continuing management of this patient?

    a. Aspirin 81 mg and Clopidogrel (Plavix) 75 mg orally daily for at least 12 months
    b. Clopidogrel (Plavix) 75 mg orally daily alone for the next 6 months
    c. Aspirin 81 mg orally daily alone for the next 6 months
    d. Aspirin 81 mg and Clopidogrel (Plavix) 75 mg orally daily for the next 1 month

21. An NP is called to assess a 76-year-old female patient who has a known history of systolic heart failure. The patient is being admitted to the hospital with complaints of couch orthopnea and declining activity tolerance. Oxygen saturations are lower than her usual baseline and a chest x-ray demonstrates pulmonary venous hypertension. Which is the initial intervention in the treatment of this patient?

    a. Referral to the cardiac catheterization lab
    b. Intravenous loop diuretic therapy
    c. Electrocardiography
    d. Intensify home dose of beta-blocker therapy

22. An AG-ACNP is caring for a male client in the ED with dull precordial chest pain and headache. He denies known past medical problems and is on no routine medications. The client is found to have a blood pressure of 240/130 and nicardipine (Cardene) infusion has been ordered. Which potential adverse effect might necessitate the addition of an esmolol (Brevibloc) infusion?

    a. Neurological changes
    b. Intensifying chest pain
    c. Reflex tachycardia
    d. Rebound hypertension

23. A 54-year-old client is being managed in the cardiac-surgical ICU, and is currently 14 hours post coronary artery bypass surgery. For the past 2 hours, the patient complains of progressive dyspnea at rest. Upon assessment, the NP notes markedly distant heart tones, diminished peripheral pulses during inspiration, and JVD to the angle of the jaw. The AG-ACNP recognizes this as:

    a. Cardiac tamponade
    b. Acute respiratory failure
    c. Fluid volume overload
    d. Recurrent myocardial ischemia

24. A critically ill client becomes hemodynamically unstable. Exam reveals muffled heart sounds and JVD. Blood pressure shows a narrowed pulse pressure with pulsus paradoxus. Which intervention is most important for the NP to urgently facilitate in the care of this client?

    a. Aggressive intravenous diuresis
    b. STAT cardiac MRI
    c. Emergent intravenous vasodilators
    d. Immediate cardiac surgical consultation

25. A 43-year-old female client with known history of congenital bicuspid aortic valve presents with complaints of substernal chest discomfort and exertional dyspnea. The NP notes that the client is volume overloaded. The echocardiogram demonstrates severe aortic stenosis with peak gradient over 60 mmHg. Which intervention would be most important for the NP to facilitate in the care of this client?

    a. Prescription for diuretic therapy
    b. Initiate vasodilator therapy
    c. Referral to interventional cardiology
    d. Recommend for participation in a cardiac rehabilitation program

26. A 19-year-old male client is brought into the ED with a 3-day history of progressive exertional dyspnea and chest pain. He has no known medical issues, but does report a recent upper respiratory infection, approximately 1 week ago, of 3 days duration, for which he did not seek treatment. After assessment suggests fluid volume overload, which diagnostic test would be most pertinent in informing the initial treatment plan for this client?

    a. Echocardiography
    b. Endomyocardial biopsy
    c. Chest radiography
    d. Serum troponin I testing

27. A patient presents with severe dyspnea, respiratory rate 32, SaO_2 84%, heart rate 112, a blood pressure of 82/50, cold extremities, and confusion. As the NP examines the patient, the patient begins to cough pink-tinged sputum. This scenario reflects:

    a. Cardiogenic shock
    b. Right-sided heart failure
    c. HFpEF
    d. Cardiac tamponade

28. A patient presents with acute on chronic HFrEF. The most likely signs and symptoms are:

    a. Bilateral crackles, increase urinary output, and peripheral edema
    b. Chest pain, JVD, and bilateral infiltrates
    c. Shortness of breath, bilateral crackles, and elevated JVD
    d. Pericardial friction rub, bilateral bruits, and systolic murmur

29. Signs of dilated cardiomyopathy include:

    a. Enlarged cardiac silhouette, PMI 2 cm left of midclavicular line, and an ejection fraction of less than 40%
    b. Enlarged cardiac silhouette and an ejection fraction greater than 55%
    c. Normal cardiac silhouette and an ejection fraction greater than 55%
    d. A sustained PMI that is 2 cm right of the midclavicular line

30. Which of the following cardiomyopathies is likely to be associated with a sustained PMI, a systolic murmur, and an enlargement of the intraventricular septum?

    a. Dilated cardiomyopathy
    b. Ischemic cardiomyopathy
    c. Hypertrophic cardiomyopathy
    d. Restrictive cardiomyopathy

31. A patient presents with a new onset of chest pain, diaphoresis, ST segment depression in two contiguous leads, and a troponin I level of 0.5. Of the following, the most likely diagnosis is:

    a. Unstable angina
    b. Prinzmetal angina
    c. Non-ST segment myocardial infarction
    d. Pericarditis

32. Current treatment for a patient who has had a non-ST elevated myocardial infarction is:

    a. Amlodipine (Norvasc)
    b. Enoxaparin (Lovenox)
    c. Thrombolytics
    d. Enoxaparin (Lovenox) and clopidogrel (Plavix)

33. For a patient who presents to a small rural ED with crushing chest pain and ST segment elevation in V1 through V4, the most appropriate immediate treatment is:

    a. Amlodipine (Norvasc)
    b. Sotalol (Betapace)
    c. Alteplase (Activase)
    d. Carvedilol (Coreg)

34. Appropriate management for a patient who has sustained an ST segment elevation MI include:

    a. A calcium channel blocker and heparin
    b. Stents, ACE inhibitor, and a loop diuretic
    c. Fibrinolytics, ACE inhibitor, beta-blocker, and stents
    d. Morphine and a beta-blocker

35. A patient returns from the OR following a three-vessel coronary artery bypass with the following vital signs: heart rate 105, respirations 12/12 on mechanical ventilation, blood pressure 88/50, CVP 14. The AG-ACNP assesses muffled heart sounds and no output from the mediastinal chest tubes. The most likely diagnosis is:

    a. Cardiac tamponade
    b. Hypovolemic shock
    c. Hemorrhagic shock
    d. Right-sided heart failure

36. The most appropriate management for a patient who is in cardiogenic shock with heart rate 102, blood pressure 92/53, respiratory rate 28, SaO_2 88%, CVP 14, cardiac index 2.1, and systemic vascular resistance 1,700 is:

    a. Dobutamine
    b. Dopamine
    c. Nitroprusside (Nipride)
    d. Nitroglycerin

37. A patient presents with palpitations. An ECG shows an irregular rhythm, without P waves and no significant Q waves and no ST segment changes and a QRS less than 0.10 seconds. The most likely diagnosis is:

    a. Atrial flutter
    b. Atrial fibrillation
    c. Premature atrial contraction
    d. Premature ventricular contractions

38. A patient who is on sotalol presents with a long QT syndrome. A potentially adverse outcome for this patient is:

    a. Sudden cardiac arrest related to ventricular arrhythmias
    b. Sudden cardiac arrest related to severe bradycardia
    c. Multifocal PVCs
    d. Third-degree heart block

39. A patient was started on lisinopril (Zestril) 3 months ago. A side effect the AG-ACNP should assess for is:

    a. Hyperkalemia and an elevated creatinine
    b. Hyperkalemia and hypomagnesemia
    c. Hypokalemia and hypomagnesemia
    d. Hypokalemia and an elevated creatinine

40. A patient presents to the ED with a severe headache and a blood pressure 220/132, heart rate 98, respirations 14, and SaO_2 94%. Serum creatinine is elevated at 2.2 mg/dL. The most appropriate diagnosis for this patient is:

    a. Hypertensive emergency
    b. Hypertensive urgency
    c. Renal insufficiency
    d. Chronic kidney disease stage II

41. A patient presents with a fasting LDL level of 142 mg/dL with a history of CAD. The most appropriate action of the NP to take in managing this patient is:

    a. Recommend the patient lose weight
    b. Recommend the patient begin a diet low in unsaturated fat
    c. Recheck the patient's LDL level in 2 weeks
    d. Begin a statin

42. Which of the following profiles best describes metabolic syndrome for female patients?

    a. Fasting blood glucose level greater than 110, triglycerides ≥150 mg/dL, HDL less than 50 mg/dL, waistline measurement greater than 35 inches, and blood pressure ≥130/85
    b. Fasting blood glucose level greater than 110, triglycerides greater than 120 mg/dL, HDL less than 40 mg/dL, waistline measurement greater than 40 inches, and blood pressure ≥130/85
    c. Fasting blood glucose level greater than 100, triglycerides greater than 180 mg/dL, HDL less than 50 mg/dL, waistline measurement greater than 35 inches, and blood pressure ≥150/90
    d. Fasting blood glucose level greater than 100, triglycerides greater than 160 mg/dL, HDL less than 40 mg/dL, waistline measurement greater than 30, and blood pressure ≥130/85

43. A 29-year-old woman presents with a recent onset of substernal chest pain that radiates to the left shoulder and back. The pain is nonexertional and is lessened when sitting up. On examination, she has stable vital signs, clear lungs, a normal S_1 and S_2, and a scratchy sound heard at the left sternal border. Her ECG is shown in the following figure.

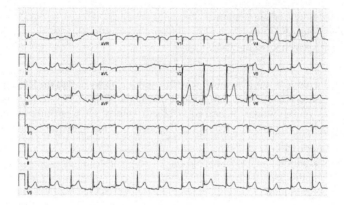

    Treatment includes which of the following?

    a. No medications
    b. Oral steroids
    c. Indomethacin (Indocin)
    d. Colchicine (Colcrys) and ibuprofen (Advil/Motrin)

44. The AG-ACNP is seeing an 86-year-old-male patient with severe aortic stenosis in a follow-up clinic visit. He has a history of severe aortic stenosis without symptoms. He recently noted decreased physical activity along with exertional lightheadedness. He had a syncopal episode while working in the yard. On examination, his blood pressure is 150/85 and his heart rate is 76. He has a grade III/VI systolic ejection murmur that radiates to the carotids. S_2 is barely audible. Carotid pulses are delayed. He has femoral and abdominal aortic bruits. Peripheral pulses are 2+ bilaterally. What is the next appropriate step in this patient's management?

    a. Improved blood pressure control

    b. Cardiac rehabilitation

    c. Aortic valve surgery

    d. End-of-life arrangements with hospice

45. The AG-ACNP is caring for a 79-year-old man who has been successfully resuscitated. He had a sudden, witnessed collapse in a shopping mall where he was found to be in pulseless VT. He has a prior history of CAD with a single coronary stent placed 2 years ago. He now has stable vital signs but remains comatose. His 12-lead ECG shows ST segment depressions in the anterior leads. Which statement regarding the role of cardiac catheterization in his care is true? Cardiac catheterization is:

    a. Contraindicated secondary to his neurologic status

    b. Advisable in the setting of ST-segment myocardial ischemia

    c. Indicated based on his presentation

    d. Advisable after the patient is stabilized

46. A 65-year-old female with known CAD and an ejection fraction of 20% undergoes placement of an ICD. One day later, her nurse calls the NP because her blood pressure has decreased to 85/60 mmHg, with complaints of severe lightheadedness and dyspnea. Examination reveals elevated JVP, bibasilar crackles, and distant heart sounds. An ECG shows low voltage and nonspecific T-wave changes. The NP recommends:

    a. Coronary artery angiography

    b. Right-sided heart catheterization

    c. Emergent pericardiocentesis

    d. A transthoracic echocardiography

47. A 30-year-old woman is found in an alley with a single stab wound to the left thorax. Vital signs are blood pressure, 60/40; pulse, 140/min; respirations, 30/min. Physical examination reveals distended neck veins, midline trachea, equal breath sounds, and a carotid pulse that disappears during inspiration. Which of the following diagnoses best fits these findings?

    a. Cardiac tamponade

    b. Hemorrhagic shock

    c. Massive hemothorax

    d. Tension pneumothorax

48. A 70-year-old woman with a history of hypertrophic cardiomyopathy is admitted to the hospital with severe exertional dyspnea and new-onset orthopnea. Over the course of her hospital stay, she is treated with metoprolol (Toprol), verapamil (Calan), and a loop diuretic. After her condition improves, she is discharged. She presents to the clinic for follow-up with continued dyspnea with less-than-ordinary activity. She has a blood pressure of 90/60 mmHg, heart rate of 75 beats/min, and on examination has a JVP of 13 cm, clear lungs, a displaced cardiac apex with an S_3 heart sound, and 2+ lower extremity pitting edema to her knees. Labs on discharge from the hospital reveal a potassium level of 4.5 mEq/L and a creatinine of 1.2 mg/dL. Which of the following medication changes would be appropriate at this time?

    a. Add an ARB and a direct renin inhibitor to maximize inhibition of the renin–angiotensin system.

    b. Increase her diuretic dosing and counsel patient on fluid and salt restriction.

    c. Consider cardiac transplantation.

    d. Start vasodilator therapy with nitroglycerin.

49. The NP is discharging a 54-year-old female patient who has newly diagnosed CAD and is status post STEMI. She underwent stent placement to her LAD artery during this admission and her hospitalization has been uncomplicated. Her ejection fraction is 35%. Which of the following is the most appropriate pharmacological regimen for discharge?

    a. Aspirin, atorvastatin (Lipitor), clopidigrel (Plavix), and nifedipine (Procardia)
    b. Aspirin, metoprolol (Toprol), lisinopril (Prinivil), and clopidigrel (Plavix)
    c. Aspirin, hydrochlorathiazide (Microzide), atorvastatin (Lipitor), and lisinopril (Prinivil)
    d. Aspirin, atorvastatin (Lipitor), furosemide (Lasix), and amlodipine (Norvasc)

50. A 58-year-old man is seen in the ED for syncope. His wife reports that she was in the kitchen when she heard him fall on the living room floor. He recalls feeling very lightheaded but remembers nothing more. Upon further questioning, he recalls feeling dizzy on several occasions over the past few months. He has a history of hypertension and a myocardial infarction 10 years earlier. He has since been well and exercises on a daily basis. In the ED, he has a blood pressure of 95/55 mmHg and a heart rate of 30 beats/min. An ECG is obtained (see the following ECG). What is the most important initial step in managing this patient?

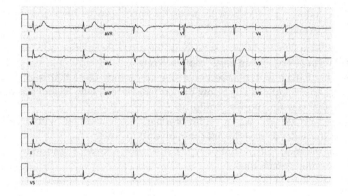

    a. Administer dopamine.
    b. Admit for further monitoring.
    c. Place a temporary pacemaker.
    d. Administer isoproterenol.

51. An 80-year-old gentleman is sent to the ED by his PCP with a blood pressure of 210/110. The patient had a blood pressure screening in the office while he was there for a flu shot. The last time the patient was seen by the PCP was 6 years ago for a sinus infection and was normotensive at the time. He currently takes no medication. To determine if this episode of hypertension is an emergency, which tests should be ordered?

    a. ECG, urinalysis, creatinine
    b. Complete blood cell count, chemistry profile
    c. Thyroid stimulating hormone, chest x-ray
    d. CT head, chest x-ray

52. A 67-year old male comes to the clinic for evaluation of leg pain. He describes the pain as aching in the muscles of his thighs while walking. The pain subsides after resting for a few minutes, is worse at night and he has noted occasional left foot numbness. He has a history of hypertension and cerebrovascular disease. During the physical examination, loss of hair in the distal

extremities and diminished dorsalis pedis and posterior tibial pulses bilaterally with a very faint left dorsal pedis pulse are noted. Which of the following findings would be suggestive of severe/critical ischemia of the left foot?

a. ABIof less than 0.3
b. ABI of less than 0.9
c. ABI of greater than 1.2
d. Presence of pitting edema of the lower extremities

53. When providing treatment for a patient with signs and symptoms of pulmonary edema, it is important to determine if the cause is noncardiogenic or cardiogenic. Which of the following would be a cause of cardiogenic pulmonary edema?

a. Severe left ventricular dysfunction that leads to pulmonary congestion
b. Direct injury to the lung mediated by aspiration
c. Indirect injury to the lung as a consequence of sepsis
d. Acute changes in pulmonary vascular pressures due to high altitude

54. Which of the following patients with aortic dissection can be managed medically, without surgical or endovascular intervention?

a. A 42-year-old male with Marfan syndrome, the distal aortic dissection beginning below the left subclavian artery, and an aortic root of 53 mm
b. a 72-year-old female with a dissection of the descending aorta that begins distal to the left subclavian artery and extends below the left renal artery, who has no symptoms and has a creatinine that is within normal limits
c. A 27-year-old male who was a victim of a motorcycle accident, with an ascending aortic dissection that extends past the left common carotid artery
d. An 80-year-old male with a chronic type B dissection with a CT scan showing advancement of that dissection at 6 months

55. A 30-year-old male patient presents with a complaint of a new onset headache that he describes as pounding that occurs throughout the day and night. He has minimal relief with NSAIDs. On physical examination, his blood pressure is 185/115 mmHg in the right arm and 188 /113 mmHg in the left arm. He has a heart rate of 70 bpm, no JVD, and no carotid or abdominal bruits. Decreased pulses in the lower extremities and a hyperdynamic PMI are noted along with a systolic murmur second ICS right sternal border. The review of systems is positive for leg fatigue. Which of the following cardiac abnormalities is this patient most likely to have?

a. Bicuspid aortic valve
b. Mitral stenosis
c. Mitral regurgitation
d. Tricuspid atresia

56. A 35-year-old Caucasian female, without significant past medical history who takes oral birth control pills, presents to the ED with shortness of breath and chest pain. She recently returned from a 2-week vacation tour of Europe. She has fatigue since returning, but this morning she became acutely short of breath. The shortness of breath is associated with some moderately sharp chest pain located along the left side of her chest. Her vital signs are 120/76, heart rate 110, respiratory rate is 16, and temperature is 99.6 F. The pain seems worse when she attempts to take a deep breath. Her breath sounds are clear. Which test will be most appropriate to aid in her diagnosis?

a. Chest radiograph
b. Arterial blood gases
c. D-dimer
d. Oxygen saturation

57. A 28-year-old woman with no significant past medical history presents to clinic with complaints of progressive shortness of breath; she becomes dyspneic with less activity than she had 1 year ago. If she exerts herself beyond a brisk walk, she becomes lightheaded, presyncopal, and feels tightness in her chest. She also notes generalized fatigue. The physical examination notes the following: heart rate of 105 bpm and blood pressure within normal range. Resting transcutaneous oximetry is 92%. BMI is 24 kg/m². She has JVD but clear lungs. A grade 2/6 mid-systolic murmur is heard over the left upper sternal border. Her ECG show right atrial enlargement, right ventricular hypertrophy, and right axis deviation. Right heart catheterization reveals a mean PA pressure of 29 mmHg. What is this patient's most likely diagnosis?

   a. Idiopathic pulmonary arterial hypertension
   b. Aortic stenosis
   c. Asthma
   d. Ischemic cardiomyopathy

58. A 24-year-old woman presents to the ED with a complaint of, "My heart is pounding out of my chest and I've been short of breath for 4 hours." She has had similar episodes, but all have spontaneously stopped. She is in good health and takes no medications. Her blood pressure is 120/80 mmHg and pulse too rapid to count. Her rhythm is shown in the following ECG.

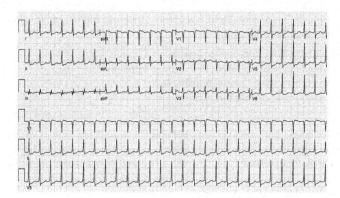

What is the most appropriate immediate management for this patient?

   a. Administer verapamil orally
   b. Immediate cardioversion after administration of a mild sedative
   c. Elicit a vagal maneuver
   d. Insert a temporary transvenous pacemaker

59. A 75-year-old man with a history of CAD, hypertension, and dyslipidemia is brought to the ED with a complaint of chest pain. He describes the pain "tearing" and radiating from his anterior chest to his back between shoulder blades. He takes metoprolol, lisinopril, and simvastatin. He is afebrile; his blood pressure in his right arm is 180/98 mmHg and 112/56 mmHg in his left arm. His heart rate is 100 beats per minute and his respiratory rate is 23/min, his cardiac monitor shows normal sinus rhythm, and his lungs are clear to auscultation. ECG shows sinus tachycardia. The most appropriate diagnostic study to order is which of the following?

   a. Myoview cardiac scan
   b. Contrast-enhanced chest CT
   c. Ventilation perfusion scan
   d. A tagged red blood cell scan

60. The AG-ACNP is treating a 79-year-old male for systolic heart failure. When prescribing medications, the AG-ACNP understands that normal age-related changes that must be considered include:

    a. Decreased body fat percentage
    b. Increased albumin
    c. Increased hepatic blood flow
    d. Decreased glomerular filtration

61. The AG-ACNP is caring for a 55-year-old male who is 2 days post-AMI. He is also known HIV-positive and is on protease inhibitors. His lipid profile is total cholesterol 242; triglycerides 156; LDL 142; HDL 30. As part of secondary prevention, the AG-ACNP would initiate which of the following medications?

    a. Omega 3FA (Vascepa/Lovaza)
    b. Rosuvastatin (Crestor)
    c. Simvastatin (Zocor)
    d. Lovastatin (Mevacor)

62. In treating a client with decompensated heart failure and acute pulmonary edema who has not previously been shown to have fluid retention, which pharmacologic intervention should be considered for immediate therapy?

    a. Morphine sulfate 4 mg intravenously now
    b. Aminophylline 0.25 mg/kg/hour intravenous infusion
    c. Furosemide (Lasix) 40 mg intravenously now
    d. Metoprolol (Lopressor) 5 mg intravenously now

63. A 65-year-old female with known PAD is being evaluated for reports of severe pain in the dorsum of her right foot and associated pallor. She endorses a history of hypertension and has a 30-pack-year smoking history. She has pain at rest, though it seems improved when walking or letting her foot dangle from the bed. Which associated finding increases this client's risk of requiring an amputation related to critical limb ischemia?

    a. Cool, atrophic skin over the foot
    b. Nonhealing ulcerations on distal toes
    c. Rubor on dependency
    d. Diminished pedal pulse amplitude

64. A patient with HFrEF is on lisinopril (Prinivil), furosemide (Lasix), and metoprolol (Loppressor). Given recent mortality data, a decision is made to start the patient on valsartan/sacubitril (Entresto). What must the AG-ACNP do prior to initiating Entresto?

    a. Nothing. Entresto can be started without changes to the current regimen.
    b. Lisinopril must be stopped one day before Entresto can be started.
    c. The patient must be off any ACI inhibitor or ARB for 36 hours before Entresto can be started.
    d. Furosemide must be stopped before Entresto can be started.

65. An AG-ACNP wishes to start a patient who has HFrEF on ivabradine (Corlanor). Criteria for starting a HFrEF patient on Corlanor are:

    a. Ejection fraction less than 35%, on maximum dosage of a beta blocker and a resting heart rate of 70 or greater
    b. Ejection fraction less than 40%, on 3.125 mg carvedilol once daily and no evidence of atrial fibrillation
    c. History of paroxysmal atrial fibrillation that is poorly controlled with metoprolol
    d. History of HFrEF well managed with an ACE Inhibitor, a diuretic, and a beta blocker

■ CARDIOVASCULAR ANSWERS AND RATIONALES

1. **a) Inferior myocardial infarction with evidence of right ventricular involvement**. This patient has ST-elevation in the inferior leads II, III, and AVF indicating inferior wall involvement. He also has elevated JVD in the setting of clear lung fields, a sign for right ventricular involvement. Although not noted in the question, confirming right ventricular involvement would be noted by changes in the placement of right ventricular V3–V4 leads with noted ST-segment changes.

2. **b) Metoprolol (Toprol/Lopressor)**. This patient is hemodynamically stable with a complaint of palpitations caused by atrial fibrillation, and thus does not require hospitalization. Beta blockers or calcium channel blockers are first-line treatment for rate control for a patient who is hemodynamically stable. Amiodarone has a relatively slow onset and is most useful as an adjunct when rate control with beta blockers or calcium channel blockers is incomplete or contraindicated or when cardioversion is planned. Procainamide, due to multiple side effects, is rarely used, and dofetilide must be initiated in the hospital due to potential risk of torsades de pointes.

3. **c) Aortic stenosis**. Aortic stenosis is a systolic murmur that is best heard at the second ICS, right sternal border and often radiates to the carotids. Mitral stenosis is a diastolic murmur best heard at the apex and radiates to the axilla. Pulmonic insufficiency is a systolic murmur. However, it is best heard at Erb's point (second ICS, left sternal boarder) and mitral insufficiency is best heard at the apex.

4. **b) Left carotid endarterectomy followed by a right carotid endarterectomy**. Patients with transient ischemic attacks or strokes from which they have recovered will benefit from carotid intervention if the ipsilateral carotid artery has a stenosis of more than 70%. In this case, his stroke was due to left (internal) carotid artery stenosis and needs initial surgical intervention.

5. **d) Administration of enoxaparin (Lovenox)**. Based upon this patient's age and lack of symptoms, she is considered a low-risk patient and can be treated on an outpatient basis. Although a venous Doppler is appropriate, the patient presents with classic history and symptoms of DVT, thus treatment needs to be started prior to diagnostic testing. Warfarin will take an average 5 days to reach a therapeutic level, thus enoxaparin injections should be initially started. Treatment with direct-acting oral anticoagulants is also an option; however, this is not provided as a distractor. This patient is hemodynamically stable without symptoms suggestive of a pulmonary embolism, thus negating further testing.

6. **d) Phentolamine (OraVerse)**. This patient presents with hypertensive emergency and thus requires parenteral treatment. In hypertensive emergencies that arise from catecholaminergic mechanisms such as cocaine use, beta-blockers can worsen the hypertension because of unopposed peripheral vasoconstriction. Calcium channel blockers or phentolamine are better choices in treating this patient.

7. **a) Cardiac tamponade**. The patient presents with classic signs of tamponade. There is no mention of bleeding, uncorrected coagulopathy, arrhythmia, or ventilator management. Thus the correct answer is tamponade that requires emergent intervention.

8. **c) Dopamine**. This patient presents with acute heart failure in the setting of systemic hypoperfusion (hypotension and oliguria). In this situation, medications that are vasodilators, such as nesiritide, nitroglycerin, and nitroprusside, might worsen the hypotension and therefore should be avoided. Since this patient has a reduced cardiac output, a positive inotropic drug such as dopamine is appropriate.

9. **c) Metoprolol (Lopressor)**. This patient has peripartum cardiomyopathy and as such needs to be treated as a heart failure patient, baring the use of ACEI/ARB therapy. Methyldopa (Aldomet) is not first-line therapy although this drug is used to treat hypertension during pregnancy. Diltiazem—a calcium channel blocker—has negative inotropic effects and may worsen the ejection fraction.

10. **b) IV fluids**. This patient is in shock, from possible blood loss or the effects of general anesthesia and needs volume replacement as first-line therapy. If fluids were unsuccessful, then vasoactive therapy would need to be administered.

11. **c) S3 gallop**. An S3 gallop in an adult arises from high pressures and abrupt deceleration of inflow across the mitral valve at the end of the rapid filling phase of diastole and can be present in heart failure, volume overload, and decreased myocardial contractility. Wait gain, ankle edema, and wheezing are nonspecific signs and can be associated with multiple disease states.

12. **c) Isoproterenol (Isuprel)**. Denervation of the transplanted heart leads to loss of autonomic nervous system modulation of the heart's electrophysiologic properties. Parasympathetic denervation causes loss of basal suppression of SA node automaticity, leading to a persistent increase in resting heart rate and a loss of normal, rapid heart rate modulation. This parasympathetic loss also causes elimination of the chronotropic effects of digoxin and atropine after heart transplantation. The most effective drug to increase heart rate is a pure beta agonist-isoproterenol.

13. **d) Pericarditis**. Diffuse ST-segment changes that are not localized to one wall suggest pericarditis, particularly in the setting of chest discomfort. Endocarditis is not associated with pleuritic pain or ECG changes and for an AMI, there would be localization to one wall of the heart, that is, changes in the inferior leads, anterior leads, and so on, and not diffuse ECG changes. Although the patient has pleuritic pain, in light of the ECG changes, the correct diagnosis is pericarditis.

14. **d) Acute pericarditis**. The symptoms described are characteristic of a classic presentation of acute pericarditis. Acute myocardial infarction is less likely in this client, given the classic pain presentation for pericarditis, and the negative troponin is reassuring. Acutely decompensated heart failure typically manifests as fluid volume overload and possibly pulmonary edema. Acute mitral chordae rupture would present as sudden onset of severe chest pain and symptoms consistent with left heart failure.

15. **c) Order metoprolol (Lopressor) 5 mg to be given slow IV push now**. This client has a stable tachycardia, as evidenced by stable mentation, lack of chest pain, and reasonably normal blood pressure. According to American Heart Association ACLS guidelines, the goal of therapy in this case would be rate control. Adenosine is indicated only for regular-rhythm supraventricular tachycardia. ACLS guidelines recommend the administration of a beta-blocker or nondihydropyridine calcium channel blocker. Synchronized cardioversion would be indicated if the client was unstable, and a transthoracic echocardiogram may be ordered, but would not be an initial therapy.

16. **c) Cessation of alcohol may improve his heart function**. Alcoholic cardiomyopathy is sometimes a reversible condition and cessation of consumption can allow for significant improvement in ventricular function. Counselling the client about his alcohol intake should be started early after diagnosis and be reiterated often during follow-up. Aerobic exercise is shown to improve functional status and diminish symptoms, so patients are encouraged to be physically active. Sexual activity is not contraindicated, but modifications may need to accommodate the client's heart function. Following a low-sodium diet will improve symptoms by reducing fluid retention, but not directly influence resolution of heart function.

17. **c) Aggressive blood pressure control**. Severe, sudden, persistent chest pain radiating down the back is characteristic of aortic dissection. Multiplanar CT scan is the immediate diagnostic test of choice, but aggressive measures to lower blood pressure should occur when a dissection is suspected, even before diagnostic studies are completed. Surgical consultation should be undertaken urgently once the diagnosis is confirmed. Transesophageal echocardiography is a valuable diagnostic tool, but is not readily available in the emergency/acute care setting.

18. **d) Lisinopril (Prinivil) 20 mg orally once per day**. According to guidelines for the management of hypertension by the Eighth Joint National Committee, patients of all ages who have evidence of kidney disease, with or without diabetes and regardless of race, should be treated

with an ACE-inhibitor or ARB, either alone or in combination with antihypertensive medications of other drug classes. For African American patients with proteinuria, the use of an ACEI or ARB is especially important given a higher likelihood of progression of renal disease to end-stage. Hydrochlorothiazide is the recommended initial treatment of clients of all ages and races without kidney dysfunction.

19. **a) Atorvastatin (Lipitor) 40 mg orally once per day.** According to 2013 ACC/AHA Guideline on the Treatment of Blood Cholesterol, patients with clinical evidence of atherosclerotic heart disease (such as CAD and MI) should be treated with high-intensity statin therapy regardless of lipid levels, unless they have a history of intolerance to the therapy or other contraindication. Examples of high-intensity statin therapy include atorvastatin (Lipitor) 40–80 mg orally once daily and rosuvastatin (Crestor) 20–40 mg daily. Daily dosing of lovastatin 40 mg, pravastatin, and simvastatin are examples of moderate-intensity statin therapy.

20. **a) Aspirin 81 mg and clopidogrel (Plavix) 75 mg orally daily for at least 12 months.** For patients receiving DES, 1 year (12 months) of DAPT is recommended.

21. **b) Intravenous loop diuretic therapy.** The client in question has evidence of pulmonary edema (pulmonary venous hypertension) with relative hypoxemia related to heart failure exacerbation and fluid volume overload. The cornerstone in the management of pulmonary edema remains diuretic therapy to mobilize excess fluid. There is no urgent indication given for referring the client to the cardiac catheterization lab, and while electrocardiography should be performed in cases of heart failure exacerbation to rule out ischemic etiology, it would not be considered an urgent therapeutic need. Finally, in acute exacerbations, depending on severity, the negative inotropic effects of beta blockers may complicate the situation. In some cases, inotropic medications such as beta agonist dobutamine, may be indicated for optimal diuresis.

22. **c) Reflex tachycardia.** Intravenous nicardipine is the most potent of parenteral calcium channel blockers, which causes arterial vasodilation, and this may precipitate reflex tachycardia. Beta-blocker infusion is often coupled with nicardipine in these patients to help manage the adverse effect. Neurological changes are an ominous sign in clients with hypertensive emergencies, but are not in itself an indication for the beta blocker. Intensifying chest pain may trigger further investigation and consideration of possible myocardial ischemia. Nicardipine is a potent vasodilator and the longest acting parenteral calcium channel blocker. For this reason, episodes of rebound hypertension are less likely than with other agents.

23. **a) Cardiac tamponade.** Diminished peripheral pulses upon inspiration (pulsus paradoxus), elevated JVP, and distant heart tones are suggestive of cardiac tamponade, a potential complication related to hemopericardium after cardiac surgery. Acute respiratory failure is a concern, but not directly indicated by the assessment findings mentioned. Fluid volume overload or recurrent ischemia will cause dyspnea, but the assessment finding of pulsus paradoxus is a highly sensitive and specific indicator for cardiac tamponade.

24. **d) Immediate cardiac surgical consultation.** Drainage of the pericardial effusion to release the compressive features of cardiac tamponade is the cornerstone of therapy in cases of hemodynamic compromise. Intravenous diuresis, MRI, and vasodilators are not helpful in addressing the situation and may sacrifice valuable time before getting the client managed surgically by either pericardiocentesis or more invasive pericardial window surgery.

25. **c) Referral to interventional cardiology.** All patients with symptomatic severe aortic stenosis should be considered for valve intervention. When symptoms begin to present, prognosis without intervention is poor. The client described should be managed closely to manage fluid volume overload and promote normal systemic blood pressure, but ultimately the valve will need to be replaced to prevent poor outcomes. Referral to a cardiac rehabilitation program is not indicated in this situation.

26. **a) Echocardiography**. In the situation described, there should be a concern for post-infective myocarditis and resultant heart failure. An echocardiogram would provide useful assessment of cardiac performance and may exclude other processes. While histologic evidence will ultimately be necessary for confirmation of myocarditis and assessment of etiology, endomyocardial biopsy would not be the initial step in treating this client. Chest radiography may provide clues suggesting heart failure, but does not provide direct assessment of cardiac function. Troponin I levels do not always correlate with the diagnosis of myocarditis, and are considered not a specific diagnostic tool.

27. **a) Cardiogenic shock**. The production of pink, frothy sputum is a sign of acute pulmonary edema and a systolic blood pressure less than 90 mmHg, with cold extremities and confusion, represents cardiogenic shock. While the right side may be failing, the signs and symptoms represent fluid backing up into the pulmonary bed, which correlates with left-sided heart failure. Cardiac tamponade is ruled out because there is no mention of a pericardial friction rub, an elevated JVD, or pulsus paradoxus.

28. **c) Shortness of breath, bilateral crackles, and elevated JVD**. Signs of HFrEF include dyspnea, rhonchi or crackles, and elevated jugular venous pressure (elevated JVD). While patients may have nocturia, their problem is fluid overload and hence not an increase in urinary output, and a pericardial friction rub correlates with cardiac tamponade or a pericardial effusion, while chest pain correlates with angina pectoris.

29. **a) Enlarged cardiac silhouette, PMI 2 cm left of midclavicular line, and an ejection fraction of less than 40%**. Signs of dilated cardiomyopathy included an enlarged heart on chest x-ray (enlarged cardiac silhouette) and cardiomegaly on physical exam (PMI left of midclavicular line) and an ejection fraction less than 40% as noted on 2D echocardiogram.

30. **c) Hypertrophic cardiomyopathy**. Hypertrophic cardiomyopathy presents on physical exam with a sustained point of maximal impulse and a systolic murmur and on an echocardiogram with "asymmetrical septal hypertrophy" or septal enlargement. Neither dilated cardiomyopathy nor restrictive cardiomyopathy have septal enlargement, nor do they have a sustained point of maximal impulse. Ischemic cardiomyopathy can be a cause of dilated cardiomyopathy.

31. **c) Non-ST segment myocardial infarction**. Unstable angina, non-STEMI and STEMI all fall under the category of ACS. With unstable angina the biomarkers are not elevated, but with a non-STEMI there is a rise in the biomarkers (troponin I or troponin T or CK-MB) but no-ST segment elevation. In comparison, a STEMI has ST segment elevation.

32. **d) Enoxaparin (Lovenox) and clopidogrel (Plavix)**. Treatment for a non-STEMI includes aspirin, enoxaparin, or unfractionated heparin, and clopidogrel as conservative treatment. Studies have indicated that enoxaparin is more effective than unfractionated heparin, and clopidogrel demonstrated a 20% reduction in death in non-STEMI, with current guidelines recommending both enoxaparin and clopidogrel. Amlodipine is a calcium channel blocker and it is not part of the non-STEMI guidelines, nor is thrombolytics.

33. **c) Alteplase (Activase)**. Guidelines recommend fibrinolytic therapy within 30 minutes of arriving to the hospital or PCI including stents. Alteplase is recombinant tissue plasminogen activator and is one of three fibrinolytic agents used in the United States. A beta-blocker such as carvedilol is recommended to be started in the first 24 hours, but alteplase is to be started within the first 30 minutes. Sotalol is not part of the management of a STEMI, nor is the calcium channel blocker amlodipine.

34. **c) Fibrinolytics, ACE inhibitor, beta-blocker, and stents**. Appropriate management of a patient who has had a STEMI includes fibrinolytics such as lteplase, an ACE inhibitor, PCI with stents, and a beta-blocker within the first 24 hours. EBP does not support the use of calcium channel blockers, nor is a loop diuretic part of the guidelines. Morphine may be given initially in the stabilization phase to relieve pain, but the ACE inhibitor should be given early in the management of a STEMI, and the beta-blocker within the first 24 hours, but after starting the ACE inhibitor.

35. **a) Cardiac tamponade**. Classic signs of cardiac tamponade include muffled or distant heart sounds, elevated jugular venous pressures (elevated CVP) and hypotension. These three signs compromise Beck's triad, and point to cardiac tamponade. One of the causes of cardiac tamponade is post heart surgery or postcardiotomy. While hypotension is common to both hemorrhagic shock and hypovolemic shock, neither an elevated venous pressure nor muffled heart sounds are associated with either form of shock. Right-sided heart failure does produce elevated venous pressures, but Beck's triad is diagnostic for cardiac tamponade.

36. **a) Dobutamine**. Dobutamine is the drug of choice for cardiogenic shock with a systolic blood pressure greater 90 mmHg because it will increase myocardial contractility and decrease afterload. Dopamine is the drug of choice if the systolic blood pressure is less than 80 mmHg.

37. **b) Atrial fibrillation**. AF is an irregular rhythm with fibrillatory waves and no P waves but with normal QRS complexes. Atrial flutter has a sawtooth baseline and one can count the number of flutter waves between each QRS. A premature atrial contraction is an early beat, not a rhythm, and a premature ventricular contraction is also an early beat with no P wave and a wide QRS.

38. **a) Sudden cardiac arrest related to ventricular arrhythmias**. Many antiarrhythmic medications including sotalol can prolong the QT interval and place the patient at risk of sudden death related to ventricular arrhythmias, including torsades de pointe.

39. **a) Hyperkalemia and an elevated creatinine**. A potential side effect of lisinopril (Zestril) is an elevated creatinine level and hyperkalemia.

40. **a) Hypertensive emergency**. While an elevated creatinine may signal renal insufficiency, the NP needs to recognize that the severe headache reflects hypertensive encephalopathy and the elevated creatinine may reflect hypertensive nephropathy. With new onset of symptoms and diastolic pressure above 130, the most appropriate diagnosis is hypertensive emergency. Hypertensive urgency is a situation in which the blood pressure should be lowered over a longer period of time, whereas hypertensive emergency reflects a situation where the blood pressure should be lowered in a timelier manner.

41. **d) Begin a statin**. The management of a patient with CAD with high LDL levels is lifestyle change and to begin a cholesterol-lowering medication such as a statin. While a patient may need to lose weight, no data was provided in the scenario to suggest the patient is overweight. Dietary recommendations are to reduce saturated fat intake and total fat intake. Because the LDL is from a fasting blood sample, the LDL does not need to be rechecked in 2 weeks; however, response to therapy should be rechecked in 6 to 8 weeks.

42. **a) Fasting blood glucose level greater than 110, triglycerides ≥150 mg/dL, HDL less than 50 mg/dL, waistline measurement greater than 35 inches, and blood pressure ≥130/85**. The criteria for metabolic syndrome for women is fasting blood glucose level greater than 110 mg/dL, triglycerides greater than 150 mg/dL, HDL less than 50 mg/dL, waistline measurement greater than 35 inches, and blood pressure ≥130/85.

43. **d) Colchicine (Colcrys) and ibuprofen (Advil/Motrin)**. This patient presents with acute pericarditis. That her symptoms of substernal chest pain improve with sitting up, together with the friction rub on exam, support this diagnosis. The ECG in the first hours to days is characterized by diffuse ST elevation with reciprocal ST depression in leads aVR and V1. Also, there may be an atrial injury, reflected by elevation of the PR segment in lead aVR and depression of the PR segment in other limb leads and in the left chest leads, primarily V5 and V6. The most likely cause in this otherwise healthy woman is viral or idiopathic. In many cases, acute pericarditis is self-limited and will resolve in 2 to 6 weeks. In the treatment of acute pericarditis, the goals of therapy are the relief of pain, resolution of inflammation, and prevention of recurrence. Acute pericarditis is painful, so acute therapy usually requires NSAIDs. She should also be treated with colchicine concurrently, because it is well tolerated, reduces symptoms, and decreases the rate of recurrent pericarditis. High-dose corticosteroids are reserved for

individuals whose pericarditis is unresponsive to nonsteroidal agents and colchicine. Corticosteroids are not usually used as first-line therapy, because individuals treated with them have a higher rate of recurrent pericarditis.

44. **c) Aortic valve surgery**. Many patients with severe stenosis are asymptomatic for a period of time. Often, a long asymptomatic period is followed by stepwise onset of symptoms starting with dyspnea followed by chest pain, then syncope, and finally signs of heart failure. Once symptoms start, mortality increases. Most patients with newly symptomatic aortic stenosis are admitted. Without surgery, 40% to 50% of patients with classic symptoms die within 1 year.

45. **c) Indicated based on his presentation**. Because of the evidence linking early PCI to improved survival outcome, the 2015 American Heart Association guidelines recommend that all patients successfully resuscitated from cardiac arrest of suspected cardiac etiology should be considered for emergent coronary angiography. The patient in this scenario has known CAD. This recommendation applies regardless of neurologic status or presenting arrest rhythm.

46. **c) Emergent pericardiocentesis**. This patient presents with acute cardiac tamponade arising as a complication from ICD placement (hemopericardium is a known complication). Her symptoms are consistent with Beck's triad: an elevated jugular venous pressure, arterial hypotension, and quiet, "muffled" heart sounds. This is a medical emergency, and urgent pericardiocentesis is the treatment of choice.

47. **a) Cardiac tamponade**. This patient presents with acute cardiac tamponade as her symptoms are consistent with Beck's triad: an elevated jugular venous pressure, arterial hypotension, and quiet "muffled" heart sounds.

48. **b) Increase her diuretic dosing and counsel patient on fluid and salt restriction**. Management focuses on treatment of symptoms and prevention of sudden death and stroke. Left ventricular outflow tract obstruction can be controlled medically in the majority of patients. Beta adrenergic blocking agents and L-type calcium channel blockers (e.g., verapamil) are first-line agents that reduce the severity of obstruction by slowing heart rate, enhancing diastolic filling, and decreasing contractility. Patients with or without obstruction may develop heart failure symptoms due to fluid retention and require diuretic therapies for venous congestion. Although her lungs are clear at the clinic visit, this patient's examination and symptoms reflect persistent volume overload, and she would benefit from further diuresis to correct this. Excessive use of multiple inhibitors of the renin–angiotensin system has not been found to be beneficial. Cardiac transplantation would not be appropriate based on her clinical presentation. Vasodilator therapy would not help correct her apparent volume overload.

49. **b) Aspirin, metoprolol (Toprol), lisinopril (Prinivil) and clopidigrel (Plavix)**. Various secondary preventive measures contribute to improvement in the long-term mortality and morbidity rates after STEMI. American Heart Association/American College of Cardiology guidelines on duration of DAPT recommend DAPT for 1 year in patients presenting with an ACS. Long-term treatment with an antiplatelet agent (usually aspirin) after STEMI is associated with a 25% reduction in the risk of recurrent infarction, stroke, or cardiovascular mortality. ACE inhibitors or ARBs should be used indefinitely by patients with clinically evident heart failure, a moderate decrease in global ejection fraction, or a large regional wall motion abnormality to prevent late ventricular remodeling and recurrent ischemic events. Beta-blocker therapy after STEMI is useful for most patients (including those treated with an ACE inhibitor) except those in whom it is specifically contraindicated.

50. **c) Place a temporary pacemaker**. This patient's ECG shows third-degree heart block. He is clearly symptomatic with syncope. In the ED, he is still not stable as his blood pressure is very low and he remains lightheaded. Urgent treatment is required, and a temporary pacemaker is the most important initial step. Management of the symptomatic patient can be with either medication and/or pacing. Nodal blocks (narrow QRS complex) may respond to atropine;

infranodal blocks (wide QRS complex) are unlikely to respond to atropine or other medications that can enhance AV nodal conduction. Patients should have transcutaneous cardiac pacer pads applied in the ED. If there is no or incomplete response to atropine, use transcutaneous (temporary) cardiac pacing, recognizing that transvenous pacing is eventually necessary in most patients.

51. **a) ECG, urinalysis, creatinine**. Formal recommendations for the evaluation of an ED patient presenting with asymptomatic but severe hypertension do not exist. However, hypertensive urgency must be distinguished from hypertensive emergency. Urgency is defined as severely elevated blood pressure (systolic blood pressure greater than 220 mmHg or diastolic blood pressure greater than 120 mmHg) with no evidence of target organ damage. A hypertensive emergency is a condition in which elevated blood pressure results in target organ damage. Hypertensive emergencies necessitate immediate therapy to decrease blood pressure within minutes to hours. Commonly ordered tests to determine if there is end-organ damage and a possible cause include complete blood count, basic metabolic panel, ECG, chest radiograph, urinalysis, and TSH.

52. **a) ABI of less than 0.3**. The primary symptom of PAD is claudication. This patient describes claudication that occurs with ambulation which is relieved with rest. In severe PAD, pain in the extremities occurs at rest. Physical findings of PAD often include diminished peripheral pulses, loss of hair in the distal extremities, and skin that is cool to the touch. Findings during the examination can determine the need for obtaining an ABI. A resting ABI of less than 0.9 is abnormal, but critical ischemia with rest does not occur until the ABI is less than 0.3 individuals with heavily calcified blood vessels may have an abnormally elevated ABI greater than 1.2 when PAD is present. Lower extremity edema may be suggestive of CHF.

53. **a) Severe left ventricular dysfunction that leads to pulmonary congestion**. The most common etiology is severe LV dysfunction that leads to pulmonary congestion and/or systemic hypoperfusion. This dysfunction leads to an increase in pulmonary venous pressure shift. Hydrostatic pressure is increased and fluid exits the capillary at an increased rate, resulting in interstitial and, in more severe cases, alveolar edema. Causes of noncardiogenic pulmonary edema are due to injury to the lung. The injury is likely to result from direct, indirect, or pulmonary vascular causes. Direct injuries are mediated via the airways (e.g., aspiration) or as the consequence of blunt chest trauma. Indirect injury is the consequence of mediators that reach the lung via the bloodstream. The third category includes conditions that may result from acute changes in pulmonary vascular pressures, possibly due to sudden autonomic discharge (in the case of neurogenic and high-altitude pulmonary edema) or sudden swings of pleural pressure as well as transient damage to the pulmonary capillaries (in the case of reexpansion pulmonary edema).

54. **b) A 72-year-old female with a dissection of the descending aorta that begins distal to the left subclavian artery and extends below the left renal artery, who has no symptoms and has a creatinine that is within normal limits**. Ascending aortic dissection requires surgical intervention, whereas descending aortic dissection that is uncomplicated maybe managed medically. Indications for intervention for descending dissections acutely include occlusion of a major aortic branch with symptoms. Once a descending dissection has been found, intensive medical management of blood pressure is imperative and should include agents that decrease cardiac contractility and aortic sheer force. Follow-up should occur every 6 to 12 months and surgical intervention should be considered if there is continued advancement despite medical management. Patients with Marfan syndrome have increased complications with descending dissections and should be considered for surgical repair, especially if concomitant disease in the ascending aorta is demonstrated by aortic root dilatation of greater than 50 mm.

55. **a) Bicuspid aortic valve**. This patient has a coarctation of the aorta presenting with hypertension proximal to the lesion. Narrowing most commonly occurs distal to the origins of left subclavian artery, explaining the equal pressures in the arms. Coarctation accounts for approximately 10% of congenital cardiac anomalies, occurring more than two times more

frequently in men, and are associated with bicuspid aortic valve. Adults will present with manifestations of hypertension in the upper body, such as headache and/or epistaxis, or leg claudication.

56. **c) D-dimer**. This patient has a history and classic presentation for a PE. Routine cardiopulmonary testing in the ED generally demonstrates nonspecific findings in patients with PE. ECG findings are often normal or nonspecific in patients with PE and thus are not the most useful in ruling out PE in this patient. Chest radiographs are also usually normal, though the Westermark sign or Hampton hump may be noted. ABG findings are often confusing, and abnormalities are usually a result of underlying pathology such as COPD or pneumonia. A low Po_2 in an otherwise healthy patient at risk for DVT/PE is more useful. O_2 saturation is rarely depressed and not very useful in the workup of PE. High-sensitivity d-dimer levels are most useful for their negative predictive value in helping to rule out PE in low-to-moderate pretest-probability patients. It is a very sensitive but nonspecific test. A normal high-sensitivity d-dimer level in a low-to-moderate pretest probability patient makes PE unlikely, and further diagnostic workup is not indicated.

57. **a) Idiopathic pulmonary arterial hypertension**. IPAH is a progressive disease that leads to right heart failure and death. It is typically seen in young women. This patient's physical examination is consistent with right ventricular pressure overload. This is supported by the ECG demonstrating right atrial enlargement, right axis deviation, and RVH. The hemodynamic definition of pulmonary arterial hypertension is a mean pulmonary artery pressure at rest greater than or equal to 25 mmHg based on a right heart catheterization. Because they have a fixed cardiac output (limited by lung vascular pressures), patients with pulmonary hypertension often get presyncopal with exertion. Ischemic cardiovascular disease is almost unheard of in a woman younger than 30 years without any risk factors. Asthma may cause her symptom complex but is not supported by her examination. Aortic stenosis causes neither resting hypoxemia nor RVH.

58. **c) Elicit a vagal maneuver**. Vagal maneuvers are often effective. If there is no response to vagal maneuvers, adenosine is recommended to convert to sinus rhythm. It is rare that the patient requires a calcium channel blocker. If the patient becomes unstable, use of electrical cardioversion may be necessary for conversion. Overdrive pacing is rarely needed for this in young adults. Paroxysmal supraventricular tachycardia is seen more frequently in females, with a peak in the late teenage and young adult years. The majority of patients are without active cardiovascular disease. Patients may be able to describe the abrupt onset of this re-entrant dysrhythmia and also note when it self-terminates. Palpitations, lightheadedness, and dyspnea are common symptoms.

59. **b) Contrast-enhanced chest CT**. This patient's history and examination are very concerning for the dissection of the thoracic aorta. If the ascending aorta is involved in a dissection, it becomes a surgical emergency. Dissections of the descending aorta can be managed medically. Therefore, whenever an aortic dissection is suspected, it is of extreme importance to determine its presence and extent. Cardiac stress test is not useful in the diagnosis of an aortic dissection and is contraindicated. A tagged red blood cell scan can be used to diagnose areas of small ongoing bleeding. Ventilation perfusion scan has no utility in the diagnosis of an aortic dissection. A chest x-ray may be the first test that suggests the diagnosis, with a finding of a widened mediastinum. Echocardiography, particularly transesophageal, can be used to assess proximal ascending aorta and descending thoracic aorta. Contrast enhanced CT, MRI, and a conventional invasive aortogram are sensitive and specific tests.

60. **d) Decreased glomerular filtration**. The kidney is the major organ for clearance of drugs from the body, thus age-related decline of renal functional capacity is very important. The decline in creatine clearance occurs in about two-thirds of the population. It is important to note that this decline is not reflected in an equivalent rise in serum creatinine because the production of creatinine is also reduced as muscle mass declines with age;

therefore, serum creatinine alone is not an adequate measure of renal function. Dosing recommendations for the elderly often include an allowance for reduced renal clearance. Dosing can be calculated by using the MDRD formula that is available online at www.niddk.nih.gov/health-information/communication-programs/nkdep/laboratory-evaluation/glomerular-filtration-rate-calculators

61. **b) Rosuvastatin (Crestor)**. PIs are extensively metabolized by CYP3A4. As a result, there is enormous potential for drug-drug interactions with other commonly used medications. HMG-co reductase or statins are recommended post-AMI as secondary prevention. Omega 3FA is not a statin and is usually given for hypertriglyceridemia. Simvastatin and lovastatin are mainly metabolized by CUP3A4. As such they would increase the area under the curve and may lead to muscle myopathy. Rosuvastatin is mediated by CUP2CP. As such there is less potential for myopathy in patients on PIs.

62. **c) Furosemide (Lasix) 40 mg intravenously now**. In pulmonary edema, the typical course of treatment would include diuretics, nitrates, and morphine. IV diuretic therapy with furosemide is indicated and should be considered first, even if the client has not previously suffered fluid retention. Loop diuretics produce venodilatory effects, reducing preload even before diuresis begins. The use of intravenous morphine can lower left heart pressures and has effects of anxiolysis, but should be used in caution given its tendency to reduce ventilatory drive. Acute use of beta-blockers in this decompensated state could exacerbate heart failure due to the immediate negative inotropic effects, and should be saved until the acute phase is managed and introduced for chronic heart failure management. Aminophylline infusion could be used, with caution, for management of bronchospasm as a complication of pulmonary edema, but will not treat the heart failure and pulmonary edema directly.

63. **b) Nonhealing ulcerations on distal toes**. In clients with known peripheral arterial disease, cool, atrophic, hairless skin; diminished peripheral pulse amplitude; and rubor on dependency are expected findings. The hallmark signs of critical limb ischemia include pain at rest and distal ulcerations. Patients with these findings are at high risk for requiring amputation.

64. **c) The patient must be off any ACI inhibitor or ARB for 36 hours before Entresto can be started**. Entresto, which contains a neprilysin inhibitor (sacubitril) "should not be administered along with an ACE inhibitor or within 36 hours of the last dose of an ACE inhibitor." This is a Class III recommendation indicating that administering a neprilysin inhibitor either in addition to an ACE inhibitor or within a 36-hour window of an ACE inhibitor places the patient at an increased risk for angioedema since Entresto is a combination drug that includes an ARB in addition to the neprilysin inhibitor.

65. **a) Ejection fraction less than 35%, on maximum dosage of a beta-blocker and a resting heart rate of 70 or greater**. According to the 2016 American College of Cardiology/American Heart Association/Heart Failure Society of America guidelines, the criteria for starting a patient on ivabradine (Corlanor) are the patient should have stable HFrEF with an ejection fraction of ≥35%, on a maximum dose of a beta-blocker and in sinus rhythm with a resting heart rate of 70 beats per minute or greater (Yancy, Jessup, Bozkurt, et al., 2016). For individuals who meet all three criteria, the data indicate that there is a reduction in heart failure hospitalizations. Important points to remember are the patient needs to be titrated up to the highest level of a beta-blocker that can be tolerated and the patient should be in sinus rhythm. It is not a drug to use for treating atrial fibrillation.

■ BIBLIOGRAPHY

American Diabetes Association. (2016). ADA standards of medical care in diabetes. *Diabetes Care, 39*(Suppl. 1), S1–2. doi:10.2337/dc16-S001

American Heart Association ACLS Project Team. (2016). *Advanced cardiovascular life support provider manual.* Dallas, TX: American Heart Association.

Bickley, L., & Szilagyi, P. (2013). *Bates' guide to physical examination and history taking.* Philadelphia, PA: Lippincott.

Callaway, C. W., Donnino, M. W., Fink, E. L., Geocadin, R. G., Golan, E., Kern, K. B., & Zimmerman, J. L. (2015). Part 8: Post-cardiac arrest care: 2015 American Heart Association guidelines update for cardiopulmonary resuscitation and emergency cardiovascular care. *Circulation, 132*(18 Suppl. 2), S465–482. doi:10.1161/CIR.0000000000000262

Crawford, M. H. (2014). *Current diagnosis & treatment in cardiology* (4th ed.). New York, NY: McGraw-Hill.

Fleisher, L. A., Fleischmann, K. E., Auerbach, A. D., Barnason, S. A., Beckman, J. A., Bozkurt, B., & Wijeysundera, D. N. (2014). 2014 ACC/AHA guideline on perioperative cardiovascular evaluation and management of patients undergoing noncardiac surgery. *A Report of the American College of Cardiology/American Heart Association Task Force on Practice Guidelines, 64*(22), e77–e137. doi:10.1016/j.jacc.2014.07.944

Godara, H., Heirbe, A., Nassif, M., Otepka, H., & Rosenstock, A. (2014). *The Washington manual of medical therapeutics* (34th ed.). Philadelphia, PA: Wolters Kluwer-Lippincott Williams & Wilkins.

Hamon, D., Taleski, J., Vaseghi, M., Shivkumar, K., & Boyle, N. G. (2014). Arrhythmias in the heart transplant patient. *Arrhythmia & Electrophysiology Review, 3*(3), 149–155.

Huff, J. (2017). *ECG workout: Exercises in arrhythmia interpretation.* Philadelphia, PA: Wolters Kluwer.

James, P. A., Oparil, S., Carter, B. L., Cushman, W. C., Dennison-Himmelfarb, C., Handler, J., Lackland, D. T., . . . LeFevre, M. L. (2014). 2014 evidence-based guideline for the management of high blood pressure in adults: Report from the panel members appointed to the Eighth Joint National Committee (JNC 8). *JAMA, 311*(5), 507–520. doi:10.1001/jama.2013.284427

Kasper, D., Hauser, S., Jameson, J., Fauci, A., Longo, D., & Loscalzo, J. (2015). *Harrison's principles of internal medicine* (19th ed.). New York, NY: McGraw-Hill.

Katzung, B., & Trevor, A. (2015). *Basic & clinical pharmacology* (13th ed.). New York, NY: McGraw-Hill.

Levine, G. N., Bates, E. R., Bittl, J. A., Brindis, R. G., Fihn, S. D., Fleisher, L. A., & Smith, S. C. (2016). 2016 ACC/AHA guideline focused update on duration of dual antiplatelet therapy in patients with coronary artery disease: A report of the American College of Cardiology/American Heart Association task force on clinical practice guidelines. An update of the 2011 ACCF/AHA/SCAI guideline for percutaneous coronary intervention, 2011 ACCF/AHA guideline for coronary artery bypass graft surgery, 2012 ACC/AHA/ACP/AATS/PCNA/SCAI/STS guideline for the diagnosis and management of patients with stable ischemic heart disease, 2013 ACCF/AHA guideline for the management of ST-elevation myocardial infarction, 2014 AHA/ACC guideline for the management of patients with non–ST-elevation acute coronary syndromes, and 2014 ACC/AHA guideline on perioperative cardiovascular evaluation and management of patients undergoing noncardiac surgery. *Circulation, 134*(10), e123–155. doi:10.1161/cir.0000000000000404

Mann, D., Zipes, D., Libby, P., & Bonow, R. (2015). *Braunwald's heart disease: A textbook of cardiovascular medicine* (10th ed.). Philadelphia, PA: Elsevier.

Papadakis, M. A., McPhee, S. J., & Rabow, M. W. (2017). *Current medical diagnosis & treatment 2017.* New York, NY: McGraw-Hill Education.

Parrillo, J., & Dellinger, R. (2013). *Critical care medicine: Principles of diagnosis and management in the adult* (4th ed.). Philadelphia PA: Elsevier.

Stecker, E. C., Strelich, K. R., Chugh, S. S., Crispell, K., & McAnulty, J. H. (2005). Review article: Arrhythmias after orthotopic heart transplantation. *Journal of Cardiac Failure, 11*464–11472. doi:10.1016/j.cardfail.2005.02.005

Stone, N. J., Robinson, J., Lichtenstein, A. H., Merz, C. N. B., Blum, C. B., Eckel, R. H., & Wilson, P. W. F. (2013). 2013 ACC/AHA guideline on the treatment of blood cholesterol to reduce atherosclerotic cardiovascular risk in adults. A report of the American College of Cardiology/American Heart Association task force on practice guidelines. *Journal of the American College of Cardiology, 63*(25), 2889–2934. doi:10.1161/01.cir.0000437738.63853.7a

Tintinalli, J. E. (2016). *Tintinalli's emergency medicine: A comprehensive study guide* (8th ed.). New York, NY: McGraw-Hill.

7

Pulmonary

DONNA LYNCH-SMITH, TRACI M. MOTES,
AND HELEN MILEY

PULMONARY QUESTIONS

1. An intubated patient is receiving enteral nutrition. Today she has a new onset fever, leukocytosis, and increased sputum production. Chest x-ray demonstrates right lower lobe (RLL) infiltrate. Which of the following interventions is most beneficial to decrease the incidence of this complication?

   a. Elevate the head of bed ≥ 30 degrees
   b. Prescribe sulcrafate (Carafate)
   c. Mouth care with oral suctioning every shift
   d. Assessment of frequent gastric residuals

2. A 24-year-old female presents with complaints of shortness of breath, chest tightness, wheezing ,and non-productive cough three to four times a week for the past month. This resolves within 30 minutes with the use of her albuterol inhaler and rest. She has a past medical history of asthma that has been well controlled with an albuterol metered dose inhaler. She states that she thought that it would improve, but has failed to do so. She denies fever, chills, chest pain, dizziness, syncope, or hemoptysis. A chest x-ray is negative for any acute processes. What would be the next step in management?

   a. Add an ICS.
   b. Add an ICS and a LABA.
   c. Add a LABA and a systemic corticosteroid.
   d. Add an ICS and a systemic corticosteroid.

3. A patient with potential asthma was referred to the AG-ACNP in the pulmonology clinic for further evaluation. To obtain the most information on her current respiratory status, the AG-ACNP orders:

   a. ABS
   b. Peak flow
   c. Pulse oximetry
   d. Pulmonary function test

4. A 59-year-old male presents with complaints of chest tightness and shortness of breath. He has a medical history of CAD, hypertension, and hyperlipidemia. Family history is positive for CAD, hypertension, hyperlipidemia, and asthma. His vital signs are: heart rate 110, blood pressure 189/106, respiratory rate 28, and SpO2 96%. On exam the AG-ACNP appreciates bilateral expiratory wheezes, but no rubs, gallops, or murmurs. Capillary refill time is less than 3 seconds. Which medication should be avoided until asthma has been ruled out?

a. Nitroglycerin
b. Morphine
c. Aspirin
d. Captopril

5. Management of asthmatics includes a 6-step process depending on level of control. Poor control is easily managed by 1 or 2 steps up in treatment. What is the least amount of time a patient must remain controlled at their current step prior to attempting a step down?

a. 2 months
b. 3 months
c. 6 months
d. 12 months

6. A 60-year-old male presents to the pulmonary clinic for exertional shortness of breath. The patient reports that he quit smoking cigarettes 3 years ago and that he smoked 1 pack of cigarettes a day for 40 years. According to the Global Strategy for the Diagnosis, Management and Prevention of Chronic Obstructive Pulmonary Disease, which of the following in most adults is needed for a confirmed diagnosis of COPD?

a. Pre-bronchodilator FEV_1/FVC less than 0.70
b. Pre-bronchodilator FEV_1/FVC greater than 0.70
c. Post-bronchodilator FEV_1/FVC less than 0.70
d. Post-bronchodilator FEV_1/FVC greater than 0.70

7. Which of the following chronic medical therapies are shown to improve survival in patients with COPD? Smoking cessation with:

a. Correction of hypoxemia with supplemental O_2
b. All inhaled medications administered via nebulizer
c. Vaccinations for influenza and pneumonia
d. Pulmonary rehabilitation

8. In addition to smoking cessation and vaccinations that include influenza and pneumococcal, which of the following should be included in the management of a patient with mild or Global Strategy for the Diagnosis, Management and Prevention of Chronic Obstructive Pulmonary Disease stage I COPD?

a. SABA, ICS, LABA, O_2
b. SABA, LABA, oral prednisone
c. SABA, ICS, oral prednisone
d. SABA

9. The gold standard for the diagnosis of OSA-hypopnea syndrome is:

a. Overnight polysomnography with direct technician observation
b. 24-hour continuous pulse oximetry with Holter monitoring
c. Physical exam including Mallampati airway classification
d. Fiberoptic laryngoscopy and nasolarynoscopy

10. Which of the following is a potential complication of untreated OSA?

    a. Hypertension
    b. Septal deviation
    c. Mandibular hypoplasia
    d. COPD

11. An unrestrained driver presents to the ED after a head-on motor vehicle crash with airbag deployment. The patient is awake and alert. GCS = 15. Vital signs: heart rate 94, blood pressure 138/78, respiratory rate 28, and SpO2 99% on room air. Chest wall is symmetrical, but tender to palpation. Breath sounds are diminished throughout related to shallow respirations. Chest x-ray is negative for any acute changes. Initial management should include which of the following?

    a. 0.09% normal saline 1,000 mL bolus
    b. 100% O2 via nonrebreather mask
    c. Pain management
    d. ABG

12. A patient presents with a report of blunt force injury to the chest wall. Upon inspection the AG-ACNP notes that a portion of the ribs are unstable, with a section moving independently of the rest of the chest wall on inspiration and expiration. Vital signs include heart rate 118; blood pressure 120/70; respiratory rate 30; O_2 saturation 90% on 60% face mask. Chest x-ray reveals multiple rib fractures. Initial management for this patient would include:

    a. Wrapping the ribs to brace the fractured area
    b. Intubation with positive pressure ventilation
    c. Chest tube insertion preventing pneumothorax from ribs puncturing lung
    d. Surgical repair of ribs

13. The AG-ACNP is managing a 68-year-old male patient with respiratory failure due to an acute exacerbation of COPD. Upon chest auscultation the patient has normal S1 and S2 heart sounds as well as clear breath sounds. The patient is on the following ventilator settings: SIMV rate 12, VT 500 mL, FiO_2 40%, PEEP 5 cmH$_2$0. The AG-ACNP examines the waveform (see the following ventilator waveform). After viewing this waveform, the AG-ACNP:

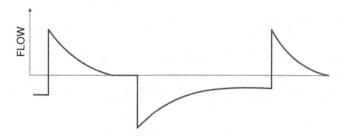

    a. Decreases the tidal volume
    b. Decreases the inspiratory flow rate
    c. Increases the tidal volume
    d. Increases the inspiratory flow rate

14. The AG-ACNP is seeing a 67-year-old female with a medical history of COPD who has experienced increasing dyspnea, which is now more prominent at rest. She has a slight increase in sputum production for the last 3 days at home. Sputum remains clear to white. The AG-ACNP notes she is short of breath, but able to speak in full sentences. The patient's last hospitalization

for COPD was 3 years ago. WBC is 8,800/mm^3, sodium 142 mmol/L, BUN 16 mg/dL, creatinine 0.9 mg/dL. Nasal swab for MRSA is negative. Based on these findings, what is the best treatment?

a. Administer supplemental oxygen, albuteral nebulizers, increase LABA, oral corticosteroids
b. Admit to ICU on levofloxacin (Levaquin), piperacillin-tazobactam (Zosyn), and ceftriaxone (Rocephin)
c. Admit to ICU for oxygen, noninvasive ventilation, and IV corticosteroids
d. Admit to observation, prescribe piperacillin-tazobactam (Zosyn) and and vancomycin

15. The AG-ACNP is reviewing the pulmonary function test result on a 72-year-old patient who has chronic respiratory failure. The pulmonary function tests reveal airflow obstruction. Which of the following pulmonary function results indicate airflow obstruction?

a. A decrease in the FEV1-to-FVC ratio
b. A FEV1 level greater than 1 L
c. A FVC level greater than 1.5 L
d. A reduction in both FEV1 and FVC with a normal FEV1/FVC

16. The AG-ACNP is preparing to intubate a 33-year-old male. Before the intubation the AG-ACNP examines the patient's airway for a Mallampati score to help predict for a difficult intubation. The AG-ACNP knows that which of the classifications predicts a difficult in intubation:

a. Class I
b. Class II
c. Class III
d. Class IV

17. A 60-year-old male who had his tracheostomy decannulated 3 weeks ago presents to the ED with stridor and shortness of breath. The patient is able to speak in sentences and clear his own secretions. His oxygen saturation is 95%. Upon auscultating the trachea, the AG-ACNP hears stridor. Which of the following diagnostics would give the quickest and most information on the etiology of this patient's stridor and dyspnea?

a. Bronchoscopy
b. CT scan of the soft tissues of the neck
c. MRI
d. Soft tissue radiography

18. The AG-ACNP is managing a 36-year-old-male with both hypercapneic and hypoxic respiratory failure. The patient has been on the ventilator for 3 days. On day 3 the patient's PIP and heart rate suddenly increase. The pulse oximeter reading is dropping. After increasing the FiO$_2$, the most appropriate next step for the AG-ACNP is to check the:

a. Breath sounds
b. Heart sounds
c. Blood pressure
d. Chest x-ray

19. The AG-ACNP is seeing a patient who is initiating breaths on SIMV. The SpO2 is 98% on 40% fraction of inspired oxygen. The AG-ACNP notices that the patient's spontaneous tidal volumes are 130 mL per breath, and the patient is getting mildly tachycardic and is complaining of fatigue. Respiratory muscle fatigue can best be reduced by:

    a. Increasing the number of ventilator breaths
    b. Adding PEEP
    c. Adding PS
    d. Increasing the flow rate

20. A 48-year-old-male is admitted to the ICU with pancreatitis. After 24 hours the patient presents with an acute onset of dyspnea with an oxygen saturation of 85%. The patient is placed on 100% and a stat chest x-ray is ordered. Based on this stat chest x-ray (see the following x-ray), the AG-ACNP diagnoses the patient with which of the following?

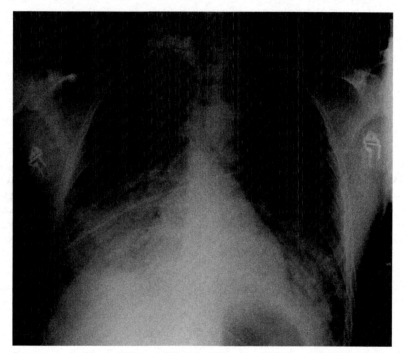

Source: van der Vaart, T.W., van Thiel, P., Juffermans, N.P., et al. (2014). Severe murine typhus with pulmonary system involvement. *Emerging Infectious Diseases, 20*(8), 1375-1377. doi:10.3201/eid2008.131421.

    a. ARDS
    b. Pneumonia
    c. Pulmonary embolism
    d. Pulmonary edema

21. A 67-year-old-male with bullous emphysema is scheduled for a bullectomy to prevent air-leak syndrome. The AG-ACNP knows which of the following patients would not be suited for a bullectomy:

    a. A patient who continues to drink alcohol
    b. A patient who continues to smoke
    c. A patient with type 2 diabetes
    d. A patient who continues to be obese

22. The AG-ACNP is managing a 30-year-old female with dyspnea and fatigue who was just diagnosed with pulmonary hypertension by echocardiogram. The AG-ACNP knows that pulmonary hypertension in young women is:

    a. Idiopathic in nature
    b. Due to left heart disease
    c. Due to chronic thrombotic or embolic disease
    d. Caused by parenchymal lung disease

23. The AG-ACNP is reviewing an ECG on a 35-year-old female who has severe pulmonary hypertension. What findings would the AG-ACNP expect to see on a patient with severe pulmonary hypertension on an ECG?

    a. Elevated T waves in II, III, aVF, and V1–V5
    b. Q1S3 pattern
    c. Left axis deviation
    d. Tall R in V1 and deep S in V6

24. In a patient with pulmonary hypertension secondary to right heart failure, the AG-ACNP should order prostanoids intravenous and:

    a. Anticholinergic
    b. Beta2 adrenergic agonist
    c. Platelet aggregation inhibitors
    d. Thrombolytics

25. The AG-ACNP is seeing a 70-year-old female patient with a significant history of COPD and 3 months status post right total knee replacement who woke up this morning with severe dyspnea. The chest x-ray was inconclusive of pertinent findings, therefore a CT of the thorax was completed. The CT angiogram of the chest was positive for a pulmonary embolism in the right upper lobe. Two hours later the patient's vital signs changed and she is now tachycardic to 130s, blood pressure 64/48, respiratory rate 30, SaO_2 80%. The AG-ACNP identifies this type of shock as:

    a. Cardiogenic shock
    b. Neurogenic shock
    c. Septic shock
    d. Obstructive shock

26. The AG-ACNP is auscultating the chest of a 53-year-old male with a pulmonary embolism. What findings should the AG-ACNP expect to hear upon auscultating the patient's chest?

    a. Bilateral clear breath sounds
    b. Pleural friction rub
    c. Rales throughout lung fields
    d. S4 at the fourth intercostal space, left sternal border

27. A 58-year-old male with a significant medical history of COPD, type 2 diabetes, and chronic alcoholism presents with complaints of increasing shortness of breath at rest and abdominal pain in the epigastric area for the past 2 days. Upon examination the patient was found to be dehydrated and a liter of lactated ringers was administered. Two hours later the patient becomes progressively more dyspneic with a respiratory rate of 35 breaths per minute. The chest x-ray demonstrates bilateral patchy infiltrates. Which of the following would confirm the diagnosis of ARDS?

    a. Blood glucose of 250 mg/dL
    b. LDH of 300
    c. PaO2 less than 60 mmHg
    d. PCWP less than 18 mmHg

28. A 48-year-old male presents with complaints of chest pain, shortness of breath, and coughing up frothy sputum for the past 2 days. The patient was discharged 1 week ago with STEMI and cardiac catheterization with stenting in the left anterior descending artery. The patient's chest x-ray shows blunting of the costophrenic angles. The decubitus chest x-ray shows free-flowing fluid collection greater than 1 cm. What is the AG-ACNP's priority action for this patient?

   a. Order a CT scan of the chest.
   b. Perform a thoracentesis.
   c. Perform a chest tube insertion.
   d. Treat the underlying condition.

29. The AG-ACNP is managing the care of 75-year-old female with significant history of COPD and systolic CHF who presented with a 1-day history of increasing shortness of breath at rest. Vital signs: temperature 36.0C, heart rate 100, repsiratory rate 24, SaO2 92%. Which diagnostic test is the highest priority for this patient?

   a. ABG
   b. Chest x-ray
   c. Noncontrast CT scan chest
   d. Right-sided heart catheterization

30. A 55-year-old-male patient is being treated for latent pulmonary tuberculosis infection. The AG-ACNP knows that the patient will need to take chemoprophylaxis treatment isoniazid 300 mg by mouth daily for:

   a. 3 months
   b. 6 months
   c. 9 months
   d. 12 months

31. A patient is in the postanesthesia care unit immediately postop from a total hip replacement. The nurse calls saying the patient is progressively more somnolent and has received multiple doses of fentanyl for severe pain. The AG-ACNP obtains the following ABG: pH 7.30, PaCO2 56, PaO2 68; HCO$_3$ 24; Sat 92%; BE 1. The next step the AG-ACNP order is:

   a. Placed on BiPAP
   b. Given flumazenil (Romazicon)
   c. Give naloxone (Narcan)
   d. Intubated immediately

32. A 78-year-old male patient is admitted with sepsis secondary to a UTI. One month prior to this hospitalization he had been treated with IV antibiotics for a wound infection. He was intubated on admission. On day 4 of hospitalization he is diagnosed with VAP. He has no known allergies. Empiric coverage for VAP in this patient should include:

   a. Piperacillin-tazobactam, cefepime, and levofloxacin
   b. Piperacillin-tazobactam, linezolid, and vancomycin
   c. Oxacillin, levofloxacin, and doxycycline
   d. Piperacillin-tazobactam, meropenem, and vancomycin

33. A 62-year-old patient with a history of COPD presents to the office with a complaint of cough and "body aches" for 3 days. He tests positive for influenza A. For this patient, the current CDC recommendation to treat influenza is to begin therapy with:

   a. Tamiflu (oseltamivir)
   b. Flumadine (rimantadine)
   c. Azithromycin (Zpak)
   d. Over-the-counter® Theraflu

34. A patient was mechanically vented for 7 days for CAP and was extubated 2 days ago. His vitals and labs have been stable, but he failed the swallow evaluation by the speech therapist. What is the most appropriate intervention?

   a. Continue ICU monitoring and management.
   b. Discharge patient to a long-term care facility.
   c. Transfer the patient to a subacute care unit.
   d. Consult GI for a PEG tube.

35. A 26-year-old male presents to the ED with complaints of shortness of breath and right-sided chest pain that began after a 2-mile run. The symptoms have been persistent for the past 3 hours. Pain is increased with inspiration. He denies any constitutional symptoms of fever, cough, chills, or sick contacts. He is an avid runner on a daily basis, but does smoke ½-pack of cigarettes per day. On physical exam he is tachypneic, with repiratory rate 30, 94% saturation on room air. Breath sounds are decreased in the left lung fields, and there is hyperresonance to percussion. The AG-ACNP obtains a chest x-ray (see the following x-ray):

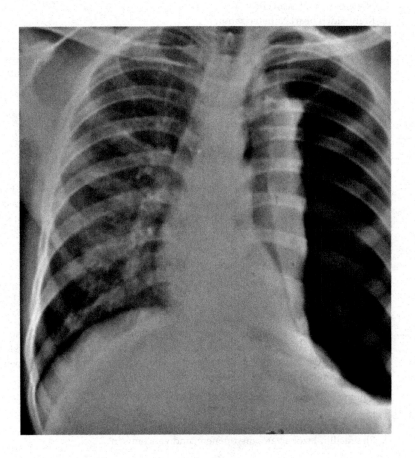

What is the diagnosis?

   a. Pneumothorax
   b. Tension pneumothorax
   c. Perihilar infiltrate
   d. Pleural effusion

36. A 42-year-old woman presents to the hospital with a probable diagnosis of CAP. Her chest x-ray shows a large pleural effusion. The AG-ACNP performs a thoracentesis, which results as follows:

    - Color: Viscous, cloudy
    - pH: 7.11
    - Protein: 5.8 g/dL
    - LDH: 285 IU/L
    - Glucose: 66 mg/dL
    - WBC: 3,800/mm^3
    - RBC: 24,000/mm^3
    - PMDs: 93%
    - Gram stain: Many PMN; no organism seen

    What is the next step in management this patient?

    a. Tube thoracostomy
    b. Diuresis with Lasix
    c. Antiviral therapy
    d. VAT

37. A patient is initiating breaths on SIMV. The patient is saturating at 98% on 40% fraction of inspired oxygen. Upon assessing the ventilator waveform (see the following figure) and the AG-ACNP's physical exam that noted the patient is showing respiratory muscle fatigue, the AG-ACNP's best action is to:

    a. Increase the number of ventilator breaths.
    b. Add PEEP.
    c. Add PS.
    d. Increase the flow rate.

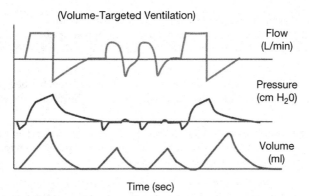

(Volume-Targeted Ventilation)

Flow (L/min)

Pressure (cm H$_2$0)

Volume (ml)

Time (sec)

■ PULMONARY ANSWERS AND RATIONALES

1. **a) Elevate the head of bed ≥30 degrees.** Head of bed elevation is a grade I recommendation for prevention of ventilator pneumonia. Carafate, H2 blockers, and PPIs are indicated to prevent gastric ulcers. Mouth care and oral suctioning should ideally be performed more often than every shift. (In addition, shift length varies by institution: Some are 8 hours, others are 12 hours.) Gastric residuals are a poor predictor in aspiration pneumonia.

2. **a) Add an ICS.** Daytime symptoms greater than 2 days per week require one step up. This patient was on step 1 with, as necessary, SABA use only, but now requires step 2 which is the addition of an ICS.

3. **d) Pulmonary function test.** Pulmonary function test can be calibrated for accuracy and will include measurements of FEV_1 and FVC and calculates the ratio that directly measures degree of obstruction present. The peak flow meters are useful to measure change from baseline, and improvement or worsening is relative to the patient's baseline with the same meter. ABS and pulse oximetry many times will not note deterioration in status until late in the decline. Asthmatics often maintain normal oxygenation for quite some time.

4. **c) Aspirin.** Aspirin, a COX-1 inhibiting NSAID, can cause severe exacerbation of asthma symptoms from an overproduction of leukotrienes.

5. **b) Three months.** Patients should be stable on the current step for 3 months before considering stepping down. If a patient is stable for at least 3 months, then it is not necessary to remain at a higher level of care if the patient improves.

6. **c) Post-bronchodilator FEV_1/FVC less than 0.70.** The results of a pulmonary function test (PFT) confirm a persistent existence of airflow restriction.

7. **a) Correction of hypoxemia with supplemental O_2.** Smoking cessation with correction of hypoxemia are the only chronic medical therapies shown to improve survival rates of COPD patients.

8. **d) SABA.** All stages need smoking cessation and vaccinations (influenza, pneumococcus). Stage I requires only a short-acting beta agonist SABA as necessary. All COPD patients should have a short-acting beta agonist for rescue use.

9. **a) Overnight polysomnography with direct technician observation.** Overnight polysomnography with direct technician observation detects true apneic episodes and physical movements. The other distractors may identify signs and symptoms of sleep apnea, but are not diagnostic.

10. **a) Hypertension.** Cardiovascular disease, especially hypertension, has been documented as an independent risk factor caused by OSA. All of the other choices are risk factors for developing OSA.

11. **c) Pain management.** Pain management facilitates patient's coughing and deep breathing to prevent hypoventilation and subsequent atelectasis and improves tachypnea. There is no indication for hydration, supplemental oxygen, or ABG.

12. **b) Intubation with positive pressure ventilation.** This patient has a flail chest. In light of the tachypnea and hypoxia, intubation with positive pressure ventilation is indicated as it also stabilizes a flailed segment. Wrapping the ribs can cause hypoventilation. A chest tube would not be inserted unless there was a present pneumothorax or hemothorax. Surgery is seldom required for rib fractures.

13. **d) Increases the inspiratory flow rate.** By increasing the inspiratory flow rate, the inspiratory time decreases, allowing the expiratory time to increase. This allows the patient more time to exhale, which will decrease the autoPEEP. There is no need to change the tidal volume. Tidal volume would be decreased for decreased lung compliance as in CHF, ARDS, consolidation, fibrosis, and lung resection. Otherwise, tidal volume is set by patient's height and ideal body weight. If the flow rate is decreased, the inspiratory time would have increased and the expiratory time would have decreased, which would decrease the time the patient has to exhale,

thus increasing the autoPEEP. If the patient had been wheezing a bronchodilator would have been given to open the airways, which would decrease the autoPEEP. This patient was not wheezing and had clear breath sounds.

14. **a) Administer supplemental oxygen, albuteral nebulizers, increase LABA, oral corticosteroids.** For mild acute exacerbation of COPD, antibiotics are not indicated. Supplemental oxygen, SABAs, LABAs, and oral corticosteroids are indicated. Noninvasive ventilation is recommended over intubation. This patient does not warrant admission to ICU or require antibiotics. Severe acute exacerbation of COPD is defined by at least two of the following: increased dyspnea, increased sputum volume, increased sputum virulence with respiratory failure, for which fluoroquinolone, antipseudomonal penicillin, and third-generation cephalosporin are the treatments of choice for 5 to 7 days.

15. **a) A decrease in the FEV1-to-FVC ratio (FEV1/FVC).** A decrease in FEV1/FVC indicates airflow obstruction. Respiratory failures are uncommon on obstructive lung diseases when the FEV1 is greater than 1 L. Respiratory failure is uncommon when the FVC is greater than 1 L in restrictive disease. Restrictive diseases are a volume issue. A reduction in both FEV1 and FVC with a normal FEV1/FVC is indicative of a restrictive lung disease.

16. **c) Class III.** Class III predicts a difficulty in intubation as only the soft palate is visible. The amount of mouth opening to the size of the tongue provides enough space for oral intubation. The soft palate, uvula, and pillars are visible. The base of the uvula is visible. Class IV predicts severe difficulty in intubation as only the hard palate is visible. (See the following figure.)

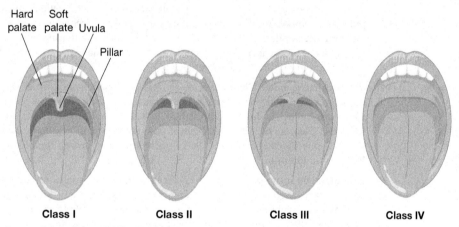

Class I Class II Class III Class IV

Source: Adapted from Walls, R. M., & Brown, C. A. Approach to the difficult airway in adults outside the operating room. In T. W. Post (Ed.), UpToDate.

17. **b) CT scan of the soft tissues of the neck.** CT scan of the soft tissues of the neck is the diagnostic of choice in the evaluation of upper airway disease, especially helical CT scan. Helical CT scans delineate precisely diffuse lesions and airway involvement. Although bronchoscopy can evaluate tracheal disorders precisely, it is an invasive procedure. An MRI will not give you the quickest information. MRI is typically used for the evaluation of the larynx and trachea when looking for infection. Anterior-posterior and lateral films of the neck will give you information about the anterior and posterior trachea wall.

18. **a) Breath sounds.** A sudden increased PIP indicates a respiratory issue, so auscultate for breath sounds. Chest x-ray can be a correct answer, but not the first step. Patient assessment is critical.

19. **c) Adding PS.** Adding PS in SIMV mode will decrease the work of breathing and augment the tidal volume, thereby decreasing respiratory muscle fatigue. Increasing the number of breaths defeats the purpose of SIMV. Adding PEEP is not needed as the patient is not having issues with oxygenation. The patient is not having flow asynchrony as evidenced in the waveform.

20. **a) Acute respiratory distress syndrome**. The chest x-ray shows bilateral infiltrates consistent with ARDS. Pneumonia usually is a homogenous pattern. Pulmonary embolism on chest x-rays depicts Hampton's hump. Pulmonary edema presents as cephalization and perihilar fullness.

21. **b) A patient who continues to smoke**. Contraindications for a bullectomy include patients who continue to smoke, patients who have pulmonary hypertension, and patients who do not have well-defined bullae on chest x-ray and computed tomography.

22. **a) Idiopathic in nature**. Idiopathic pulmonary hypertension is often seen in young women. Pulmonary hypertension is due to left heart disease as seen in LV systolic dysfunction, LV diastolic dysfunction, valvular disease, and cardiomyopathies. Pulmonary hypertension can also be due to chronic thrombotic or embolic disease, which is not stated in the stem of the question. Pulmonary hypertension due to parenchymal lung disease occurs in older adults with chronic obstructive lung disease or interstitial lung disease.

23. **d) Tall R in V1 and deep S in V6**. In severe pulmonary hypertension the electrocardiogram may show a tall R in V1 and deep S in V6 that is indicative of RV hypertrophy. In severe hypertension it will show inverted T waves in II, III, aVF, and V1 to V5. In severe pulmonary hypertension the electrocardiogram will show sinus tachycardia. Q1S3 is a pattern seen with acute pulmonary embolism. RVH is associated with right axis deviation.

24. **c) Platelet aggregation inhibitors**. Pulmonary vasodilators (prostanoids) decrease PAPs by decreasing RV afterload. Platelet aggregation inhibitors, such as clopdidogrel, are administered to prevent platelet adhesion in pulmonary hypertensive patients as they are at risk for pulmonary embolism. While a patient may be on beta2 adrenergic agonist and anticholinergics for bronchodilation, the supportive care for patients with pulmonary hypertension due to right heart failure is intravenous prostanoids and platelet aggregation inhibitors. Thrombolysis is used to dissolve an existing clot.

25. **d) Obstructive shock**. Obstructive shock caused by inadequate cardiac output as a result of impaired ventricular filling, which is most often caused by a massive pulmonary embolism. Cardiogenic shock is due to pump failure with acute myocardial infarction most often being the cause. Neurogenic shock is a loss of vasomotor tone most often caused by spinal cord injury. Septic shock is caused infective organisms that get into the blood stream and alter vascular motor tone.

26. **a) Bilateral clear breath sounds**. Clear breath sounds are usually auscultated in patient with a pulmonary embolism. Pulmonary infarction may produce crackles over the affected lung. Pleural friction rubs are heard when the visceral and parietal pleura are inflamed, commonly appreciated after a viral illness. Pulmonary infarction may produce crackles over the affected lung. RV S3 may be heard in a patient with pulmonary embolism.

27. **d) PCWP less than 18 mmHg**. PCWP of less than 18 mmHg would indicate ARDS over pulmonary edema. PCWP greater than 18 mmHg would indicate pulmonary edema. This patient likely went into ARDS due to pancreatitis. Elevated blood glucose is one of five Ranson's criteria for pancreatitis. Ranson's criteria predict the severity of pancreatitis and not ARDS. Lactate dehydrogenase of 300 is one of five Ranson's criteria for pancreatitis. While hypoxemia is present in ARDS, it is diagnosed based on the PaO2:FiO_2 ratio. A PaO_2 is also a less specific finding than PCWP.

28. **d) Treat the underlying condition**. Treating the underlying condition of CHF is the priority action. Although a CT scan of the thorax may be done prior to deciding to perform a thoracentesis, it is not the priority action. Performing a thoracentesis may be indicated for pleural effusion greater than 1 cm. Performing a chest tube insertion would be indicated in a pneumothorax or a hemothorax.

29. **b) Chest x-ray**. A chest x-ray will show more about what is going on in the lungs. Chest x-ray is essential in the diagnosis of dyspnea and can assess for abnormalities such as infiltrates, hyperinflation, and heart failure. A CT scan will provide much information, but a better option would be to have IV contrast to also assess for a pulmonary embolus. A CT

scan may not be needed as the answer may be found on the chest X-ray. A right-sided heart catheterization is not routine in diagnostic cardiac catheterization. A few indications for right heart catheterization are for unexplained dyspnea, valvular heart disease, pericardial disease, and congenital heart disease. ABS are useful in assessing acid–base status, oxygenation and hypercarbia, and making ventilator changes. It can help distinguish between hypoxic respiratory failure and hypercapneic respiratory failure or both. In this case the patient is tachypneic, thus hypercarbia is less likely. An echocardiogram will give information about blood flow patterns, valvular defects, wall motion, chamber size, and presence of pericardial effusion, but would not identify a pulmonary process.

30. **b) 6 months**. A 6-month course of isoniazid is adequate for all patients with latent tuberculosis infection. Patients who are at risk for relapse include cavitary pulmonary disease or positive TB cultures after taking two months of therapy. Nine months is indicated for patients with HIV and/or immunocompromised patients. Tuberculosis is treated with a 6-month or 9-month regimen.

31. **a) Placed on BiPAP**. This patient needs supportive therapy to correct the respiratory acidosis. Flumazenil is indicated for benzodiazepine excess. Narcan is not the best answer as the patient will have her pain return. Intubation can be avoided with supportive therapy.

32. **d) Piperacillin-tazobactam, meropenem, and vancomycin**. In a patient with hospital associated pneumonia (HAP) who is at high risk for ventilator associated pneumonia (VAP), coverage with two antipseudomonal agents plus coverage for Staphylococcus aureus is recommended. If the patient is at high risk for MRSA, then coverage with vancomycin or linezolid is recommended. Patients who are at high risk for MRSA are patients who have been treated with antibiotics within the past 30 days, patients in units with prevalence of MRSA isolates greater than 20%, or previous positive culture for MRSA.

33. **a) Tamiflu (oseltamivir)**. The CDC recommends beginning antiviral therapy in patients with diseases that put them at high risk for complications from influenza. Oseltamivir is FDA-approved for treatment of influenza in people aged 2 weeks and older. Recently, widespread amantadine resistance among influenza virus strains has made this class of medications less useful clinically. Therefore, amantadine and rimantadine are not recommended for antiviral treatment or chemoprophylaxis of currently circulating influenza A virus strains. Azithromycin is a macrolide antibiotic and has no impact on the influenza virus.

34. **c) Transfer the patient to a subacute care unit**. This patient has had a long stay in the ICU, and has been extubated 2 days ago with demonstrated hemodynamic stability. Though he has failed the swallow evaluation, transfer to a subacute is appropriate. The patient does not need ICU management. Transfer to a long-term care facility is premature. Consulting GI for a PEG tube is premature as well. Reevaluation of swallowing in a few days is appropriate.

35. **b) Tension pneumothorax**. Primary spontaneous pneumothorax is typically noted in young males with a history of smoking. The symptoms of shortness of breath and chest pain that persist are common findings. The fact that there is desaturation and abnormal pulmonary findings makes this a more urgent situation. This film demonstrates trachial deviation to the unaffected side with shifting of the heart and great vessels, indicative of a tension pneumothorax. The perihilar density is the collapsed lung. If this was an infiltrate, the patient would also likely have a cough, fever, and sputum production. Pleural effusion is not likely due to the abruptness of the symptom onset and no history to suggest an etiology for pleural effusion.

36. **a) Tube thoracostomy**. All large pleural effusions complicated by pneumonia are most likely to be exudative. A tube thoracotomy includes loculated pleural fluid, pH below 7.2, pleural glucose less than 60 mg/dL, Gm+ or culture of pleural fluid, and the presence of pus. Diuresis would not help, as this is an inflammatory process, not a fluid issue. Antivirals are not indicated since this is a bacterial infection. VAT is not appropriate at this time.

37. **c) Add PS**. Adding PS in SIMV mode will decrease the work of breathing and augment the tidal volume, thereby decreasing respiratory muscle fatigue. Increasing the number of

breaths may decrease muscle fatigue if the patient is pulling in enough volume. Adding PEEP is not needed, as the patient is not having issues with oxygenation. The patient is not having flow asynchrony as evidenced in the waveform. There is no scooping in during inspiration.

■ BIBLIOGRAPHY

Al-Qadi, M. O., Artenstein, A. W., & Braman, S. S. (2013). The "forgotten zone": Acquired disorders of the trachea in adults. *Respiratory Medicine, 107*(9), 1301–1313. doi:10.1016/j.rmed.2013.03.017

Broderick, S. R. (2013). Hemothorax: Etiology, diagnosis, and management. *Thoracic Surgery Clinics, 23*(1), 89–96, vi–vii. doi:10.1016/j.thorsurg.2012.10.003

Centers for Disease Control and Prevention. (2014). *Latent TB infection: A guide for primary health care providers.* Retrieved from www.cdc.gov/tb/publications/ltbi/diagnosis.html

Centers for Disease Control and Prevention. (2017). *Antiviral drugs for seasonal influenza.* Retrieved from https://www.cdc.gov/flu/professionals/antivirals/links.htm

Doherty, G. (2015). *Current diagnosis and treatment: Surgery.* New York, NY: McGraw-Hill Education.

Global Initiative for Chronic Obstructive Lung Disease. (2017). *Global initiative for chronic obstructive lung disease: Pocket guide to COPD diagnosis, management, and prevention: A guide for health care professionals 2017 report.* Retrieved from http://goldcopd.org/wp-content/uploads/2016/12/wms-GOLD-2017-Pocket-Guide.pdf

Godara, H., Heirbe, A., Nassif, M., Otepka, H., & Rosenstock, A. (2014). *The Washington manual of medical therapeutics* (34th ed.). Philadelphia, PA: Wolters Kluwer-Lippincott Williams & Wilkins.

Halter, J. B., Oslander, J., Studenski, S., High, K. P., Asthana, S., Supiano, M. A., & Ritchie, C. (2017). *Hazzard's geriatric medicine and gerontology* (7th ed.). New York, NY: McGraw-Hill.

Hellyer, T. P., Ewan, V., Wilson, P., & Simpson, A. J. (2016). The Intensive Care Society recommended bundle of interventions for the prevention of ventilator-associated pneumonia. *Journal of the Intensive Care Society, 17*(3), 238–243. doi:10.1177/1751143716644461

Hess, D. R., & Kacmarek, R. M. (2014). *Essentials of mechanical ventilation* (3rd ed.). New York, NY: McGraw-Hill Education.

Kalil, A. C., Metersky, M. L., Klompas, M., Muscedere, J., Sweeney, D. A., Palmer, L. B., & Brozek, J. L. (2016). Management of adults with hospital-acquired and ventilator-associated pneumonia: 2016 clinical practice guidelines by the Infectious Diseases Aociety of America and the American Thoracic Society. *Clinical Infectious Diseases, 63*(5), e61–e111. doi:10.1093/cid/ciw353

Kasper, D., Hauser, S., Jameson, J., Fauci, A., Longo, D., & Loscalzo, J. (2015). *Harrison's principles of internal medicine* (19th ed.). New York, NY: McGraw-Hill.

Kosmoski-Goepfert, K. (2014). *Integrating adult-gerontology acute care skills & procedures into nurse practitioner curricula.* Washington, DC: National Organization of Nurse Practitioner Faculties.

Marx, J. A., Hocksberger, R. S., Walls, R. M., Biros, M. H., Ling, L. J., Danzl, D. F., & Jagoda, A. (2014). *Rosen's emergency medicine concepts and clinical practice* (8th ed.). Philadelphia, PA: Saunders.

Oropello, J., Kyetan, V., & Pastores, S. (2017). *Critical care.* New York, NY: McGraw-Hill Education.

Papadakis, M. A., McPhee, S. J., & Rabow, M. W. (2017). *Current medical diagnosis & treatment 2017.* New York, NY: McGraw-Hill Education.

Tintinalli, J. E. (2016). *Tintinalli's emergency medicine: A comprehensive study guide* (8th ed.). New York, NY: McGraw-Hill.

Tobin, M. H., S. & Hubmayr, R. (2013). *Principles and practice of mechanical ventilation* (3th ed.). New York, NY: McGraw-Hill.

8 Neurological

HOPE MOSER AND DAWN CARPENTER

NEUROLOGICAL QUESTIONS

1. A homeless, uninsured patient with a past medical history of hypertension presents with new onset confusion, change in vision, headaches, nausea, and vomited once. Vital signs: temperature 98.6°F (37.0°C), heart rate 88, blood pressure 224/118, respiration rate 22; SaO2 95%. The AG-ACNP diagnoses his change in mental status as:

   a. Hypertensive urgency
   b. Essential hypertension
   c. Meningitis
   d. Hypertensive encephalopathy

2. A patient with a past medical history of hypertension and CHF presents with complaints of headache, nausea and vomiting, and progressive confusion over the past 3 days. Physical exam reveals blood pressure 196/124, S1S2, regular rate with an S3. Fundoscopic exam reveals papilledema. Urinalysis shows proteinuria. What is the most likely diagnosis?

   a. Hypertensive urgency
   b. Hypertensive emergency
   c. Primary hypertension
   d. Secondary hypertension

3. An unrestrained driver presented to the shock trauma ICU after being involved in a motor vehicle crash. At the scene of the accident, the patient was found with initial Glasgow Coma Scale of 12 (eyes 3, verbal 4, motor 5). En route, he became more responsive and oriented. While in the CT scanner, the patient progressed into a somnolent state, requiring intubation for a Glasgow Coma score of 8. Upon repeat exam, his left pupil was 7 mm and unreactive. This presentation is characteristic of:

   a. Intracerebral hemorrhage
   b. Subdural hematoma
   c. Epidural hematoma
   d. Subarachnoid hemorrhage

4. The Cushing's triad is a phenomenon often seen in the setting of critically elevated ICP and is more commonly seen in the later phase of increased ICP, often when the patient is close to brain death. Cushing's triad includes:

a. Hypotension, bradycardia
b. Arrhythmias, apnea
c. Bradycardia, severe hypertension
d. Hyperglycemia, hyperreflexia

5. The AG-ANCP is caring for a 20-year-old man who sustained a severe traumatic brain injury. She is explaining elevated ICP to the patient's mother. Which of the following is a correct explanation of why ICPs become elevated?

a. The pressure volume relationship between intracranial pressure, cerebral spinal fluid, and blood determines the amount of cerebral blood volume.
b. An intermittent outflow of venous blood from the cranial cavity is necessary to make room for the intermittent incoming arterial blood.
c. The brain volume, cerebral spinal fluid, and intracranial blood are variable and always fluctuating.
d. The brain is encased in a confined space, and any increased volume of intracranial components can lead to elevated ICP.

6. An elderly patient presents with acute right-sided weakness, aphasia, and facial droop. The initial order needed to make a treatment decision is for the AG-ACNP to order a/an:

a. CT head without contrast
b. CT head and neck with/without contrast
c. MRI brain with contrast
d. MRI brain and neck with/without contrast

7. A young woman presents with complaints of weakness, paresthesias, sensory loss, and optic neuritis. The AG-ACNP is most concerned these symptoms represent:

a. MS
b. MG
c. GBS
d. MD

8. A 24-year-old cachectic and disheveled-appearing woman with unknown past medical history presents after a witnessed generalized tonic-clonic seizure. The AG-ACNP understands the cause of this seizure is most likely related to:

a. A viral illness
b. A fever
c. Encephalopathy
d. Illicit drug use

9. A 38-year-old male, who is 80 kg, presents with tonic-clonic seizures. Family reports he stopped taking his medication 2 months ago due to financial issues. He has been actively seizing for 30 minutes. He has received a total of 8 mg of lorazepam (Ativan) in two doses and 1,600 mg loading dose of (phenytoin) Dilantin. The AG-ACNP anticipates which of the following orders will be needed next:

a. Fosphenytoin (Cerebyx) 100 mg TID
b. Valproic acid (Depakene) 1600 mg IV × 1
c. Midazolam (Versed) 1 mg/hr infusion
d. Pentobarbital (Nembutal) infusion 2 mg/kg/hr

10. An elderly patient who sustained a large right MCA territory ischemic stroke remains with a facial droop and expressive aphasia. She has failed a bedside screen by the nursing staff. The AG-ACNP explains to the family she needs a formal swallow evaluation to prevent aspiration because:

    a. Dysphagia is due to impaired vascular function.
    b. Dysphagia can lead to aspiration and pneumonia.
    c. The risk of aspiration related to dysphagia increases over time.
    d. A swallow evaluation is required in all stroke patients.

11. An AG-ACNP caring for a recent stroke patient ensures the patient's risk factors are addressed in the plan of care, including aspirin, atorvastatin, blood pressure control, and:

    a. Carotid duplex scan
    b. Smoking cessation
    c. Noncontrast MRI
    d. Warfarin (Coumadin)

12. An AG-ACNP is examining a patient and notices one pupil is slightly larger than the other by 0.5 mm. The left pupil is 3.5 mm and the right pupil is 3 mm. The size difference does not change in different lighting. Review of systems for vision changes and headaches are negative. The most likely cause of this is:

    a. Physiologic anisocoria
    b. Horner's syndrome
    c. Marcus Gunn pupil
    d. Epidural hematoma

13. An 88-year-old female is brought to the ED by her daughter for confusion. The AG-ACNP ascertains from the daughter that this confusion developed over the past 3 to 4 days with no previous episodes of confusion or memory impairment. She denies injury. Review of systems is negative except for recent urinary incontinence. The patient's medical history is positive for dyslipidemia which is controlled with diet and hypertension which is controlled with lisinopril 10 mg daily. The AG-ACNP explains to the daughter that her mother is experiencing:
    a. Delirium
    b. Dementia
    c. Alzheimer's disease
    d. Lewy body disease

14. A 22-year-old college football player is brought to the ED after 4 days of an intermittent fever, headache, and stiffness in his neck. He has become confused, and his parents are at the bedside. The AG-ACNP requests consent from the parents to obtain which of the following diagnostic tests:

    a. CT scan of the cervical spine
    b. Brudzinski's and Kernig's signs
    c. Lumbar puncture
    d. MRI/magnetic resonance angiography of the brain

15. A 50-year-old African American man was admitted 2 days ago for ACS. Troponins and EKG were negative for MI. A rapid response team is activated because he is suddenly experiencing left-sided weakness and expressive aphasia, repeating "okay" in response to all questions. Vital signs:

    • Temperature 98.6°F (37.0°C)
    • Heart rate 110

- Blood pressure 200/110
- Respiration rate 20
- O_2 saturation 94% on RA

What is the AG-ACNP's first course of action?

a. Recheck the patient's vitals and apply supplemental O_2.
b. Order tPA to be hung stat.
c. Obtain a stat glucose finger stick.
d. Order labetalol (Trandate) 10 mg IV stat.

16. A 21-year-old male is brought into the ED from a large, loud dance party and is experiencing a focal seizure of the right hand. Recent use of which drug of abuse would the AG-ACNP consider to be the most likely cause of his condition?

a. Marijuana
b. Heroin
c. Nicotine
d. Cocaine

17. A 54-year-old male presents with right-arm weakness. His wife reports that patient had decreased strength in that arm since yesterday and subsequently dropped a dinner plate he was holding in his right hand. He also reported clumsiness in his right foot. The patient has a medical history of hyperlipidemia and takes atorvastatin 40 mg daily. Vital signs include heart rate 78, blood pressure 137/91, temperature 98.9°F, O_2 sat 94% on 2L NC. CT scan reveals a small ischemic stroke in the left MCA territory. What is the AG-ACNP's next order?

a. Aspirin 324 mg orally
b. Alteplase (tPA) 0.9 mg/kg IV infusion over 60 minutes
c. Heparin 5000 units IV push with infusion per protocol
d. Clopidogrel (Plavix) 75 mg orally

18. A 41-year-old male presents after a motor vehicle crash. The patient was the restrained driver going 45 mph when he hit a tree head on. The airbag did not deploy and the windshield was starred. He is unconscious with a Glasgow Coma Score is 5, and has decorticate posturing. The patient was intubated and an ICP monitor was placed. Vital signs:

- Heart rate 54
- Blood pressure 120/64
- Respiration rate 12

02 Saturation 95% on the following settings:

- Volume control, assist control TV 450, respiration rate 12, 60% + 5 PEEP
- ABG on these settings: pH 7.40, $PaCO_2$ 37, PaO_2 100, Sat 99%. BE -1

In the unit, the ICP is noted to be 24 mmHg sustained × 5 minutes. What is the AG-ACNP's next step?

a. Increase the ventilator rate to 16.
b. Decrease the HOB to 25 degrees.
c. Prescribe mannitol 1 gm/kg over 20 min.
d. Call neurosurgery for decompressive craniotomy.

19. An older adult male patient is admitted after a fall. Physical therapy is assessing the patient to determine rehabilitation needs. The AG-ACNP observes the patient is ambulating slowly, has a stiff gait with minimal arm swing, and his face appears "mask-like." The occupational therapist note informs the AG-ACNP of hand tremors when at rest, micrographia, and microphonia. Both therapists recommend inpatient rehabilitation for strength training and help with activities of daily living. The AG-ACNP is concerned he has:

   a. Parkinson's disease
   b. Alzheimer's disease
   c. Huntington's disease
   d. MG

20. A young adult woman presents with complaints of facial weakness. She reports that she has normal strength upon awakening. As the day progresses, she notes continued weakness. Her eyes are mainly affected with diplopia and difficulty opening her eyelids. In addition she states she has difficulty chewing and swallowing dinner. The AG-ACNP suspects:

   a. Bell's palsy
   b. MS
   c. GBS
   d. MG

21. A middle-aged adult presented with bilateral lower extremity weakness. He reports a viral illness about two weeks prior and recently developed neck and back pain. He says his feet were weak at first and then noticed the weakness increased to his knees and into his hips. He is now unable to stand. The AG-ACNP's examination reveals reduced deep tendon reflexes in the Achilles and patellar tendons. The AG-ACNP admission orders:

   a. Glucocorticoids
   b. Physical therapy
   c. Vital capacity
   d. Antiviral therapy

■ NEUROLOGICAL ANSWERS AND RATIONALES

1. **d) Hypertensive encephalopathy.** In hypertensive encephalopathy, the blood pressure exceeds cerebral autoregulation limits which allows for proportionate increases in cerebral blood flow and volume. Hypertensive urgency does not have the target-organ damage that is occurring in this scenario. Meningitis typically has a fever, nuchal rigidity, or positive Kernig's and/or Brudzinski's signs.

2. **b) Hypertensive emergency.** Hypertensive emergency is an elevated blood pressure with evidence of end-organ damage. This patient already has a given history of hypertension and secondary hypertension can be due to pheochromocytoma, excess catecholamines related to cocaine or amphetamine use, clonidine withdrawal, or interactions between tyramine-containing substances and monamine oxidase inhibitors.

3. **c) Epidural hematoma.** The patient likely has an epidural hematoma, caused when a fractured temporal bone lacerates the middle cerebral artery. As arterial blood accumulates, the pressure "dissects" the dura away from the skull. A classic sign of an epidural hematoma is a "lucid interval" between head trauma and decline in consciousness. The arterial blood must reach a certain volume/pressure to overcome the adherence of the dura to the skull, and when it does, the hematoma rapidly expands, raising intracranial pressure. Intracerebral, subdural, and subarachnoid hemorrhages do not have the lucid interval in their presentation.

4. **c) Bradycardia, severe hypertension.** Cushing's reflex involves severe hypertension, bradycardia, and respiratory irregularity due to medullary dysfunction. While these patients are critically ill, hyperglycemia and arrhythmias may be present but are not part of Cushing's triad.

5. **d) The brain is encased in a confined space, and any increased volume of intracranial components can lead to elevated ICP.** The brain, cerebral spinal fluid, and blood are contained in a nonenlargeable vault. Any space-occupying lesion or increased volume of these intracranial components may lead to elevated ICP.

6. **a) CT head without contrast.** A noncontrast head CT is immediately needed to rule out intracerebral hemorrhage, mass lesion, or subacute stroke. If these are absent, then the patient can be evaluated for administration of tPA. Further work-up, including CT angiography of the head/neck or MRI, may be subsequently performed to identify the cause of the stroke and base further treatment decisions or prognostications.

7. **a) MS.** Initial symptoms of MS include sensory loss, optic neuritis, weakness, and paresthesia. GBS presents with ascending paralysis with legs being affected before arms with subsequent loss of reflexes over a few days. In MG, the facial muscles, especially the eyelids, demonstrate ptosis and extraocular muscles gradually weaken with fatigue as the day progresses. Muscular dystrophies are present with proximal and symmetric limb weakness with preserved reflexes and sensation.

8. **d) Illicit drug use.** The most common causes of seizures in the young adults are head trauma, central nervous system infections, brain tumors, congenital central nervous system lesions, illicit drug use, or alcohol withdrawal. Viral illnesses and fever are seen in children, whereas encephalopathy is commonly seen in neonates or after an anoxic event in an adult. Central nervous system tumors are more common agents in older adults.

9. **b) Valproic acid (Depakene) 1,600 mg IV × 1.** Valproic acid (Depakene) and/or phenobarbital can be used early management of status epilepticus at a dose of 20 mg/kg IV bolus. Fosphenytoin dosing will be based off a repeat Dilantin level. Lorazepam dose has already been maximized for his weight, in addition he's already had twice the dose without effect. Versed infusion is indicated, but will need doses of 0.2 to 0.6 mg/kg/hr. Propofol can also be given next. Lastly, pentobarbital is used as a last resort, after other agents have failed.

10. **b) Dysphagia can lead to aspiration and pneumonia**. Dysphagia is a common complication after stroke due to laryngeal dysfunction and requires dedicated evaluation by specially trained SLP. Aspiration pneumonia carries a grave risk of adverse outcomes. Dysphagia is due to impaired motor function. The risk of aspiration related to dysphagia decreases over time.A formal swallow evaluation is required in all stroke patients with aphasia or who fail a bedside screen. A negative screen can negate the need for a formal swallow evaluation.

11. **b) Smoking cessation**. Smoking cessation is a modifiable risk factor. There is no demonstrated benefit of using warfarin over aspirin in patients with symptomatic intracranial atherosclerosis. In addition, warfarin has higher rates of bleeding complications. Carotid duplex scan will identify a potential source of the stroke and an MRI can help with prognostication; they do not address risk factors.

12. **a) Physiologic anisocoria.** Anisocoria is a normal physiological variation as long as it does not change with changes in ambient lighting. Horner's syndrome results from a lesion to the sympathetic pathway resulting in ptosis, miosis, and anhidrosis. Marcus Gunn pupil is a relative afferent pupillary defect that is elicited with a swinging-flashlight test. A significantly dilated pupil in the setting of cranial trauma could be an epidural hematoma that, when enlarging, can cause pressure on the optic nerve, causing dilation.

13. **a) Delirium**. Delirium is an acute, fluctuating disturbance of consciousness, associated with a change in cognition or development of perceptual disturbances. Dementia is a persistent and progressive impairment in intellectual function, with compromise of memory and at least one other cognitive domain. Dementia with Lewy bodies may be confused with delirium, as fluctuating cognitive impairment is frequently observed. Rigidity and bradykinesia are the primary signs of Lewy body dementia. Alzheimer's disease typically presents with early problems in memory and visuospatial abilities, but is gradual in onset and progression.

14. **c) Lumbar puncture**. The most likely diagnosis is meningitis. Thus, a lumbar puncture and the associated testing will confirm the diagnosis of meningitis. A CT scan of the cervical spine will not confirm diagnosis of meningitis. But it can rule out bony injury of the spine; however, there is no history in the stem indicating an injury occurred. An MRI would confirm presence of an abscess or tumor as the cause of the symptoms, but these are not the most likely diagnosis. An MRI or magnetic resonance angiography will not confirm diagnosis of meningitis. Eliciting Brudzinski's and Kernig's signs are assessments and, when positive, leads the diagnostician toward the diagnosis of meningitis, but do not confirm diagnosis. Furthermore, these do not warrant consent to perform.

15. **d) Order labetalol (Trandate) 10 mg IV stat**. From these signs and symptoms, this patient is likely having an ischemic stroke. African Americans have the highest rate of strokes in the United States. A stat noncontrast CT head is the diagnostic test required to rule out hemorrhagic stroke so that tPA can be considered. But in order to safely administer tPA, the goal blood pressure must be below 185/110 if the patient is going to receive tPA. Supplemental O2 is required only if the patient falls below 94%. Exclusion criteria for administering tPA includes systolic blood pressureBP greater than 185 mmHg and diastolic blood pressure ≥110 mmHg. The patient's blood glucose should be assessed prior to tPA administration; however, this is not the best answer.

16. **d) Cocaine**. Cocaine can cause seizure due to alteration of neuronal excitability and can therefore lower the seizure threshold in a patient. Marijuana would be concerning for the potential to be laced with another drug of abuse, but itself is not a cause of seizures. Heroin withdrawal could cause seizures, but use of heroin itself does not cause seizures. Nicotine usage is has numerous long-term effects on the body, but recent usage is not a trigger for seizure activity.

17. **a) Aspirin 324 mg orally**. Aspirin has been proven as a safe and effective antiplatelet drug for an ischemic stroke. Since his stroke is over 6 hours old, TPA is contraindicated. If his stroke was within the past 4.5 hours, he could have been a candidate for alteplase. Heparin and Plavix are not indicated for ischemic stroke.

18. **c) Prescribe mannitol 1 gm/kg over 20 min**. Mannitol is the first-line agent for increased ICP. This bolus dose of mannitol is an osmotic diuretic which will treat the elevated ICP. Preferred administration is through a central line. Hyperventilation is not indicated as it causes vaso-constriction and reduced blood flow, thus causing a secondary injury. HOB is recommended to be elevated 30 to 45 degrees. Craniotomy is done once other therapies (HOB, osmolality therapy, and hypertonic saline) have been maximized.

19. **a) Parkinson's disease**. Classic signs of Parkinson's disease are resting tremor, rigidity, and bradykinesia. Other common features are hypomimia or mask-like face, sleep disorders, micrographia, and microphonia. Myasthenia gravis typically affects women in their early 20s and 30s and men in their 50s and 60s. Hallmark features include weakness later in the day or with repeated usage.

20. **d) MG**. Myasthenia gravis typically affects women in their early 20s and 30s and men in their 50s and 60s. Hallmark features include weakness later in the day or with repeated usage. Cranial and facial muscles, including eyelids, extraocular muscles with diplopia, ptosis, and chewing and swallowing muscles commonly affected early in the course of exacerbations. Symptoms typically improve after sleep or rest. Bell's palsy affects a unilateral facial nerve, causing muscle paralysis that does not get better with rest. GBS is a polyradiculoneuropathy that causes ascending paralysis with the legs being more affected than the arms, but may cause complete paralysis and ventilator dependence.

21. **c) Vital capacity**. This patient has Guillain-Barre syndrome. Classic precursors include recent infections, viral illness, or immunizations. Classic presentation is neuropathic pain in the neck and back, and ascending paralysis with loss of deep tendon reflexes. Thirty percent of patients require ventilator support, including tracheostomy. Treatment is intravenous immunoglobulin. Glucocorticoids are not indicated. Physical therapy can be beneficial for the patient, but is not the highest priority at this time.

■ BIBLIOGRAPHY

Amin, H. P., & Schindler, J. L. (2016). *Vascular neurology board review*. New York, NY: Springer Science+Business Media.

Berkowitz, A. L. (2017). *Clinical neurology and neuroanatomy: A localization-based approach*. New York, NY: McGraw-Hill.

Kasper, D., Hauser, S., Jameson, J., Fauci, A., Longo, D., & Loscalzo, J. (2015). *Harrison's principles of internal medicine* (19th ed.). New York, NY: McGraw-Hill Education.

Lee, K. (2012). *The neuro ICU book*. New York, NY: McGraw-Hill.

Marino, P. (2014). *Marino's the ICU book* (4th ed.). Philadelphia, PA: Wolters Kluwer Health | Lippincott Williams & Wilkins.

McKean, S. C., Ross, J., Dressler, D. D., & Scheurer, D. B. (2017). *Principles and practice of hospital medicine* (2nd ed.). New York, NY: McGraw-Hill.

Papadakis, M. A., McPhee, S. J., & Rabow, M. W. (2017). *Current medical diagnosis & treatment 2017*. New York, NY: McGraw-Hill Education.

Powers, W. J., Derdeyn, C. P., Biller, J., Coffey, C. S., Hoh, B. L., Jauch, E. C., . . . American Heart Association-American Stroke Association. (2015). 2015 American Heart Association/American Stroke Association focused update of the 2013 guidelines for the early management of patients with acute ischemic stroke regarding endovascular treatment: A guideline for healthcare professionals from the American Heart Association/American Stroke Association. *Stroke, 46*(10), 3020–3035. doi:10.1161/STR.0000000000000074

Prabhakaran, S., Ruff, I., & Bernstein, R. (2015). Acute stroke intervention. *JAMA, 313*(14), 1451. doi:10.1001/jama.2015.3058

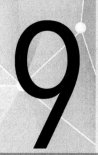

9 Renal Genitourinary

CARLA C. TURNER

RENAL GENITOURINARY QUESTIONS

1. A 58-year-old male with a past medical history of gouty arthritis presents to the emergency with complaints of acute onset of flank pain with radiation to the groin. He reported the pain appears to be worse with movement. Other associated symptoms are painful urination and blood-tinged urine. The clinical exam reveals a distressed male who grimaced while moving to try to find a comfortable position. He complained of severe pain in the costovertebral angle with palpitation, and abdominal exam was negative. A urinary analysis revealed the following: color = cloudy, pH = 4.5, 10 red blood cells per high power field, 0 WBCs, and positive uric acid crystals. Considering examination findings and urinary analysis results, the most likely diagnosis is:

   a. Cystitis
   b. Nephrolithiasis
   c. Pyelonephritis
   d. Prostatitis

2. A 68-year-old male complains of difficulty urinating. Which of the following medications could be contributing to his chief complaint?

   a. Hytrin (terazosin)
   b. Norvasc (amlodipine)
   c. Proventil (albuterol)
   d. Atrovent (ipratropium)

3. A 21-year-old female presents with complaint of 3-day history of fever 101.4°F and pain in the left lower abdomen and pelvis. The history reveals multiple sexual partners. The patient decided to have an IUD placed 6 months ago. Physical exam revealed cervical motion tenderness and adnexal tenderness. A saline microscopy of vaginal fluid analysis indicated numerous white blood cells. No tenderness was noted at McBurney point. Surgical history is significant for laparoscopic examination 6 months ago, because she was having difficulty getting pregnant. No abnormalities were noted. The most likely diagnosis is:

   a. Interstitial cystitis
   b. Appendicitis
   c. Pelvic inflammatory disease
   d. Endometriosis

4. A 60-year-old male with a history of type 2 DM and systolic heart failure presents to the ED with complaints of fatigue, painful urination and urinary frequency with urgency, and acute onset of fever and chills. He reported that he underwent a prostate needle biopsy 10 days ago. Vital signs obtained in triage were blood pressure 80/40, heart rate 130, respiration 28, temperature 102°F, and oxygen saturation 88% on room air. He received Levaquin (levofloxacin) 6 months ago for similar urinary symptoms and again as a pre-procedure prophylaxis. What is the most appropriate initial course of action for the AG-ACNP?

a. Obtain blood and urine cultures, initiate the sepsis bundle, and admit to the hospital
b. Obtain urinalysis and culture; outpatient management with Bactrim-DS (trimethoprim–sulfamethoxazole)
c. Consult urology
d. Consult infectious disease services

5. A possible cause of prerenal AKI includes which of the following?

a. Nephrolithiasis
b. Prostate hyperplasia
c. Hypovolemia due to hemorrhage
d. Acute glomerulonephritis

6. The AG-ACNP is seeing a 58-year-old male with a history of type 2 DM, hypertension, and AF on chronic anticoagulation therapy. Laboratory data revealed the following:

• Sodium 138

• Chloride 102

• Potassium 4.8

• Bicarbonate 22

• BUN 64

• Creatinine 6.9

• Creatinine clearance less than 10

• Glucose 298

Based on these values, which of the following medications should the AG-ACNP discontinue?

a. Apresoline (hydralazine) 100 mg by mouth every 8 hours
b. Xarelto (rivaroxaban) 15 mg by mouth daily
c. Isordil (isosorbide) 10 mg by mouth every 8 hours
d. Coreg (carvedilol) 25 mg every 12 hours

7. A 62-year-old patient is admitted to the ICU with a serum potassium level 7.5 mEq/L and abdominal pain. An electrocardiogram now reveals peaked T waves. Hemodialysis has been ordered. The dialysis catheter was placed and hemodialysis will be initiated when the on-call staff arrives. What is the AG-ACNP's most appropriate first line intervention?

a. Dextrose 50% 25 g, insulin 10 units IV, sodium bicarbonate 50 mEq
b. Sodium bicarbonate 50 mEq IV × 1 and ipratropium bromide (Atrovent) 2 puffs STAT
c. Calcium gluconate 2 g IV over 1 hour and calcium acetate (PhosLo) 667 mg PO
d. Sodium polystyrene (Kayexalate) 60 g PO × 1 and Kayexalate enema 60 g PR × 1

8. A 68-year-old patient presents to the hospital from the local dialysis facility with complaints of shortness of breath and chest pain. Considering the most common cause of death in patients with chronic kidney disease, the AG-ACNP orders which of the following laboratory tests?

a. Complete blood cell count with differential
b. Cardiac enzymes with troponins
c. Prothrombin time with international normalized ratio
d. Sputum culture with Gram stain

9. A frail elderly patient presents with acute change in mental status. She is found to have a WBC count of 22,000 with 26% bands and a lactate level of 4.2 mmol/L. Urinalysis is positive for 3+ leukocyte esterase, 3+ nitrites, and 100 WBCs. Chest x-ray is clear. The patient has received 4 L of normal saline and the blood pressure is 70/40. A central line is placed and norepinephrine (Levophed) is started. The AG-ACNP identifies which of the following diagnoses as the patient's admitting diagnosis:

a. UTI
b. Pyelonephritis
c. Severe sepsis
d. Septic shock secondary to UTI

10. A 64-year-old male unrestrained driver was admitted to the trauma unit after a head-on automobile collision while returning home from his 3-times-per-week hemodialysis. He is mechanically intubated, but there are reports that he responds to simple commands. He sustained multiple bone fractures and right hemothorax requiring chest tube placement. The current vital signs are blood pressure 90/48, heart rate 128, and temperature 98.4°F. What is the most appropriate method for management of his end-stage renal disease?

a. Hemodialysis
b. Peritoneal dialysis
c. Continuous renal replacement therapy
d. Considering his condition, dialysis is contraindicated

11. A 48-year-old with a past medical history of type 2 DM and end-stage kidney disease with a 6-month history of live-donor renal transplant from a relative presents with complaints of generalized swelling and decreased urinary output. On clinical examination the AG-ACNP notices facial grimacing with palpation over the graft site. A urine sample is noticeably hematuric. Renal work-up, including urine protein measurements, are consistent with acute rejection. The next appropriate intervention is to:

a. Begin normal saline for aggressive rehydration.
b. Schedule a computed tomography scan with intravenous contrast.
c. Notify the transplant team and schedule for a renal biopsy.
d. Discontinue corticosteroid therapy.

12. The AG-ACNP is seeing a patient who was referred for chronic kidney disease with a GF rate of less than 10 mL per minute per 1.73 m² and potassium of 5. The patient has a history of systolic heart failure, hypertension, and type 2 DM. Which of the following medications should the AG-ACNP immediately discontinue considering the patient's GF rate?

a. Insulin detemir (Levemir)
b. Apresoline (hydralazine)
c. Lasix (furosemide)
d. Aldactone (spironolactone)

13. The AG-ACNP is performing an initial evaluation of a 42-year-old male whose hypertension has been difficult to manage and who has progressively worsening chronic kidney disease. He was diagnosed with hypertension at age 26, and is currently prescribed five antihypertensive medications for blood pressure control. He has smoked two packs of cigarettes daily for the past 10 years. Clinical examination reveals an abdominal bruit and an abnormal ABI. A renal ultrasound indicated renal asymmetry with the right kidney being 2.0 cm smaller than the left kidney. Considering the patient's history and diagnostic and clinical examination findings, the AG-ACNP suspects which of the following abnormalities:

    a. Amyloidosis
    b. Renal artery stenosis
    c. Medication noncompliance
    d. Contrast nephropathy

■ RENAL GENITOURINARY ANSWERS AND RATIONALES

1. **b) Nephrolithiasis**. The classic presentation for a patient with acute renal colic is the sudden onset of severe pain that originates in the flank and radiates inferiorly and anteriorly. The abdominal examination was negative, and unlike patients with an acute abdomen, patients with renal colic are often repositioning to try to get comfortable. The urinary analysis revealed a pH of 4.5, which suggests uric acid stones. The lack of WBCs does not support the diagnosis of a UTI. Pain involving the prostate is usually located in the perineum and radiates to the lumbosacral inguinal canals or legs.

2. **d) Atrovent (ipratropium)**. Atrovent (ipratropium) is an anticholinergic and may cause urinary retention. Prescribers should administer Atrovent with caution, and monitor patients with a history of prostate hyperplasia or bladder neck obstruction closely for a postvoid residual greater than 250 to 300 mL. Hytrin (terazosin) is an effective treatment for moderate to severe lower urinary tract symptoms due to benign prostate hyperplasia. Amlodipine can cause an increase in micturition, and albuterol has been associated with urinary tract symptoms in a very small population of patients.

3. **c) Pelvic inflammatory disease**. The CDC recommends presumptive treatment for pelvic inflammatory disease in sexually active young women at risk for sexually transmitted diseases who are experiencing pelvic or lower abdominal pain. This is especially true if no other cause for the symptoms can be identified and if one or more of the following criteria are present: cervical motion tenderness, uterine tenderness, or adnexal tenderness. Appendicitis usually presents with right lower quadrant tenderness in the majority of cases, and tenderness on palpation over the McBurney point is concerning for appendicitis. The patient underwent a laparoscopic exam of the abdomen, which was negative and which excludes endometriosis. The patient was febrile, which excludes the diagnosis of interstitial cystitis.

4. **a) Obtain blood and urine cultures, initiate the sepsis bundle, and admit to the hospital**. The most common complication following prostate biopsy is infection. This includes prostatitis, epididymitis, bacteremia, and sepsis. This patient presented with symptoms consistent with bacteremia and sepsis. The most common cause of infection after transrectal prostate biopsy is fluoroquinolone-resistant Escherichia coli. This is particularly the case for patients who are immunocompromised and who have received antimicrobial therapy within the past 6 months prior to biopsy. Considering the patient's risk factors and high suspicion of sepsis, the most appropriate initial course of action is to begin treatment for sepsis.

5. **c) Hypovolemia due to hemorrhage**. Prerenal causes are due to three mechanisms: decrease in extracellular fluid volume, decreased renal blood flow, or altered intrarenal hemodynamics. Nephrolithiasis and prostate hyperplasia are postrenal causes of acute kidney injury. Acute glomerulonephritis is an intrarenal cause of acute renal failure.

6. **b) Xarelto (rivaroxaban) 15 mg by mouth daily**. For patients with nonvalvular AF, Xarelto can be prescribed to reduce stroke risk for patients with a creatinine clearance of 15 to 50 mm/min and must be discontinued for creatinine clearance less than 15. The remaining medications can be prescribed and safely administered for patients with chronic and end-stage renal disease.

7. **a) Dextrose 50% 25 g, insulin 10 units IV, sodium bicarbonate 50 mEq**. Serum potassium levels greater than 6.5 mEq/L requires immediate aggressive treatment. Administration of dextrose 50% 25 g IV followed by regular insulin 5 to 10 units IV is the first-line agent as it works quickly to push potassium back into the cells. Sodium bicarbonate and albuterol are both immediate first-line agents, but not Atrovent. Kayexalate takes time to work and more urgent treatment is required at this point. If electrocardiogram changes are present, including widening of the QRS complex or loss of P waves, additional treatment with calcium is required to antagonize the effect of potassium on the cardiac muscles.

8. **b) Cardiac enzymes with troponins**. The most common cause of death among patients with end-stage renal disease on long-term hemodialysis is predominately cardiovascular. This patient population has a high prevalence of CAD, which contributes to the occurrence of sudden cardiac death among patients with end-stage renal disease. Therefore, in addition

to performing an electrocardiogram, cardiac enzymes with troponins are important in risk stratification of patients with chest pain and suspected coronary syndrome.

9. **d) Septic shock secondary to UTI.** This patient meets the definition of septic shock and the source is the urinary tract. Septic shock is the highest of the acuity levels and, as such, will draw the higher reimbursement for the admission. Urosepsis is no longer a term in the *International Statistical Classification of Diseases and Related Health Problems, 10th Revision* codes. While UTI and severe sepsis are not totally incorrect, they are not the best answer. There are not sufficient data to diagnose pyelonephritis.

10. **c) Continuous renal replacement therapy.** Continuous renal replacement therapy is the most frequently utilized method for the management of chronic kidney disease and acute kidney injury in critically ill patients.

11. **c) Notify the transplant team and schedule for a renal biopsy.** Initial treatment of suspected acute rejection is biopsy before treating acute rejection unless the biopsy cannot be readily performed in a timely manner and will substantially delay treatment. Obtaining a biopsy will aid in determining if the patient is experiencing acute cellular rejection versus antibody mediated rejection to guide treatment. Patient presented with generalized swelling and decreased urinary output, and excessive hydration could contribute to fluid volume overload. Receiving intravenous contrast dye is nephrotoxic and contraindicated for this patient. Corticosteroid therapy is recommended for the initial treatment of acute cellular rejection, and it is recommended that corticosteroid therapy be added or restored in patients not on steroids who are experiencing a rejection episode.

12. **d) Aldactone (spironolactone).** Spironolactone should be discontinued with a glomerular filtration rate (GFR) less than 10 mL per minute per 1.73 m^2 and potassium greater than 5. No dose adjustment or discontinuation is warranted in cases of chronic kidney disease for Levemir, hydralazine, or furosemide.

13. **b) Renal artery stenosis.** Patients with renal artery stenosis may present with one or more of the following: abdominal bruit, difficult to manage hypertension requiring three or more antihypertensive agents, worsening renal function. Patients with early-onset hypertension usually have other atherosclerotic disease, such as PAD. Physical examination may indicate an abdominal bruit.

■ BIBLIOGRAPHY

American Urological Association. (2010). *Management of priapism.* Retrieved from https://www.auanet.org/guidelines/priapism-(2003-reviewed-and-validity-confirmed-2010)#x3010

American Urological Association. (2014). *Management of benign prostatic hyperplasia.* Retrieved from https://www.auanet.org/guidelines/benign-prostatic-hyperplasia-(2010-reviewed-and-validity-confirmed-2014) #x2513

American Urological Association. (2016). *The prevention and treatment of the more common complications related to prostate biopsy update.* Retrieved from https://auanet.org/guidelines/prostate-needle-biopsy-complications

Anderson, S., Eldadah, B., Halter, J. B., Hazzard, W. R., Himmelfarb, J., Horne, F. M., . . . O'Hare, A. M. (2011). Acute kidney injury in older adults. *Journal of the American Society of Nephrology, 22*(1), 28–38. doi:10.1681/ASN.2010090934

Centers for Disease Control and Prevention. (2015a). *2015, Sexually transmitted diseases treatment guidelines.* Retrieved from https://www.cdc.gov/std/tg2015/default.htm

Centers for Disease Control and Prevention. (2015b). *Sexually transmitted disease treatment guidelines: Pelvic inflammatory disease.* Retrieved from https://www.cdc.gov/std/tg2015/pid.htm

Chan, M., Patwardhan, A., Ryan, C., Trevillian, P., Chadban, S., Westgarth, F., & Fry, K. (2011). Evidence-based guidelines for the nutritional management of adult kidney transplant recipients. *Journal of Renal Nutrition, 21*(1), 47–51. doi:10.1053/j.jrn.2010.10.021

Connor, M. J., Jr., & Karakala, N. (2017). Continuous renal replacement therapy: Reviewing current best practice to provide high-quality extracorporeal therapy to critically ill patients. *Advances in Chronic Kidney Disease, 24*(4), 213–218. doi:10.1053/j.ackd.2017.05.003

Crane, C. M., & Bennett, N. E. (2011). Priapism in sickle cell anemia: Emerging mechanistic understanding and better preventive strategies. *Anemia*, vol. 2011, article ID 297364, 6 pages. doi:10.1155/2011/297364

Dellinger, R. P., Levy, M. M., Rhodes, A., Annane, D., Gerlach, H., Opal, S. M., . . . Jaeschke, R. (2013). Surviving sepsis campaign: International guidelines for management of severe sepsis and septic shock, 2012. *Intensive Care Medicine, 39*(2), 165–228. doi:10.1007/s00134-012-2769-8

Kasiske, B. L., Zeier, M. G., Chapman, J. R., Craig, J. C., Ekberg, H., Garvey, C. A., . . . Balk, E. M. (2010). KDIGO clinical practice guideline for the care of kidney transplant recipients: A summary. *Kidney International, 77*(4), 299–311. doi:10.1038/ki.2009.377

Piraino, B., Bernardini, J., Brown, E., Figueiredo, A., Johnson, D. W., Lye, W.-C., . . . Szeto, C.-C. (2011). ISPD position statement on reducing the risks of peritoneal dialysis–related infections. *Peritoneal Dialysis International, 31*(6), 614–630. doi:10.3747/pdi.2011.00057

Plau, A., & Knauf, F. (2016). Update of nephrolithiasis: Core curriculum. *American Journal of Kidney Disease 68*(6), 973–985. doi:10.1053/j.ajkd.2016.05.016

Porter, R. S., & Kaplan, J. L. (2011). *The Merck manual* (19th ed.). West Point, PA: Merck, Sharp, & Dohme.

Renal Association, British Cardiovascular Intervention Society, & Royal College of Radiologists. (2013). *Prevention of contrast induces acute kidney injury (CI-AKI) in adult patients*. Retrieved from https://renal.org/wp-content/uploads/2017/06/Prevention_of_Contrast_Induced_Acute_Kidney_Injury_CI-AKI_In_Adult_Patients-1.pdf

Saravanan, P., & Davidson, N. C. (2010). Risk assessment for sudden cardiac death in dialysis patients. *Circulation: Arrhythmia and Electrophysiology, 3*(5), 553–559. doi:10.1161/CIRCEP.110.937888

Sharp, V. J., Kieran, K., & Arlen, A. M. (2013). Testicular torsion: Diagnosis, evaluation, and management. *American Family Physician, 88*(12), 835–840.

10

Gastrointestinal

MARY ANNE McCOY, STEPHANIE BLACKWELL PRUITT, AND JENNIFER ADAMSKI

GASTROINTESTINAL QUESTIONS

1. A 49-year-old male sustains a stab wound to the left upper quadrant of his abdomen. He complains of minimal pain and is alert, oriented x3, and hemodynamically stable. The results of his abdominal examination show no abnormalities. Which of the following statements is true?

   a. The focused assessment with sonography for trauma examination reliably rules out intra-abdominal injury.
   b. Local wound exploration revealing fascial penetration is an absolute indication for an exploratory laparotomy.
   c. Intra-abdominal injury is highly unlikely in this patient.
   d. The patient should be admitted for a 24-hour observation period.

2. A 33-year-old male comes to the unit with an 8-day history of vomiting "large amounts of blood." Which of the following is the most appropriate first step in the treatment of this patient?

   a. Obtaining a history and performing a physical exam
   b. Fluid resuscitation
   c. Inserting a nasogastric tube
   d. Determining hemoglobin and hematocrit levels

3. An 18-year-old restrained female was involved in a car crash involving a head-on collision. Upon arrival to the ED, she was obtunded and intubated in the field, along with hemodynamically instability as evidenced by tachycardia, and hypotension. Upon primary exam, the AG-ANP observes a seatbelt sign and performs a focused assessment with sonography for trauma (FAST). The focused assessment with sonography for trauma showed evidence of free fluid, what is the most appropriate next intervention?

   a. CT scan
   b. Transport immediately to the operating room for surgical intervention
   c. Fluid and electrolyte replacement
   d. Monitor and reassess

4. The AG-ACNP is caring for an 87-year-old patient in the ICU with past medical history of CHF and morbid obesity who was in a recent motor vehicle accident with subsequent cardiac arrest from hemorrhagic shock and is intubated and on two vasopressor therapies: Levophed and

vasopressin. Lab data reveals a worsening aminotransferase/alanine aminotransferase elevation, so an abdominal ultrasound is ordered. The ultrasound reveals pericholecystic fluid and gallbladder distention with associated "sludge." She is febrile, despite antimicrobial therapy with meropenem. She has normal renal function. A STAT CT of the abdomen and pelvis with contrast is obtained and found an abscess to the gallbladder area without obstructing stones. The best treatment option for her currently would be to:

a. Change to pipracillin/tazobactam and mitronidazole (Flagyl)
b. Percutaneous cholecystostomy tube placement for drainage of abscess
c. Consult general surgery for an emergency cholecystectomy
d. Continue oral diet and gentle hydration with intravenous fluids

5. A 68-year-old male with past medical history of sarcoidosis on chronic steroid therapy, cirrhosis, CAD, chronic cholecystitis, and DMII is a patient in the ICU and develops abdominal rigidity, severe right upper quadrant abdominal pain, and acute rebound tenderness and guarding on abdominal exam. He becomes hypotensive and tachycardic. Laboratory data reveal a rising lactic acidosis, leukocytosis, hyperbilirubinemia, and a normal serum creatinine. An ultrasound is done with nonspecific findings, except for some pericholecystic fluid. A STAT CT of the abdomen and pelvis reveals free intraperitoneal fluid, pericholecystic fluid, and a gallbladder wall defect. The most appropriate next action is:

a. Start vasopressor therapy to maintain MAP of 65 mmHg.
b. Start broad-spectrum antimicrobial therapy.
c. Give intravenous fluid boluses with normal saline.
d. Consult general surgery for emergency laparotomy with cholecystectomy.

6. The treatment for patients with *Helicobacter pylori* infection should aim to achieve high eradication rates in the setting of ever-increasing antibiotic resistance. Therefore, the evidence-based, first-line treatment for a patient with a prior exposure to a macrolide antibiotic is:

a. A PPI, clarithromycin, and amoxicillin or metronidazole for 14 days
b. A PPI, bismuth, tetracycline, and a nitroimidazole for 10 to 14 days
c. A PPI and clarithromycin, tetracycline, and a nitroimidazole for 10 to 14 days
d. Sequential therapy consisting of a PPI and amoxicillin for 5 days, followed by clarithromycin and a nitroimidazole for an additional 5 days

7. The prevalence of GERD is about 18% to 28% in adults in the U.S. Symptoms commonly include heartburn, epigastric pain, and dyspepsia. Weight loss is often key to symptom relief, but many patients take PPIs such as Omeprazole to treat GERD. What are the long-term complications of PPIs?

a. Psychological dependence
b. Stained teeth with receding gum
c. Development of clostridium difficele infection (CDI) and osteoporosis
d. Gastric atrophy

8. A 59-year-old male admitted with a 3-day history of initial diffuse abdominal pain. He relays anorexia, nausea, and constipation since symptom onset. Today he awoke with fever 38.4°C and localization left lower quadrant pain and abdominal distention. Labs reveal hemoglobin 13.5; CRP 52 mg/L; WBC 12,000. Workup included a CT of the abdomen which showed bowel wall thickening and fat stranding. The next step in the management plan should be:

a. Surgical consult for exploratory laparoscopy
b. Nothing by mouth, IV fluid resuscitation, and IV antibiotics
c. Gastric decompression, IV fluids
d. Colonoscopy

9. A 35-year-old male with a history of Crohn's disease since age 20, recently managed on azathioprine, presents to the colon-rectal clinic this morning with complaints of malodorous diarrhea, lower left quadrant abdominal pain, weakness, and malaise. Concerned, the AG-ACNP orders which test to rule out a common complication from Crohn's disease management:

   a. Stool for occult blood, and a CBC
   b. Stool culture for *Clostridium difficile*
   c. A barium enema to evaluate for fistula
   d. A CT with oral and IV contrast

10. The criteria for the diagnosis of irritable bowel syndrome is:

   a. History of GI intolerance to dairy products
   b. Abdominal pain with distention, and constipation with straining
   c. Abdominal pain associated with change in stool consistency and frequency and related to a bowel movement
   d. A change in bowel habit to looser and/or more frequent stools persisting for more than 6 weeks

11. A 43-year-old female admitted with CAP and dehydration. She had been ill for 3 days and had been seen in an urgent care 48 hours before admission. She had been taking amoxicillin which had been prescribed. She was unable to get out of bed this morning by herself due to feeling faint, so her husband took her to the ED. Her admission vitals: temperature 38.8°C, heart rate 106; blood pressure 94/56; respiration rate 22. A CBC revealed WBC 13.4; hemoglobin 6.8; platelets within normal limits. From the patient's history and review of symptoms, the AG-ACNP suspects that the patient has celiac disease. Besides her orders for her community acquired pneumonia (CAP), rehydration, and a consult to gastroenterologist, the AG-ACNP should order which of the following to support the diagnosis of celiac disease:

   a. Calcium, vitamin D, vitamin K, iron, folate, B12 levels
   b. One unit of packed red blood cells to treat her anemia
   c. A gluten-free diet to improve her symptoms
   d. Immunoglobulin A tissue transglutaminase

12. A 45-year-old-male presents to the unit with colicky abdominal pain, abdominal distention, and protracted vomiting that has been occurring for the last 6 days. His last bowel movement was 4 days ago, and he is not passing flatus per rectum. On physical exam he has high-pitched bowel sounds and no signs of peritoneal irritation. He has a well-healed midline scar from an exploratory laparotomy for a gunshot wound done 3 years ago. Abdominal x-rays show dilated loops of small bowel with air-fluid levels. The best management plan would include:

   a. Antibiotics, anticholinergic, and gentle laxatives
   b. H2 blockers, antacids, and gastric lavage
   c. Nothing taken orally, nasogastric suction, IV fluids, and careful observation
   d. Rectal tube and colonic irrigation and exploratory laparotomy

13. A 56-year-old woman is recovering from a subtotal gastrectomy for gastric cancer with a gastroduodenal anastomosis. A penrose drain has been left in the area. On the fifth postoperative day, she began to drain about 2 L per day of green fluid. She has no abdominal pain, fever, or signs of peritoneal irritation. At this time, the AG-ACNP knows the management should be:

   a. Emergency reclosure of the abdominal incision
   b. Fluid replacement, nutritional support, and protection of the abdominal wall
   c. Fluid restriction and oral intake of mostly solid foods
   d. Intensive medical management with H2 blockers, PPIs, and steroids

14. A 50-year-old woman is brought in to the unit in extreme abdominal pain, which came on suddenly and is generalized all over her abdomen. Upon examination, she has a rigid abdomen with muscle guarding and rebound on all quadrants and no bowel sounds. A CT scan was done and shows free air under the diaphragm. The diagnosis is:

    a. An acute inflammatory process in the abdomen
    b. Rupture of a fluid collection requiring emergent antibiotics
    c. Acute obstruction of some intraabdominal viscera
    d. Acute abdominal perforation somewhere in the GI tract

15. A 30-year-old male with previous medical history of chronic pain presents to the ED with abrupt onset of abdominal pain, nausea, vomiting, and encephalopathy, several hours after ingestion of acetaminophen for his pain. There is no known history of liver disease. Comprehensive labs are ordered and revealing of coagulopathy with an international normalized ratio of 3.0, AKI with creatinine of 2.0, severe transaminitis, lactic acidosis with lactate of 4, and a metabolic acidosis. A urine drug screen revealed acetaminophen level of 200 mg/kg. Serum alcohol level negative. The AG-ACNP understands that the best initial treatment for this patient is:

    a. Reversal of coagulopathy with FFP
    b. Nephrology consult to begin continual renal replacement/dialysis therapy
    c. Order N-acetylcysteine (Mucomyst)
    d. Admission to ICU and consult liver transplant surgery/transfer to liver transplant hospital

16. A 28-year-old female with history of seizure disorder on antiepileptic therapy and recent pregnancy presents with a several-day history of progressing acute encephalopathy, jaundice, nausea, emesis, fatigue, and generalized abdominal pain. Abdominal ultrasound with no evidence of cirrhosis, but revealing a fatty liver. Urine drug screen (UDS) was negative on admit. Lab data with severe transaminitis, hyperbilirubinemia, hyperammonemia, and coagulopathy. Given her history and presentation, you are most concerned that her diagnosis is:

    a. Cirrhosis
    b. Acute liver failure
    c. Autoimmune hepatitis
    d. Ischemic cholecystitis

17. A 47-year-old female with medical history of factor VII deficiency and chronic liver disease who recently traveled overseas for a mission trip where she worked in an orphanage presents with a 2-week history of malaise, headache, myalgias, anorexia, pruritis, fever, jaundice, and nausea. An ultrasound and CT of the abdomen was ordered with no reported abnormalities outside of hepatomegaly. Labs revealing of elevated aminotransferase elevations. Based on the patient's history and clinical presentation, the AG-ACNP suspects the patient most likely has:

    a. Hepatitis A
    b. Gastroenteritis
    c. Hepatitis D
    d. Chronic hepatitis B

18. A 38-year-old male with history of of type 2 diabetes and IV drug abuse presents to the ED with a 7-month history of fatigue, arthralgias, pruritis, anorexia, myalgias, and nausea and vomiting. His acute serum hepatitis panel reveals a positive hepatitis C virus (HCV) RNA and anti-hepatitis C virus antibody (anti-HCV) with serum genotype of 4. His HIV antibody is negative. The best treatment for this patient is:

    a. Tenofovir
    b. Lamivudine
    c. Supportive care
    d. Lediposvir/sofosbuvir (Harvoni)

19. A 78-year-old male with a past medical history of dementia and CVA with right-sided paralysis presents to the ED from the nursing home with hypotension, tachycardia, and altered mental status from baseline. CT of brain negative for new acute abnormalities. Labs with a leukocytosis of 25K, metabolic acidosis, and AKI. Chest x-ray concerning for right lower lobe pneumonia (RLL PNA). Started on broad spectrum antimicrobial therapy and intubated in the ED for airway protection. He was volume resuscitated adequately with normal saline, but remains hypotensive, so vasopressors started and transferred to the ICU for further critical care management of septic shock. Upon transfer, develops pulseless electrical activity (PEA) arrest from a severe metabolic acidosis with return of spontaneous circulation after 10 minutes. Stat echocardiogram revealing of acute biventricular heart failure. Over the next few days, he has a rapid continual increase in his aspartate aminotransferase (AST), alanine aminotransferase (ALT), and lactate acid dehydrogenase (LDH) with an ALT greater than 1,000 mg/dL. His total billirubin (TBili) and international normalized ratio (INR) are initially normal, but then later become elevated. The AG-ACNP is concerned he has developed:

    a. Fulminant liver failure
    b. Ischemic hepatitis
    c. Hepatorenal syndrome
    d. Portal vein thrombosis

20. A 50-year-old female with chronic hepatitis B virus on treatment with tenofovir presents to the hospital with a 3-week history of an enlarging abdominal girth, generalized weakness, abdominal pain, and progressive altered mental status. On exam, she has severe ascites. Upon admission an ultrasound is obtained revealing of segmental hypertrophy and atrophy with surface nodularity concerning for fibrotic tissue and also revealing of portal hypertension. The AG-ACNP recognizes that the patient has developed this complication from her chronic hepatitis B infection:

    a. Hepatomegaly
    b. Hepatic steatosis
    c. Cirrhosis
    d. Gilbert's syndrome

21. An elderly woman was admitted with intracerebral bleeding. The best way to assess for malnutrition or undernutrition risk in this neuro ICU patient is:

    a. Calculate the patient's BMI and compare it to national norms.
    b. Order serum albumin, pre-albumin, and total protein levels or interleukin-6 level.
    c. Use the nutritional risk screening (NRS) 2002 (>5) or nutritional risk in the critically ill (NUTRIC) score of ≥5 to determine the patient is high risk.
    d. Assess a CT scan, which will provide a precise quantification of skeletal muscle and adipose tissue depots.

22. A 57-year-old male driver with a history of COPD and hypertension is postoperative day 3, a survivor of a drive-by shooting. The bullet grazed his head, but he lost control of his car and hit a tree. He had left-sided thoracic injuries including a flail chest. He has undergone a left main stem bronchial tear repair and thoracotomy tube placement. He is on a ventilator, due to left lower lobe extensive pulmonary contusion and flail chest. The patient weighs 75 kg. The AG-ACNP is placing orders for EN. Given his current injury and medical history, what rationale for EN formula is the best for this patient?

    a. EN calculated to receive a protein goal of 0.8 g/kg/d
    b. Choice of EN should include a high-carbohydrate, low-fat formula
    c. Selected EN formula should deliver nutrients in the range of 20 to 35 kcal/kg/d
    d. Isocaloric feeding formula that meets recommended dietary allowance for his age group

23. A 75-year-old male with metastatic prostate cancer and chronic kidney disease was discharged 2 days prior, after an admission for sepsis due to a UTI and significant anemia. He had been having dysphagia with both solids and liquids, regurgitation, dry mouth, and significant weight loss. An endoscopy performed during that admission revealed a delayed swallow with dysmotility and reflux. A gastrostomy tube had been placed and the patient sent home with tube feedings. He returned feeling generally unwell and weak. Lab work reveals the following abnormalities: lbumin 2.9, CRP 229, phosphate less than 1.0, potassium 3.2. What is of most concern to the management of this patient?

    a. The patient is at risk for malnourishment.
    b. The patient is at risk for refeeding syndrome.
    c. The patient has an underlying inflammatory condition.
    d. The patient could still be anemic.

24. A 60-year-old male with past medical history of hypertriglyceridemia and alcohol abuse presents with dyspnea, diaphoresis, and fever, with a 5-day history of nausea and emesis that is worse with oral intake of food. In addition, he has epigastric abdominal pain that radiates to the left upper quadrant and to the flank region that is worse with lying supine and improves with knees sitting up and flexed. Upon exam, he displays abdominal guarding and sinus tachycardia. Labs notable for elevated serum lipase at 10,000. The AG-ACNP diagnoses the patient with:

    a. Perforated duodenal ulcer
    b. Acute appendicitis
    c. Acute pancreatitis
    d. Acute mesenteric ischemia

25. A 55-year-old male with past medical history of cholelithiasis and bilateral lung transplant due to idiopathic pulmonary fibrosis is on chronic immunosuppression with azothioprine therapy. He presents with a 3-day history of nausea, emesis, diaphoresis, and severe epigastric pain that radiates to the back. CT of the abdomen and pelvis reveals diffuse parenchymal enlargement, retroperitoneal fat stranding, and pancreatic edema. The most appropriate treatment includes which of the following:

    a. Consult GI surgery
    b. Aggressive intravenous fluid administration
    c. Pancreatic enzyme replacement
    d. Continue azothioprine

26. A 48-year-old male with past medical history of decompensated alcoholic cirrhosis who recently underwent a large volume therapeutic paracentesis is being treated in the ICU for acute pancreatitis and hepatic encephalopathy. He has complaints of acute worsening generalized abdominal pain. His labs are notable for worsening coagulopathy, anemia, thrombocytopenia, and leukocytosis. Overnight he has become hypotensive requiring vasopressor therapy of norepinephrine (Levophed) with a new onset fever of 102°F, worsening sinus tachycardia with a heart rate in the 120s, and has become more encephalopathic. Ammonia level within normal range on lactulose therapy, and his liver function panel remains elevated with no remarkable changes overnight. On exam the AG-ACNP notes a positive Cullen's sign and Grey Turner's sign. The AG-ACNP is concerned that he has most likely developed:

a. Perforated peptic ulcer
b. Peritonitis
c. Abdominal compartment syndrome
d. Necrotizing hemorrhagic pancreatitis

■ GASTROINTESTINAL ANSWERS AND RATIONALES

1. **d) The patient should be admitted for a 24-hour observation period.** Asymptomatic stab wounds should be observed for the development of symptoms or instability. The initial abdominal exam may be relatively normal even with significant intra-abdominal injuries, for example, colon perforation with contamination would not produce peritoneal irritation until peritonitis develops after several hours. The sensitivity of a focused assessment with sonography for trauma is only 50%.

2. **b) Fluid resuscitation.** Fluid resuscitation is the first priority to maintain sufficient intravascular volume to perfuse vital organs. Assessment of volume status is best accomplished clinically; acutely the hemoglobin and hematocrit levels do not fall and do not reflect volume depletion.

3. **b) Transport immediately to the operating room for surgical intervention.** In patients where focused assessment with sonography for trauma ultrasound shows free fluid and evidence of hypovolemic shock and hemodynamic instability, transport immediately to the operation room for surgical intervention without CT imaging. Fluid and electrolyte replacement and monitoring will not resolve the principal cause of her hemodynamic instability.

4. **b) Percutaneous cholecystostomy tube placement for drainage of abscess.** Early cholecystectomy is the gold standard for the management for certain patient populations. However, the surgical management of elderly and critically ill patients is thought to be associated with poor outcomes with high rates of morbidity and mortality. Current guidelines, including the Tokyo guidelines, recommend gallbladder drainage by percutaneous cholecystostomy tube placements in this patient population of those who are critically ill. Given this patient's critical condition, she will have very poor outcomes if taken to the operating room. The percutaneous cholecystectomy tube with conservative management of nasogastric tube (NGT) to low wall suction (LWS), gentle intravenous hydration given her history of CHF, pain medications, antiemetics, and appropriate antimicrobial therapy are all most appropriate at this time, until she is more stable for surgical intervention. She should stay on appropriate antimicrobial therapy with guidelines recommending second- or third-generation cephalosporins or carbapenems, or metronidazole with a Fluoroquinolone like Ciprofloxacin.

5. **d) Consult general surgery for emergency laparotomy with cholecystectomy.** This patient has acute perforated cholecystitis based on his history, presentation, labs, and imaging findings. Perforation of intra-abdominal organs is an emergency. Clinical symptoms can range from pain to the right upper abdomen to a severe picture of acute abdomen with guarding and rebound tenderness with abdominal sepsis. The most important goal of treatment is management of abdominal sepsis with surgical removal of the gallbladder. It is rarely diagnosed preoperatively; however, imaging can help aid in appropriate diagnosis. Final diagnosis is usually confirmed at the time of an exploratory laparotomy. Perforation of gallbladder occurs in approximately 3% of cases of acute cholecystitis, and is usually associated with the presence of stones. Infection, trauma, steroids, malignancy, and systemic diseases like DM and atherosclerosis are predisposing factors. The best treatment is early surgery. Early diagnosis of gallbladder perforation and immediate surgical intervention are crucial in order to decrease morbidity and mortality.

6. **b) A PPI, bismuth, tetracycline, and a nitroimidazole for 10 to 14 days.** In North America the incidence of *H. pylori* infection is in general lower than people born outside of North America (United States and Canada). In general the incidence is lower in non-Hispanic Whites than among other racial/ethnic groups. In addition, immigrants from Asia and other parts of the world have a higher incidence. Therefore, the first-line treatment for *H. pylori* patients with no previous history of macrolide exposure, who reside in areas where clarithromycin resistance among *H. pylori* isolates is known to be low (<15%), can be clarithromycin triple therapy (PPI, clarithromycin, and amoxicillin or metronidazole for 14 days). However, in cases in which resistance patterns may not be known, or in patients who may have had macrolide antibiotic exposure in the past, *most* of these patients will be better served by first-line treatment with

the addition of bismuth quadruple therapy (PPI, bismuth, tetracycline, and a nitroimidazole for 10–14 days), concomitant therapy (PPI, clarithromycin, moxicillin, and metronidazole for 10–14 days), or sequential therapy (PPI and amoxicillin 5–7 days, followed by PPI and clarithromycin + nitroimidazole for 5–7 days).

7. **c) Development of clostridium difficele infection (CDI) and osteoporosis.** The risks associated with long-term use of PPIs include chronic kidney disease, dementia, bone fractures, small intestinal bacterial overgrowth, spontaneous bacterial peritonitis, CDI, and nutritional deficiency.

8. **b) Nothing taken orally, IV fluid resuscitation, and IV antibiotics.** Complicated diverticulitis is symptoms of inflammation and potential abscess, phlegmon, fistula development, or peritonitis. CT scan is the preferred mode of imaging to complicated diverticulitis, although ultrasound can be used for uncomplicated symptoms. Although it is unusual for patients to vomit, they should receive nothing by mouth and given fluid hydration and IV antibiotics until surgical need has been cleared. If conservative treatment is able to clear symptoms, colonoscopy may be considered 4 to 6 weeks after the episode to evaluate.

9. **b) Stool culture for *C difficile*.** Patients with inflammatory bowel disease may be more prone to infectious complications based on their underlying inflammatory disease and variations in their microbiome. Immunosuppressant medications commonly used to treat patients with Crohn's play a role in predisposing these patients to acquire these infections. The most common infections of the gastrointestinal tract in patients with inflammatory bowel disease are CDI and CMV.

10. **c) Abdominal pain associated with change in stool consistency, frequency, and related to a bowel movement.** The diagnostic Rome IV criteria clearly delineates that irritable bowel syndrome is defined as recurrent abdominal pain on average at least 1 day a week in the last 3 months associated with two or more of the following: (a) related to defecation, (b) associated with a change in a frequency of stool, (c) associated with a change in form (consistency) of stool, and (d) symptoms must have started at least 6 months ago.

11. **d) Immunoglobulin A tissue transglutaminase.** An overwhelming majority of people with celiac disease will remain undiagnosed. Those who are not avoiding gluten risk developing a host of debilitating complications, including anemia, peripheral neuropathies, osteopenia and bone pain, and even cancer. The single best serology testing for celiac disease is the IgA-based TTG with a sensitivity and specificity of approximately 98%. Although the patient should have nutrient, vitamin, and trace mineral levels checked and replaced (in this case malabsorption most likely cause of her anemia), they do not diagnose celiac disease. Diagnosis is made easier while the person is still ingesting gluten, although the popularity of gluten-free diets has made necessary adjustments to the diagnosis process. Treating her anemia with packed red blood cells may be required but that is a treatment for anemia, not a diagnostic aid.

12. **c) Nothing taken orally, nasogastric suction, IV fluids, and careful observation.** Mechanical intestinal obstruction is typically caused by adhesions in those who have had a prior laparotomy. There is usually colicky abdominal pain and protracted vomiting, progressive abdominal distention (if a low obstruction), and no passage of gas or feces. Early on, high-pitched bowel sounds coincide with the colicky pain and after a few days there will be silence. X-rays show distended loops of small bowel with air-fluid levels. Treatment starts with nothing by mouth, NG suction, and IV fluids, while watching for early signs of strangulation. Surgery is performed if conservative management is unsuccessful, within 24 hours in cases of complete obstruction or within a few day of partial obstruction

13. **b) Fluid replacement, nutritional support, and protection of the abdominal wall.** Fistulas of the GI tract cause bowel contents to leak out through a wound or drain site. If they do not empty directly and completely to the outside, but leak into a "cesspool" that then leaks out, the problem will be sepsis requiring surgical drainage. If they drain freely and the patient is afebrile, with no signs of peritoneal irritation, then there are three potential problems to

prevent: fluid and electrolyte loss, nutritional depletion, and erosion and digestion of the abdominal wall.

14. **d) Acute abdominal perforation somewhere in the GI tract**. Acute abdominal pain caused by perforation has sudden onset and is constant, generalized, and very severe. Except in the very elderly or very sick, impressive generalized signs of peritoneal irritation are found with tenderness, muscle guarding, rebound, and silent abdomen. If present, free air under the diaphragm confirms the diagnosis. Perforated peptic ulcer is the most common example and emergency surgery is needed.

15. **c) Order N-acetylcysteine (Mucomyst)**. This patient is in acute liver failure. Acute liver failure is an abrupt onset of liver failure, characterized by hepatic encephalopathy, jaundice, and coagulopathy in the absence of any pre-existing liver disease with an illness less than 26 weeks. Acetaminophen toxicity is the most common cause. Other causes include idiosyncratic drug reactions from meds (antimicrobials, antituberculosis drugs, antiepileptics), viral or autoimmune hepatitis, malignancy/lymphoma, poisonous mushrooms (*Amanita phalloides*), shock, Budd-Chiari syndrome, Wilson disease, Reye syndrome, hyperthermia, or fatty liver of pregnancy. Liver transplantation is the only definitive therapy for those who are unable to maintain life with supportive care alone. Therefore, early transfer to a liver transplantation center is essential for close monitoring by the hepatology and liver transplant team. In acute liver failure, unless actively bleeding, reversal of coagulopathy is not necessary. While a nephrology consult is important, the patient may not need dialysis right away. This is not the most pressing need of the patient. N-acetylcysteine will be an appropriate treatment for this patient; however, admission to the ICU setting of a tertiary center with liver transplant abilities is essential and is first priority.

16. **b) Acute liver failure**. Acute liver failure is an abrupt onset of liver failure, characterized by hepatic encephalopathy, jaundice, and coagulopathy in the absence of any pre-existing liver disease with an illness less than 26 weeks. This patient has two risk factors for acute liver failure: recent pregnancy with resultant fatty liver and a seizure disorder on chronic antiepileptic therapy. Her symptoms and presentation are classic for that of acute liver failure. The symptoms of acute liver failure can vary depending on the cause and how severe the disease is at the time of admission. With acetaminophen toxicity, the onset is more rapid with abdominal pain, nausea and vomiting, and encephalopathy several hours after this medication. For other causes of acute liver failure the onset of symptoms may be more gradual, and also include nonspecific symptoms like fatigue, malaise, changes in behavior, new-onset ascites, and/or asymptomatic jaundice.

17. **a) Hepatitis A**. The patient has a clotting disorder, chronic liver disease and recent travel to another country, and worked in an orphanage with kids, which are all risk factors for hepatitis A. Her symptoms are classic symptoms for hepatitis. So a serum acute hepatitis panel will need to be ordered, which will reveal a positive anti-hepatitis A virus (HAV) IgM antibody. The recovery phase and immunity phase are indicated by anti-HAV IgG antibodies. Hepatitis A is transmitted by the fecal-oral route and is the most common cause of viral hepatitis worldwide. Handwashing and bottled water are important things for prevention. Treatment is supportive care with immunization as prevention. If fulminant hepatic failure occurs, liver transplantation is needed. In this clinical scenario, the history is key to diagnosis. Immunoglobulin can be given for postexposure prophylaxis, which allows for passive transfer of antibodies. hepatitis A vaccine is used for pre-exposure prophylaxis. Acute hepatitis may also be clinically silent.

18. **d) Lediposvir/sofosbuvir (Harvoni)**. Lediposvir/sofosbuvir (Harvoni) may also be used in combination with ribavirin. Harvoni is an antiviral medication that prevents the hepatitis C virus from multiplying in the body. This medication should not be taken in those with a history of hepatitis B. It can cause worsening liver disease associated with that other than hepatitis and can also affect the kidneys, so close monitoring of labs is important and should be used with caution in these patients. It is used in treatment for genotypes 1, 4, 5, or 6 and in some with genotype 3. It can be used in adults and children who are at least 12 years

old with a weight of 35 kg or greater. This patient's history of IV drug abuse is a risk factor for the development of hepatitis C. The fact that the patient has had these symptoms for a prolonged length of time and that the anti-HCV is positive lead to a diagnosis of chronic infection. Anti-HCV labs may be undetectable for the first 8 weeks after infection.

19. **b) Ischemic hepatitis**. This patient has undergone pulseless electrical activity (PEA) arrest and hypotension with decreased perfusion to his liver. He also has the risk factor of heart failure. With ischemic hepatitis there is an acute and transient elevation of liver enzymes in the thousand. There will be a rapid rise and fall in aspartate aminotransferase (AST), alanine aminotransferase (ALT) greater than 1000 mg/dL and lactate acid dehydrogenase (LDH) within 1–3 days of insult. Initially the total billirubin (Tbili), alkaline phosphatase level (ALP), and international normalized ratio (INR) will be normal, but then will rise, as a result of reperfusion injury. The treatment is supportive care and to treat the underlying cause. Ischemic hepatitis may lead to fulminant liver failure; however, it usually resolves itself with time and proper perfusion to the liver.

20. **c) Cirrhosis**. The abdominal imaging findings are those classic of cirrhosis, as well as the patient's history and presentation. Those with any type of chronic hepatitis or alcohol abuse are at risk of developing cirrhosis. During the asymptomatic period of the disease, normal liver parenchyma may slowly be replaced by fibrotic tissues, causing scarring, which can then lead to cirrhosis. Complications of cirrhosis include ascites, spontaneous bacterial peritonitis, hepatic encephalopathy, hepatorenal syndrome, and abdominal pain. The management of cirrhosis is supportive care and to treat any of the complications if present.

21. **c) Use the nutritional risk screening (NRS) 2002 (>5) or nutritional risk in the critically ill (NUTRIC) score of ≥ 5 to determine the patient is high risk**. Nutrition risk can be defined and more readily determined by an evaluation of baseline nutrition status and assessment of disease severity. Many screening and assessment tools are used to evaluate nutrition status; however, only the NRS 2002 and the NUTRIC score determine both nutrition status and disease severity. Although both scoring systems are based on retrospective analysis, they have been used to define nutrition risk in RCTs in critically ill patients. Patients at "risk" are defined by an NRS 2002 greater than 3 and those at "high risk" with a score ≥ 5 or a NUTRIC score ≥ 5 (if interleukin-6 is not included, otherwise >6) (McClave et al., 2016)

22. **c) Selected EN formula should deliver nutrients in the range of 20 to 35 kcal/kg/d**. Energy requirements vary depending on numerous factors. REE peaks over 4 to 5 days and continues to remain high for 9 to 12 days. Approximately 16% of total body protein is lost in the first 21 days, with 67% of that protein loss coming from skeletal muscle alone. Energy goals should be in the range of 20 to 35 kcal/kg/d, depending on the phase of trauma. Lower energy provision is suggested early in the resuscitative phase, unless that patient is at risk from malnutrition or his injuries are severe. Requirements for protein are similar for other ICU patients but may be at the higher end of the provision range, from 1.2 to 2 g/kg/d. Enteral formulas for respiratory compromised patients, such as COPD and lung injury, should use high-fat, low-carbohydrate to decrease CO_2. Finally, EN should be calculated on current energy expenditures and needs and not on recommended dietary allowances when critically ill.

23. **b) The patient is at risk for refeeding syndrome**. The greatest concern for this patient is the potential lethal complication of the metabolic and hormonal changes caused by rapid refeeding, whether enteral or parenteral. The under-recognition of the patients who are at risk (in this case chronic malnutrition, cancer, and elder age, along with pre-existing hypophosphatemia and hypokalemia) requires a through nutritional assessment, careful reintroduction of EN, and a close management of electrolyte replacement.

24. **c) Acute pancreatitis**. Acute pancreatitis occurs due to inflammation of the pancreas and peripancreatic tissue, due to activation of pancreatic enzymes, especially trypsin. The most common causes of pancreatitis are gallstone disease and alcohol abuse. Other causes includeabdominal trauma, medications, hypertriglyceridemia, and hypercalcemia. The patient has the risk factors of alcohol abuse and hypertriglyceridemia. The patient expresses common

symptoms of epigastric abdominal pain, especially to the left upper quadrant and to the flank region that is worse with lying supine and improves with knees sitting up and flexed; diaphoresis; sinus tachycardia; nausea and emesis that may be worse with oral intake of food; fever; anemia; altered mental status; and dyspnea. Labs show elevated serum lipase, usually two to three times the upper limits of normal. The serum amylase may also be elevated, but this is less sensitive than the serum lipase.

25. **b) Aggressive intravenous fluid administration**. The patient's symptoms, history, and imaging findings are consistent with that of acute pancreatitis. Appropriate treatment for acute pancreatitis includes nothing taken orally until inflammation, pain, nausea, and emesis improves; if unable to tolerate oral intake within a week, then begin jejunal enteral feedings, which is safer and preferred over total pareneral nutrition, if patient tolerates; aggressive intravenous fluid administration; low-fat, low-cholesterol, bland diet once oral intake resumed, with frequent small meals; antimicrobial therapy if an abscess or concerns for sepsis are identified; antiemetics; pain control and nasogastric tube to low wall suction with protracted emesis; and acid suppression for those at risk for stress ulcer bleeding. Ranson criteria for severity assessment in acute pancreatitis may provide prognostic information. A surgical consult is not indicated at this time. Azothioprine is a medication that can cause acute pancreatitis. Therefore, azathioprine needs to be held; however, this is his immunosuppression for the lung transplant and as such the transplant team should be consulted for recommendations for alternative therapy. Enzyme replacement is not indicated in acute or chronic pancreatitis.

26. **d) Necrotizing hemorrhagic pancreatitis**. Hypotension, sinus tachycardia, fever, and worsening encephalopathy are all indications of developing septic shock. Necrotizing hemorrhagic pancreatitis is a severe form of pancreatitis and can usually be diagnosed through CT imaging with contrast. Necrotizing pancreatitis has a higher morbidity and mortality rate than acute pancreatitis alone. Common presenting symptoms and signs are increasing abdominal pain, increasing leukocytosis, bacteremia, and fever. A patient may also develop Cullen's sign, which is blue discoloration around the umbilicus that signifies a hemoperitoneum. Grey Turner's sign, which is a reddish-brown discoloration along the flank, may also be present. This represents a retroperitoneal bleed or extravasation of pancreatic exudate. The fact that this patient is a liver patient and more coagulopathic increases his risk for hemorrhagic pancreatitis. This patient should not be on any type of anticoagulation medications.

■ REFERENCE

McClave, S. A., Taylor, B. E., Martindale, R. G., Warren, M. M., Johnson, D. R., Braunschweig, C., ... Gervasio, J. M. (2016). Guidelines for the provision and assessment of nutrition support therapy in the adult critically ill patient: Society of Critical Care Medicine (SCCM) and American Society for Parenteral and Enteral Nutrition (ASPEN). *Journal of Parenteral and Enteral Nutrition, 40*(2), 159–211.

■ BIBLIOGRAPHY

American Gastroenterology Associate Institute. (2017). A technical review on initial testing and management of acute liver disease. *Gastroenterology, 152*(3), 648–664. doi:10.1053/j.gastro.2016.12.027

Badillo, R., & Francis, D. (2014). Diagnosis and treatment of gastroesophageal reflux disease. *World Journal of Gastrointestinal Pharmacology and Therapeutics, 5*(3), 105–112. doi:10.4292/wjgpt.v5.i3.105

Bickley, L., & Szilagyi, P. (2013). *Bates' guide to physical examination and history taking*. Philadelphia, PA: Lippincott.

Chey, W. D., Leontiadis, G. I., Howden, C. W., & Moss, S. F. (2017). ACG clinical guideline: Treatment of Helicobacter pylori infection. *American Journal of Gastroenterology, 112*(2), 212–239. doi:10.1038/ajg.2016.563

Chiara, O., Cimbanassi, S., Boati, S., & Bassi, G. (2011). Surgical management of abdominal compartment syndrome. *Minerva Anestesiologica, 77*(4), 457–462.

Freedberg, D. D., Kim, L. S., & Yang, Y-X. (2017). The risks and benefits of long-term use of proton pump inhibitors: Expert review and best practice advice from the American Gastroenterological Association. *Gastroenterology, 152*(4), 706–715. doi:10.1053/j.gastro.2017.01.031

Friedli, N., Stanga, Z., Sobotka, L., Culkin, A., Kondrup, J., Laviano, A., . . . Schuetz, P. (2017). Revisiting the refeeding syndrome: Results of a systematic review. *Nutrition, 35*, 151–160. doi:10.1016/j.nut.2016.05.016

Fullwood, D., & Sargent, S. (2014). Complications in acute liver failure: Managing hepatic encephalopathy and cerebral oedema. *Gastrointestinal Nursing, 12*(3), 27–34. doi:10.12968/gasn.2014.12.3.27

Gans, S. L., Pols, M. A., Stoker, J., Boermeester, M. A., & Expert Steering Group. (2015). Guideline for the diagnostic pathway in patients with acute abdominal pain. *Digestive Surgery, 32*(1), 23–31. doi:10.1159/000371583

Godara, H., Heirbe, A., Nassif, M., Otepka, H., & Rosenstock, A. (2014). *The Washington manual of medical therapeutics* (34th ed.). Philadelphia, PA: Wolters Kluwer-Lippincott Williams & Wilkins.

Gralnek, I. M. (2015). Diagnosis and management of nonvariceal upper gastrointestinal hemorrhage: European Society of Gastrointestinal Endoscopy Guideline. *Endoscopy, 47*(10), a1–a46. doi:10.1055/s-0034-1393172

Grass, F., Pache, B., Martin, D., Hahnloser, D., Demartines, N., & Hübner, M. (2017). Preoperative nutritional conditioning of Crohn's patients—Systematic review of current evidence and practice. *Nutrients, 9*(6), 562. doi:10.3390/nu9060562

Heidari, K., Taqhizadeh, M., Mahmoudi, S., Panahi, H., Ghaffari Shad, E., & Asadollahi, S. (2017). FAST for blunt abdominal trauma: Correlation between positive findings and admission acid-base measurement. *American Journal of Emergency Medicine, 35*(6), 823–829. doi:10.1016/j.ajem.2017.01.035

Jansen, S., Doerner, J., Macher-Heidrich, S., Zirngibl, H., Ambe, P., & Ambe, P. C. (2017). Outcome of acute perforated cholecystitis: A register study of over 5000 cases from a quality control database in Germany. *Surgical Endoscopy, 31*(4), 1896–1900. doi:10.1007/s00464-016-5190-5

Kasper, D., Hauser, S., Jameson, J., Fauci, A., Longo, D., & Loscalzo, J. (2015). *Harrison's principles of internal medicine* (19th ed.). New York, NY: McGraw-Hill.

Landsman, M. J., Sultan, M., Stevens, M., Charabaty, A., & Mattar, M. C. (2014). Diagnosis and management of common gastrointestinal tract infectious diseases in ulcerative colitis and Crohn's disease patients. *Inflammatory Bowel Diseases, 20*(12), 2503–2510. doi:10.1097/MIB.0000000000000140

Macaluso, C. R., & McNamara, R. M. (2012). Evaluation and management of acute abdominal pain in the emergency department. *International Journal of General Medicine, 5*, 789–797. doi:10.2147/IJGM.S25936

Maluso, P., Olson, J., & Sarani, B. (2016). Abdominal compartment hypertension and abdominal compartment syndrome. *Critical Care Clinics, 32*(2), 213–222. doi:10.1016/j.ccc.2015.12.001

Maung, A. A., Johnson, D. C., Piper, G. L., Barbosa, R. R., Rowell, S. E., Bokhari, F., . . . Eastern Association for the Surgery of Trauma. (2012). Evaluation and management of small-bowel obstruction: An Eastern Association for the Surgery of Trauma practice management guideline. *Journal of Trauma and Acute Care Surgery, 73*(5 Suppl. 4), S362–S369. doi:10.1097/TA.0b013e31827019de

McClave, S. A., Martindale, R. G., Vanek, V. W., McCarthy, M., Roberts, P., Taylor, B., . . . Cresci, G., American Society for Parenteral and Enteral Nutrition Board of Directors; American College of Critical Care Medicine, Society of Critical Care Medicine. (2009). Guidelines for the provision and assessment of nutrition support therapy in the adult critically ill patient: Society of Critical Care Medicine and American Society for Parenteral and Enteral Nutrition. *JPEN: Journal of Parenteral and Enteral Nutrition, 33*(3), 277–316. doi:10.1177/0148607109335234

McStay, C., Ringwelski, A., Levy, P., & Legome, E. (2012). Hollow viscus injury. *Journal of Emergency Medicine, 37*(3), 293–299. doi:10.1016/j.jemermed.2009.03.017

Nirula, R. (2014). Esophageal perforation. *Surgical Clinics of North America, 94*(1), 35–41. doi:10.1016/j.suc.2013.10.003

Oropello, J., Kyetan, V., & Pastores, S. (2017). *Critical care.* New York, NY: McGraw-Hill Education.

Oxentenko, A. S., & Murray, J. A. (2015). Celiac disease: Ten things that every gastroenterologist should know. *Clinical Gastroenterology and Hepatology, 13*(8), 1396–1404. doi:10.1016/j.cgh.2014.07.024

Papadakis, M. A., McPhee, S. J., & Rabow, M. W. (2017). *Current medical diagnosis & treatment 2017.* New York, NY: McGraw-Hill Education.

Rostas, J., Cason, B., Simmons, J., Frotan, M. A., Brevard, S. B., & Gonzalez, R. P. (2015). The validity of abdominal examination in blunt trauma patients with distracting injuries. *Journal of Trauma and Acute Care Surgery, 78*(6), 1095–1100; discussion 1100–1091. doi:10.1097/TA.0000000000000650

Rubio-Tapia, A., Hill, I. D., Kelly, C. P., Calderwood, A. H., Murray, J. A., & American College of Gastroenterology. (2013). ACG clinical guidelines: Diagnosis and management of celiac disease. *American Journal of Gastroenterology, 108*(5), 656–676; quiz 677. doi:10.1038/ajg.2013.79

Runyon, B. A. (2013). Introduction to the revised American Association for the Study of Liver Diseases Practice Guideline management of adult patients with ascites due to cirrhosis 2012. *Hepatology, 57*(4), 1651–1653. doi:10.1002/hep.26359

Shogilev, D. J., Duus, N., Odom, S. R., & Shapiro, N. I. (2014). Diagnosing appendicitis: Evidence-based review of the diagnostic approach in 2014. *Western Journal of Emergency Medicine, 15*(7), 859–871. doi:10.5811/westjem.2014.9.21568

Simren, M., Palsson, O. S., & Whitehead, W. E. (2017). Update on Rome IV criteria for colorectal disorders: Implications for clinical practice. *Current Gastroenterology Reports, 19*(4), 15. doi:10.1007/s11894-017-0554-0

Thrumurthy, S. G., Chaudry, M. A., Hochhauser, D., & Mughal, M. (2013). The diagnosis and management of gastric cancer. *BMJ, 347*(347), f6367. doi:10.1136/bmj.f6367

Tintinalli, J. E. (2016). *Tintinalli's emergency medicine: A comprehensive study guide* (8th ed.). New York, NY: McGraw-Hill.

Wilkins, T., Embry, K., & George, R. (2013). Diagnosis and management of acute diverticulitis. *American Family Physician, 87*(9), 612–620.

Wyers, M. C. (2010). *Acute mesenteric ischemia: Diagnostic approach and surgical treatment.* Paper presented at the Seminars in Vascular Surgery.

11

Hematology, Oncology, and Immunology

GAIL LIS AND KIMBERLY LANGER

HEMATOLOGY, ONCOLOGY, IMMUNOLOGY QUESTIONS

1. A 37-year-old female was brought to the emergency department (ED) after a postsyncopal episode at work. Physical exam was unremarkable. Initial laboratory studies revealed a normal electrolyte panel and negative cardiac workup, but her complete blood count (CBC) showed white blood cells (WBC) 4.6×10^3, hemoglobin 10.7 g/dL (normal 12–14 g/dL), mean corpuscular volume (MCV) 72 m3 (normal: 80–100 m^3), hematocrit (Hct) 33% (37%–48% for women), and mean corpuscular hemoglobin (MCH) 24 picograms/cell (27–33 picograms/cells). Based on this information, her anemia would be classified as:

   a. Microcytic, normochromic
   b. Microcytic, hypochromic
   c. Macrocytic, hyperchromic
   d. Normocytic, hypochromic

2. A 69-year-old female with a known medical history of hypertension, CAD, stage II chronic kidney disease, and hypothyroidism is admitted to the medical unit for weakness. Upon further workup: WBC 6.5, hemoglobin 10.8, platelets 250,000, and MCV 85. As the AG-ACNP managing her care, your next step should include:

   a. Transfusion of a unit of packed red blood cells
   b. Epogen injection 30,000 units once
   c. Management of chronic diseases
   d. Vitamin B$_{12}$ injection

3. A 52-year-old female is admitted to the hospital with a 3-day history of nausea and vomiting. She has a past medical history of hypertension, hyperlipidemia, and obesity, currently 3 months status post Roux-en-Y bypass surgery. Upon initial evaluation of the patient, the AG-ACNP learns that the patient is experiencing numbness of her hands and feet, difficulty walking and maintaining balance, and weakness. On physical exam, the patient is found to have positive Romberg's and Babinski's signs. Initial laboratory studies included a CBC, which revealed: WBC 6.7×10^3, hemoglobin, 10.5 g/dL, MCV 115 fl, and platelets 250,000. Given these results and the findings on physical exam, the next appropriate laboratory study would be:

   a. Bone marrow biopsy
   b. Vitamin B$_{12}$ level
   c. Peripheral smear
   d. Electrolyte panel

4. A 45-year-old male is admitted to the medicine service for elective hip replacement. He has a known history of HIV but his CD4 count previously was 450 cells/μL. His CD4+ count upon admission is now 180 cells/μL. This patient should receive prophylaxis against which of the following:

   a. *Pneumocystis jiroveci* with sulfamethoxazole/trimethoprim (Bactrim)
   b. Pseudomonas with levofloxacin (Levaquin)
   c. Mucor with fluconazole (Diflucan)
   d. VZV with acyclovir (Zovirax)

5. A 70-year-old male is admitted to the hospitalist service for severe left-sided pain of the temporal region, headache, and diplopia/visual impairment. A head CT report indicated arterial narrowing of the temporal artery. The AG-ACNP's next immediate step would be to:

   a. Administer IV methylprednisolone 1 g IV now.
   b. Obtain a biopsy of the left temporal artery.
   c. Obtain laboratory studies including ESR and CRP.
   d. Monitor the patient's clinical symptoms.

6. The leading cause of cancer deaths in both men and women in the United States is:

   a. Colorectal cancer
   b. Leukemia
   c. Lung cancer
   d. Pancreatic cancer

7. A 55-year-old patient was admitted to the hospitalist service for side effects from his chemotherapy treatment for colon cancer. As the AG-ACNP is reviewing the medical record, the oncology history is reviewed to gain a better understanding of the extent of the patient's cancer. The tumor is staged at T2, N1, M0. The AG-ACNP interprets this to mean:

   a. Tumor invades muscle, 1 to 3 regional lymph nodes are affected, no distant metastasis
   b. Tumor is within the inner layer of the mucosa, no regional lymph nodes are affected, no distant metastasis
   c. Tumor penetrates muscle, greater than 3 lymph nodes are affected, no distant metastasis
   d. Two tumors are present, 1 lymph node is affected, no distant metastasis

8. A 74-year-old male with a history of prostate cancer is admitted to the hospital with progressive back pain which has progressively worsened over the past weeks. It is suspected that the patient has spinal cord compression secondary to vertebral metastasis. Common assessment findings associated with spinal cord compression are:

   a. Pain improves when the patient is supine
   b. Deep tendon reflexes are hypoactive
   c. Pain is relieved with straight leg raises
   d. Tingling sensation down the back when neck is flexed

9. A 60-year-old female with a history of metastatic breast cancer presents to the ED with shortness of breath, cough, and facial swelling. On physical exam, the patient is found to be ill appearing, andtachypneic, with left arm swelling and left JVD. The AG-ACNP anticipates which of the following findings on a STAT chest x-ray:

   a. Cavitary lesion right upper lobe
   b. Postobstructive pneumonia
   c. Pneumothorax
   d. Mediastinal widening

10. The AG-ACNP is caring for a patient with CML and understands that a genetic marker is used to diagnosis this illness. The genetic diagnostic marker for CML is:

    a. Reed-Sternberg cells
    b. Philadelphia chromosome
    c. Auer rods
    d. M protein

11. An AG-ACNP is discussing colon cancer treatment with a 45-year-old male. The patient is status post colon resection with metastasis to the liver. The AG-ACNP's response will be based upon which of the following statements regarding colon cancer treatment:

    a. Chemotherapy is typically not initiated post colon resection as the surgery has likely cured the cancer.
    b. Chemotherapy, if required, will likely be combined with endocrine therapy.
    c. Chemotherapy, if required, will likely be combined with genetic based targeted therapy.
    d. Radiation therapy without chemotherapy will likely be the treatment of choice.

12. A patient with a history of small cell lung cancer is admitted with progressive shortness of breath and dry cough. The patient was discharged post thoracentesis 2 weeks ago for similar presentation. Upon assessment, the patient is awake, alert, oriented, and tachypneic, with a respiratory rate of 28 and dyspneic with speaking. Oxygen saturation is 89% on 2 L on oxygen. A recurrent large pleural effusion is noted on chest x-ray. The best treatment for this patient is STAT:

    a. Two-dimension echocardiogram
    b. Intubation with ventilator support
    c. Thoracentesis without pleurex catheter placement
    d. Thoracentesis with pleurex catheter placement

13. A 36-year-old male is admitted to the hospital with an open ulcer to his right foot with purulent drainage. The patient states that he scratched his foot after falling off his motorcycle 2 days ago. Upon exam the AG-ACNP notes an open wound with surrounding erythema that travels proximal to the ankle and lower leg in addition to frank purulence. The remainder of the exam is normal with the exception of mild oral thrush to the upper palate. The patient denies any medical treatment to the injury and denies past medical history. Abnormal lab values include a WBC of 3.2. Patient's vital signs are stable with a low-grade temperature. In addition to a wound culture, determine the diagnostic that would be important to order:

    a. ESR
    b. HIV antigen/antibody test
    c. Hepatitis panel
    d. CRP

14. Common manifestations associated with HIV acute retroviral syndrome include which of the following assessment findings:

    a. Goiter
    b. Cervical lymphadenopathy
    c. Janeway lesions
    d. Kaposi sarcoma

15. A 44-year-old male with a history of HIV and not on any treatment verbalizes severe substernal burning without radiation and odynophagia. Upon exam the AG-ACNP notes oral thrush. The AG-ACNP suspects which of the following diagnoses:

    a. GERD
    b. Candida esophagitis
    c. Gastric ulcer perforation
    d. Esophageal cancer

16. A female patient with a history of HIV is admitted to the hospital for an unrelated medical issue. The patient indicates that her family members are not aware of the HIV diagnosis and tells the nurse that she does not want this information disclosed. The nurse queries the AG-ACNP on the unit for assistance in this matter. The best advice to provide the nurse would be to:

    a. Inform the patient that family members have a right to know this diagnosis.
    b. Inform the health department that a patient is admitted to the unit with a diagnosis of HIV and family members need to be contacted.
    c. Inform the patient that her request for confidentiality will be respected.
    d. Inform the nurse that the AG-ACNP will meet with the patient and family to discuss this diagnosis.

17. An AG-ACNP evaluates a 44-year-old patient who has HIV disease. The patient has painful linear vesicular lesions distributed over the posterior thorax. The vesicles do not cross the midline of the thorax. This presentation is most consistent with:

    a. Nonbullous impetigo
    b. Herpes zoster
    c. Atopic dermatitis
    d. Folliculitis

■ HEMATOLOGY, ONCOLOGY, IMMUNOLOGY ANSWERS AND RATIONALES

1. **b) Microcytic, hypochromic**. The classification of microcytic, hypochromic anemia refers to smaller than normal size red blood cells (based on MCV) and pale red blood cells (based on MCH). Based on the laboratory findings, the patient's hemoglobin is below the range of an adult female (normal: 12–14 g/dL). MCV is low at 72 m^3 (80–100 m^3 normal). This would constitute a microcytic anemia.

2. **c) Management of chronic diseases**. Patients with known chronic kidney disease are likely to have anemia, typically being anemia of chronic disease. This patient's hemoglobin may be stable in the current range it is in, thus no interventions are necessarily needed. If the disorder is reversible, then anemia should resolve. If the patient should require further management, specifically, if her chronic kidney disease were to worsen, you could consider Epogen injections, especially if the need for hemodialysis develops. A red blood cell transfusion is not warranted as the hemoglobin is slightly out of normal range but not within parameters of warranting a blood transfusion. A vitamin B$_{12}$ injection would not be warranted as the patient does not have a clinical diagnosis of vitamin B$_{12}$ deficiency.

3. **b) Vitamin B$_{12}$ level**. Given the patient's recent history of Roux-en-Y bypass, she is at increased risk for vitamin deficiency. Most commonly seen with this type of procedure is vitamin B$_{12}$ deficiency. Additionally, the patient presents with neurological findings consistent with those of vitamin B$_{12}$ deficiency. A bone marrow biopsy is not warranted now. A peripheral smear could be considered but would not shed much light on the current situation. An electrolyte panel could be helpful but, again, is not fitting the picture of the patient's current situation.

4. **a) *Pneumocystis jiroveci* with sulfamethoxazole /trimethoprim (Bactrim)**. Patients with a CD4+ cell count less than 200 cells/μL are at increased risk for opportunistic infections, most commonly those of pneumocystis, cryptosporidium, and candida. Bactrim is the correct drug to cover for this specific opportunistic infection found in patients with AIDS. Levaquin can cover for pseudomonas but this is not considered an opportunistic infection. Fluconazole does not have antifungal coverage for mucor. Acyclovir is indicated postexposure to sick contacts. Varicella-zoster immune globulin 125 international units per 10 kg intramuscular, administered as soon as possible and within 10 days after exposure is preferred VZV postexposure recommendation.

5. **a) Administer IV methylprednisolone 1 gram IV now**. This patient is presenting with giant cell arteritis of the left temporal artery. The gold standard is to get a biopsy but given his clinical symptomology including visual impairment, treatment should not be delayed. The most immediate management step would be administration of IV methylprednisolone 1 g. A biopsy can be obtained up to 2 weeks after steroid initiation. Laboratory studies will not be beneficial as the both ESR and CRP can be elevated but do not give a definite clinical diagnosis. The patient does need ongoing monitoring, but the priority is administering the steroids to decrease the risk of further visual damage.

6. **c) Lung cancer**. Lung cancer is the leading cause of cancer specific mortality, accounting for approximately 30% of cancer deaths in both genders. Colorectal cancer is third leading cause of cancer deaths, at 9%; pancreatic cancer is fourth (6% in males and 7% in females); and leukemia is ranked sixth, occurring at 4% in both males and females.

7. **a) Tumor invades muscle, 1 to 3 regional lymph nodes are affected, no distant metastasis**. The staging system for colorectal cancer is based upon the American Joint Committee on Cancer TNM staging. In this case, T2 the cancer has gone through the submucosa (T1) to the mucosa and into the muscle, has spread to 1 to 3 regional lymph nodes, and there is no distant metastasis. Tumors within the inner layer of the mucosa at staged at Tis (carcinoma in situ) and will likely have no lymph node or organ metastasis. Tumors penetrating the muscle would be staged as T4 with additional coding for organ involvement. The staging system does not differentiate the amount of tumors present; however, there could be multiple stages for multiple tumors.

8. **d) Tingling sensation down the back when neck is flexed**. Spinal cord compression is the second most common neurologic complication associated with cancers of the prostate, breast, and lung. Cord compression manifests with gradually worsening back pain around the level of involvement. Lhermitte's sign is a tingling sensation down the back and upper and lower limbs upon flexing or extending the neck and often an early sign of cord compression. Spinal cord compression pain worsens when the patient is supine (unlike disk disease) and with straight leg raises. Deep tendon reflexes are likely to be brisk with motor involvement.

9. **d) Mediastinal widening**. Superior vena cava syndrome can occur secondary to flow obstruction by either external compression or intravascular thrombosis. Signs and symptoms are related to the degree of flow obstruction and include shortness of breath, cough, and facial swelling. Plain chest radiographs support mediastinal widening in 64% of cases. Cavitary lesions, post obstructive pneumonia, and pneumothorax would all cause cough and shortness of breath but would not cause left arm swelling or JVD.

10. **b) Philadelphia chromosome**. Detection of Philadelphia chromosome is used for diagnosis of CML. In addition, the BCR/ABL fusion gene is used to monitor disease and response to therapy. Reed-Sternberg cells characterize the lymphoid malignancy in Hodgkin's lymphoma. Auer rods are present in acute myeloid leukemia and are formed by the aggregation of myeloid granules. The M protein is a monoclonal immunoglobulin that is produced in plasma cell disorders (multiple myeloma).

11. **c) Chemotherapy, if required, will likely be combined with genetic based targeted therapy**. Targeted drug therapy can increase the efficacy of chemotherapy through various mechanisms. The introduction of targeted therapy (antiangiogenic agents, antiepidermal growth factor receptor antibodies) has improved clinical outcomes in patients with metastatic colorectal cancer. Patients with colorectal cancer should have tumor tissue genotyped for RAS (KRAS and NAS) and BRAF mutations. Surgical resection is the treatment of choice but adjunctive therapy is necessary with metastasis. Endocrine therapy is only used in cancers originating from tissues regulated by hormones. If radiation therapy is used it will likely be combined with chemotherapy.

12. **d) Thoracentesis with pleurex catheter placement**. Patients with lung cancer often develop malignant pleural effusions; the presence often indicates a poor prognosis. Most patients with malignant pleural effusions have recurrent fluid within 30 days of initial drainage. Indwelling pleural catheter placement is a feasible palliative choice for patients with recurrent pleural effusion and allow for the pleural fluid to be drained at home versus hospital readmission. This would support a better palliative care outcome for the patient as life expectancy is limited. While a thoracentesis is indicated, it is likely that the patient will need to be readmitted for recurrent fluid buildup without an indwelling pleural catheter placement. Oxygen support via intubation is not necessary at this time. While the patient is experiencing respiratory distress, the patient remains awake, alert, and oriented with a respiratory rate less than 30 breaths per minute. An echocardiogram is not indicated as this is not an effusion related to heart failure.

13. **b) HIV antigen/antibody test**. This is a healthy patient with no clear reason to have oral thrush. Oral thrush is often the earliest recognized opportunistic infection. The patient has explicit signs and symptoms of infection with erythema and purulence, but does not have leukocytosis. Sepsis could be a reason that the WBC count is low except that the patient's vital signs are stable. The presence of oral thrush and leukopenia suggest that the patient could be immunocompromised. The patient has an infected wound with surrounding cellulitis, therefore, the ESR and CRP are likely to be elevated and will not likely provide any additional diagnostic capacity. While a hepatitis panel may be done in conjunction with HIV testing, it is not the best answer to address the clinical scenario.

14. **b) Cervical lymphadenopathy**. Following acute HIV infection, high viral replication occurs in a variety of lymphatic sites and tissues. This will cause lymphadenopathy. Acute retroviral syndrome typically occurs 2 to 6 weeks post initial exposure. Patients will also experience rash, arthralgias, fever, and pharyngitis. A goiter is an enlarged thyroid gland the result of

dysfunctional thyroid synthesis or thyroid adenoma or carcinoma. Janeway lesions are small vascular lesions found in patients with endocarditis. Kaposi sarcoma is an AIDS-associated malignancy and not typically associated with acute retroviral syndrome.

15. **b) Candida esophagitis.** Pain on swallowing and substernal burning are common symptoms with candida esophagitis. This is especially true when oral thrush is present. Patients with GERD have complaints of "heartburn" and could have dysphagia but oral candida would not be present. Patients with gastric ulcer perforation will present with severe abdominal pain that begins in the epigastrium and radiates throughout the entire abdomen. Patients with esophageal cancer typically have progressive dysphagia as an early symptoms and odynophagia with more advanced disease. Advanced esophageal will also present with pain radiating to chest and back with regurgitation and vomiting. Esophageal cancer is typically not a malignancy associated with HIV.

16. **c) Inform the patient that her request for confidentiality will be respected.** While discussion of the patient's illness should include family members, the patient's desire for confidentiality must be respected. There should be no discussion related to the patient's HIV status or other medical-related illnesses unless the patient has provided permission. HIPAA protects patients from having any type of health information disclosure without a patient's permission.

17. **b) Herpes zoster.** Herpes zoster is painful vesicular lesions that are distributed over the dermatomes. Impetigo usually presents with a single erythematous macule that evolves into a vesicle or pustule and ruptures, leaving a crusted, honey-colored exudate over the erosion. Skin on any part of the body can be involved, but the face and extremities are affected most commonly. Lesions are usually asymptomatic. Primary findings of atopic dermatitis include xerosis, lichenification, and eczematous lesions that are typically pruritic. Folliculitis presents as a papulopustular eruption and typically occurs on the face, scalp, chest, and upper back and is often associated with pruritus, pain, and desquamation.

■ BIBLIOGRAPHY

AIDSinfo, A. (2017). Guidelines for the prevention and treatment of opportunistic infections in HIV-infected adults and adolescents. *Progressive.* Retrieved from https://aidsinfo.nih.gov/contentfiles/lvguidelines/adult_oi.pdf

Benjamin, I. J., Griggs, R. C., Wing, E. J., & Fitz, J. G. (2010). *Andreoli and Carpenter's Cecil essentials of medicine* (8th ed.). Philadelphia, PA: Elsevier Saunders.

Grippi, M. A., Elias, J. A., Fishman, J. A., Kotloff, R. M., Pack, A. I., Senior, R. M., & Siegel, M. D. (2015). *Fishman's pulmonary diseases and disorders* (5th ed.). New York, NY: McGraw Hill.

James, W. D., Berger, T. G., & Elston, D. M. (2016). *Andrews' disease of the skin: Clinical dermatology* (12th ed.). Philadelphia, PA: Saunders.

Kasper, D., Hauser, S., Jameson, J., Fauci, A., Longo, D., & Loscalzo, J. (2015). *Harrison's principles of internal medicine* (19th ed.). New York, NY: McGraw-Hill

McCance, K. L., & Huether, S. E. (2014). *Pathophysiology: The biologic basis for disease in adults and children* (7th ed.). St. Louis, MO: Elsevier.

McKean, S. C., Ross, J. J., Dressler, D. D., & Scheurer, D. B. (2017). *Principles and practice of hospital medicine* (2nd ed.). New York, NY: McGraw-Hill.

National Comprehensive Cancer Network. (2017). *Clinical practice guidelines in oncologyguidelines: Colon cancer.* Retrieved from NCCN.org

U.S. Department of Health and Human Services. (2018). *Immune reconstitution inflammatroy syndrome.* Retrieved from https://aidsinfo.nih.gov/understanding-hiv-aids/glossary/787/immune-reconstitution-inflammatory-syndrome

12

Infectious Disease

DAWN CARPENTER

▦ INFECTIOUS DISEASE QUESTIONS

1. An older adult patient who was admitted after a fall down a flight of stairs, sustaining multiple rib fractures, was admitted to the ICU for pain control and respiratory support with noninvasive ventilation. On hospital day 7, he developed a fever and increased oxygen requirements, and was intubated. Repeat CBC shows a rising white count to 16.5 with a bandemia, up from 11 yesterday. Chest x-ray shows worsening atelectasis with new air bronchograms in the right lower and middle lung fields. The AG-ACNP diagnoses this as:

   a. Progressive atelectasis
   b. Hospital-acquired pneumonia
   c. Healthcare-associated pneumonia
   d. CAP

2. A middle-aged man presents with a fever, shaking chills, and malaise. He denies cough, shortness of breath, nausea, vomiting, and urinary symptoms. Past medical history is significant for hypertension, hyperlipidemia, DM, and sick sinus syndrome for which he had a permanent pacemaker implanted 6 months ago. Upon exam, the AG-ACNP notes dark areas on the tip of one finger and under two toenails and a murmur. The AG-ACNP expects which of the following is the causative organism:

   a. Streptococcus
   b. Enterococcus
   c. Staphylococcus
   d. Corynebacterium

3. A young adult woman presents with progressive shortness of breath. She appears unkempt and disheveled, having not bathed in a few days. She admits to smoking a pack of cigarettes a day, drinking six beers with a few shots daily, and IV heroin use for the past 4 months. She reports being homeless as her parents have kicked her out of the home. Vital signs: temperature 100.0°F, heart rate 100, blood pressure 100/60, respiration rate 24, and O_2 saturation 93%. Exam reveals grade IV/VI murmur heard best by the left sternal border at the fifth intercostal space. The AG-ACNP educates the patient that she needs:

   a. A peripherally inserted central catheter (PICC) line placed tomorrow
   b. IV antibiotics for 4 to 6 weeks

    c. A cardiac surgery consult for valve replacement
    d. To keep vancomycin trough 5 to 10 µg/mL

4. An adult woman was admitted for severe CAP. She had dehydration upon presentation for which she received 2 L lactated ringers over the first 24 hours. She is on day 3 of 7 of ceftriaxone and azithromycin. She is requiring less oxygen. Her BUN-to-creatinine ratio and WBC normalized on hospital day 2. She had three loose stools yesterday and today and is now complaining of abdominal pain. Her WBC is backup to 18,000 µ/L. The AG-ACNP suspects she is experiencing:

    a. *Clostridium difficile* infection
    b. Side effects from antibiotics
    c. Gastroenteritis
    d. Treatment failure of pneumonia

5. A 40-year-old woman presents with a 5-day history of a "cold" and today developed purulent yellow sinus drainage. She reports having clear nasal drainage, watery eyes, sneezing, and nonproductive cough. She denies fever, chills, and myalgias. Vital signs: temperature 98.6, heart rate 80, respiratory rate 16, blood pressure 124/76. On exam the AG-ACNP notes pharyngeal erythema and nasal passages. Palpation and percussion of sinuses reveal maxillary sinus tenderness. The treatment plan for this patient include:

    a. Prescribe amoxicillin 500 mg orally, three times a day
    b. Nasal saline lavage and decongestants
    c. Obtain culture of sinus drainage
    d. Obtain maxillofacial CT scan

6. A Nigerian immigrant presents with a persistent fever, cough, and 20-pound weight loss over 2 months. Chest x-ray shows right upper lobe infiltrate with an air-fluid level. CT scan is pending. The AG-ACNP's first step is to:

    a. Consult infectious disease
    b. Prescribe isoniazid, eifampin, pyrazinamide
    c. Obtain tuberculin skin testing and HIV testing
    d. Place on droplet precautions in negative pressure isolation room

7. An older adult presents with a sudden onset of rash that rapidly progressed on his right lower leg. The patient has severe peripheral vascular disease with 3+ pitting edema bilaterally. A 1 cm open area, draining serous fluid, is noted on the lateral aspect of the left calf. Erythema and hyperthermia is noted on exam and the patient reports tenderness to palpation. The AG-ACNP initiates:

    a. Penicillin
    b. Unna boot bilaterally
    c. Enoxaparin (Lovenox) 1 mg/kg BID
    d. Vancomycin and piperacillin/tazobactam (Zosyn)

8. A 55-year-old man is 8 weeks post liver transplant presents with back pain for 2 days that evolved into a painful rash. Upon exam, the AG-ACNP notes the rash started on his back and tracked around the left 10th rib. The rash is vesicular with open areas and oozing serous fluid. The most likely diagnosis is:

    a. Herpes zoster
    b. Atypical measles
    c. Echovirus
    d. Coxsackievirus

9. A 20-year-old college student presents with change in mental status, fever, chills, and a petechial rash. Vital signs: temperature 102.4°F, heart rate 120, respiratory rate 24, blood pressure 90/60. Upon exam, the AG-ACNP notes he is disoriented, lethargic, shows signs of dehydration, and has positive Kernig's and Bbrudzinski's signs. Blood cultures are sent, and lumbar puncture is performed. Results of the lumbar puncture demonstrated cloudy cerebrospinal fluid, with low glucose and high protein. The most likely diagnosis is:

   a. Viral meningitis
   b. Viral encephalitis
   c. Subarachnoid hemorrhage
   d. Bacterial meningitis

10. A 50-year-old woman with a medical history of obesity, hypertension, and diabetes, is post-operative day 3 following an elective total hip replacement. Her foley catheter was removed on postoperative day 1. She is now mildly confused and incontinent of urine. The urinalysis shows: 3+ leukoesterase, 3+ nitrates, 200 WBCs. The AG-ACNP treats this with:

   a. Sulfamethoxazole/trimethoprim (Bactrim)
   b. Nitrofurantoin (Macrobid)
   c. Ceftriaxone (Rocephin)
   d. Phenazopyridine (Pryidium)

11. The AG-ACNP covering the bone marrow transplant unit is called by the nurse reporting a patient who had a transplant 5 days ago has a temperature of 100.4°F (38.0°C) and an absolute neutrophil count (ANC) less than 500/μL. The most important intervention to prevent death is for the AG-ACNP to:

   a. Order blood cultures
   b. Prescribe broad spectrum antibiotics
   c. Prescribe filgrastim (Neupogen)
   d. Transfer the patient to the ICU

12. A patient admitted with septic shock related to CAP received the sepsis bundle, including central line placement, fluid resuscitation, vasopressor therapy, and broad spectrum antibiotics. The patient has resolved sepsis, weaned off vasopressors, and is completing 7-day course of antibiotics. On hospital day 7 the patient spiked a new fever to 103.3°F (39.6°C), heart rate 120, respiration rate 24, blood pressure 86/40. Chest x-ray shows resolving pneumonia, urinalysis is normal. Upon exam, the patient is warm and flushed; lungs are clear; abdomen (ABD) soft, nontender, nondistended. The most likely cause of this new fever is:

   a. Catheter-related urinary tract infection
   b. *Clostridium difficile*
   c. Catheter-related blood stream infection
   d. Hospital acquired pneumonia

13. A patient admitted with ESLD complicated by large volume of ascites and hepatic encephalopathy due to rapidly worsening ascites and decreasing mental status. Paracentesis was performed upon arrival. The peritoneal fluid was cloudy, the PMN cell count was 500/μL, and cultures are pending. The AG-ACNP's next treatment is to:

   a. Prescribe ceftriaxone (Rocephin)
   b. Obtain blood, urine, and sputum cultures
   c. Prescribe vancomycin and piperacillin/tazobactam (Zosyn)
   d. Consult interventional radiology for a transjugular intrahepatic portal shunt (TIPS) procedure

14. An older woman admitted 2 weeks ago to the ICU in septic shock has received broad spectrum antibiotics of piperacillin/tazobactam (Zosyn), levofloxacin (Levaquin), and vancomycin for 10 days. She received fluid resuscitation and vasopressor therapy for 5 days. Her recovery has been slow due to failure to respond to treatments and failure to wean off the ventilator. Her WBC remains steady at $12,000/\mu L$ and she remains afebrile. Blood cultures are negative; chest x-ray is clear. Urinalysis demonstrates WBCs, 3; negative for ketones, nitrates, and leukoesterase; but positive for hyphae. The AG-ACNP prescribes:

   a. Fluconazole (Diflucan)
   b. Amphotericin B bladder irrigation
   c. Imipenim (Primaxin) and vancomycin
   d. Ceftriaxone

■ INFECTIOUS DISEASE ANSWERS AND RATIONALES

1. **b) Hospital acquired pneumonia**. HAP is defined as pneumonia that is not incubating at the time of hospital admission and occurs 48 hours or more after admission. VAP is defined as a pneumonia occurring greater than 48 hours after endotracheal intubation. While this patient may have atelectasis, the presence of leukocytosis, bandemia, and air bronchograms are indicative of consolidation or an inflammatory process that is associated with pneumonia. CAP is defined as pneumonia that incubates within 48 hours of admission. The concept of healthcare associated pneumonia was removed in the 2016 HAP & VAP guidelines.

2. **c) Staphylococcus**. This patient has endocarditis likely related to the CEID which can occur up to 12 months after implantation of the device. Staphylococcus aureus is most common organism. Streptococcus is associated with recent upper respiratory infections, whereas enterococcus species originate from the gastrointestinal tract. Corynebacterium is an unusual organism to cause endocarditis.

3. **c) A cardiac surgery consult for valve replacement**. Endocarditis from IV drug abuse typically causes tricuspid regurgitation and is caused by staphylococcus aureus. Given the severity of her murmur, she needs to be assessed by cardiac surgery for possible valve replacement. Treatment typically requires 4 to 6 weeks of IV antibiotics, but may need longer depending on the surgical findings. A peripherally inserted central catheter (PICC) line in this patient could be considered once blood cultures are negative, but assessment of her intravenous drug use (IVDU) must be taken into consideration and thus not the best option for this patient. Vancomycin trough for MRSA bacteremia should be 15 to 20 μg/mL. Only 25% to 40% of patients will go on to need a valve replacement for left-sided endocarditis. This patient likely has left-sided endocarditis, but the severity has not been assessed, nor has the compliance with treatment been assessed yet.

4. **a) *Clostridium difficile* infection**. This patient likely has *C. diff*. Manifestations of *C. diff* infection include more than three loose stools per day and abdominal pain and leukocytosis greater than 15,000 μ/L, although patients can have a dynamic ileus, causing no stool. Side effects of antibiotics can cause diarrhea or loose stools; they would not cause a recurrent leukocytosis. Treatment failure of the pneumonia would not demonstrate improved oxygenation. Gastroenteritis is a less likely diagnosis in the inpatient setting.

5. **b) Nasal saline lavage and decongestants**. Diagnosis of acute bacterial rhinosinusitis is uncommon when duration of symptoms is less than 10 days. upper respiratory infections (URIs) are common causes of viral sinusitis, whereas bacterial sinusitis occurs in 0.2% to 2% of viral infections. Thick purulent or discolored nasal discharge is common in viral sinusitis and makes distinguishing from bacterial sinusitis difficult. Thus duration of symptoms of greater than 10 days is used to guide appropriate antibiotic prescribing. Symptom management is the mainstay of treatment for viral sinusitis, including topical and oral decongestants and nasal saline lavage. CT scans are not recommended because radiological signs are unable to differentiate between viral and bacterial sinusitis. Obtaining cultures of sinuses is done by an otolaryngologist and typically reserved for immunocompromised patients who may have fungal sinusitis.

6. **d) Place on droplet precautions in negative pressure isolation room**. The highest priority is prompt recognition and detection of cases and prevention of further transmission. Infectious disease team will be consulted but not before the patient is placed into isolation and appropriate precautions are implemented. African countries have high prevalence of HIV-associated tuberculosis, and HIV testing is indicated along with culture and sensitivity to confirm mycobacterium tuberculosis. Multidrug resistances are common, thus obtaining sensitivities are important, but not the highest priority. Treatment of active tuberculosis typically begins with four agents due to the high prevalence of multidrug resistant organisms.

7. **a) Penicillin**. A rapidly progressive rash is seen with streptococcal infections, for which penicillin is the best treatment option for this cellulitis. If the patient had systemic signs of infection such as fever, leukocytosis, or bandemia then vancomycin and piperacillin/tazobactam

would be indicated to cover for sepsis and provide MRSA coverage. Other treatment options would include penicillin, ceftriaxone, or clindamycin. Unna boots are indicated for venous stasis ulcers; however, this is not sufficient treatment for this patient's cellulitis. Lovenox is indicated in DVT.

8. **a) Herpes zoster**. Unilateral vesicular rash that follows a dermatome pattern is classic of herpes zoster. Herpes zoster in an immunocompromised patient, which includes transplant patients, should be admitted for IV acyclovir or valacyclovir. Atypical measles, echovirus, and coxsackievirus are typically morbilliform with hemorrhagic components more so than vesicular or vesiculopustular rash.

9. **d) Bacterial meningitis**. This scenario is consistent with bacterial meningitis. Viral meningitis and encephalitis will have similar presentations, however will not have cloudy cerebrospinal fluid and glucose will be normal and the Gram stain will be negative. SAH may have change in mental status and neck pain and headache. SAH will have blood in the CSF and typically does not have fever or chills or petechial rash.

10. **c) Ceftriaxone (Rocephin)**. This is a complicated UTI and recommended treatment for a complicated UTI is a fluoroquinolone or beta-lactam agent. Nitrofurantoin and Bactrim are used to treat simple UTIs and Pyridium is used to manage discomfort. Women who have diabetes are more prone to UTIs.

11. **b) Prescribe broad spectrum antibiotics**. This is a febrile patient with neutropenia, who is becoming septic. Prompt recognition and initiation of broad spectrum antibiotics is essential to prevent death. Blood cultures are important and will aid in determining the causative organism, but will not prevent death. Neupogen is indicated, but will not treat the source of infection. There is not sufficient data in the stem to determine if the patient meets ICU admission criteria.

12. **c) Catheter-related blood stream infection**. Catheter-related blood stream infection is the most likely cause of this patient change of condition. The patient has a new episode of sepsis. Chest x-ray is improving, urinalysis is normal, and abdominal exam is benign, thus lowering the possibility of catheter-related UTI, *Clostridium difficile* infection, and hospital acquired pneumonia.

13. **a) Prescribe ceftriaxone (Rocephin)**. This patient has SBP, which is presumed to occur from translocation of bacteria from the gastrointestinal tract. Patients with SBP frequently present with change in mental status, fever, and leukocytosis. The diagnosis is made when the absolute neutrophil count in the peritoneal fluid has PMN cell count of $250/\mu L$. Blood cultures should be obtained at the time, but treatment with a third-generation cephalosporin is needed. Third-generation cephalosporin is recommended if a TIPS procedure may be indicated for this patient, but is not the highest priority to treat the SBP.

14. **a) Fluconazole (Diflucan)**. This patient has a fungal urinary tract. Hyphae represent budding yeast. Candida infections are common in ICU patients who have received broad spectrum antibiotics. They are usually asymptomatic or may not be able to communicate symptoms due to intubation and ventilator use. Amphotericin bladder irrigation is not indicated. Ceftriaxone is indicated for complicated bacterial UTIs. This patient does not need imipenim or vancomycin.

■ BIBLIOGRAPHY

Kalil, A. C., Metersky, M. L., Klompas, M., Muscedere, J., Sweeney, D. A., Palmer, L. B., & Brozek, J. L. (2016). Management of adults with hospital-acquired and ventilator-associated pneumonia: 2016 clinical practice guidelines by the Infectious Diseases Society of America and the American Thoracic Society. *Clinical Infectious Diseases, 63*(5), e61–e111. doi:10.1093/cid/ciw353

Kasper, D., Hauser, S., Jameson, J., Fauci, A., Longo, D., & Loscalzo, J. (2015). *Harrison's principles of internal medicine* (19th ed.). New York, NY: McGraw-Hill.

Kauffman, C. A., Fisher, J. F., Sobel, J. D., & Newman, C. A. (2011). Candida urinary tract infections—diagnosis. *Clinical Infectious Diseases, 52*(Suppl. 6), S452–S456. doi:10.1093/cid/cir111

Runyon, B. A. (2013). Introduction to the revised American Association for the Study of Liver Diseases Practice Guideline management of adult patients with ascites due to cirrhosis 2012. *Hepatology, 57*(4), 1651–1653. doi:10.1002/hep.26359

Stevens, D. L., Bisno, A. L., Chambers, H. F., Dellinger, E. P., Goldstein, E. J., Gorbach, S. L., & Wade, J. C. (2014). Practice guidelines for the diagnosis and management of skin and soft tissue infections: 2014 update by the Infectious Diseases Society of America. *Clinical Infectious Diseases, 59*(2), e10–e52. doi:10.1093/cid/ciu444

13

Endocrine

HELEN MILEY

■ ENDOCRINE QUESTIONS

1. The patient is a 73-year-old male with past medical history of bacterial pneumonia 2 weeks ago. He now presents with generalized weakness, but otherwise asymptomatic. The relevant laboratory data demonstrate sodium of 118 mEq/L, serum osmolarity of 270 mOsm/kg, and urine osmolality of 170 Osm/kg. How should the AG-ACNP treat this patient?

   a. Begin 3% normal saline and increase the sodium level to 2 mEq/L per hour.
   b. Begin normal saline and increase the sodium level by 15 mEq/L in the next 4 hours.
   c. Begin normal saline and give furosemide 20 mg IV.
   d. Do nothing and monitor, as the patient is asymptomatic.

2. A 78-year-old male is admitted with a non-STEMI. On hospital day 2, he develops AF. As part of the workup for the AF, the AG-ACNP notes that the thyroid-stimulating hormone level is normal and T4 is low. The AG-ACNP begins levothyroxine. Which comorbidity should be monitored for?

   a. Ischemia and infarction
   b. Pulmonary edema
   c. RAF
   d. DVT

3. A 73-year-old female is complaining of fatigue, lethargy, weakness, and paresthesias. On physical exam, the AG-ACNP notes a decrease in her deep tendon reflexes and bradycardia. What diagnostic test would provide a prompt diagnosis?

   a. Electrocardiogram
   b. Thyroid studies
   c. Echocardiogram
   d. Comprehensive metabolic panel and hemoglobin A1C

4. A common symptom that accompanies the Somogyi effect and dawn phenomenon is:

   a. 7 p.m. hyperglycemia
   b. 7 a.m. hypoglycemia
   c. 7 p.m. hypoglycemia
   d. 7 a.m. hyperglycemia

5. The AG-ACNP is conducting an evaluation for heart failure in a patient with a past medical history of DM and hypertension. The AG-ACNP elicits the additional findings: deepening of the voice over the past 10 years, weight gain, thickening of the skin with skin tags, and cystic acne. What comorbidity will need to be evaluated?

   a. Hypothyoidism
   b. Pituitary adenoma
   c. Hyperprolactinemia
   d. Myedema

6. The AG-ACNP is called to the ED to evaluate a young adult patient with complaints of generalized weakness and fatigue. He is also complaining of polydipsia, nausea, and vomiting. He has no past medical history. Laboratory data reveals the following: serum glucose of 628 mg/dL, pH of 7.21, potassium 5.4 mEq/L, bicarbonate of 12 mEq/L, and with a white blood cells of 18,000 µ/L. The AG-ACNP's initial loading dose of insulin is:

   a. 0.1 to 0.15 unit/kg
   b. 3 unit/kg
   c. 5 unit/hr
   d. 10 unit single dose IV

7. The AG-ACNP is monitoring a patient with HHS, with an initial glucose of 780 mg. The nurse informs the AG-ACNP that after the first hour, the glucose is 748 mg/dL. What is the most appropriate action?

   a. Continue current therapy.
   b. Increase the drip by 2 unit/kg/hr.
   c. Administer an additional bolus dose of insulin and increase the drip.
   d. Increase the drip by 5 unit/hr.

8. The outcome for discontinuation of an insulin drip is:

   a. Closure of the anion gap
   b. Blood glucose less than 250 mg/dL
   c. Normal potassium levels
   d. Hydration has been accomplished

9. A mildly obese patient with DMII, hypertension, and depression presents to the hospital with a pulmonary embolus. As part of the history, the patient reports hirsutism and fragility of the skin. The AG-ACNP would suspect:

   a. Conn's syndrome
   b. Cushing's syndrome
   c. Adrenal hyperplasia
   d. Syndrome of inappropriate diuretic syndrome (SIADH)

10. A patient presents to the ED with tachycardia and laboratory findings of low TSH and normal free T3. She has been on amiodarone for the past 3 years. The AG-ACNP suspects type 2 amiodarone-induced thyrotoxicosis. What is the course of treatment is of highest priority?

    a. Thionamide therapy
    b. Glucocorticoids
    c. Beta-blockers
    d. Levothyroxine (Synthroid)

11. A patient presents to the ED with the symptoms of agitation and delirium. Vital signs include temperature 103°F and heart rate 110 with new onset AF. Upon examination, the AG-ACNP appreciates crackles in bilateral bases, with mild JVD. An echocardiogram is performed and the ejection fraction is 40%. The AG-ACNP's highest differential diagnosis is:

    a. Thyroid storm
    b. Sepsis
    c. Hypothyroidism
    d. Cardiomyopathy

12. The AG-ACNP is seeing a patient with the following findings: normal T3 and T4, small nodule on the thyroid with regional lymph node enlargement. The patient reports a deepening of the voice and some dysphagia. The AG-ACNP suspects this is:

    a. Myxedema
    b. Thyroid storm
    c. Thyroid carcinoma
    d. Hyperthyroidism

13. A patient presents with metastatic breast cancer and is currently receiving palliative treatment. She complains of continued weight loss and states she has no desire to eat and the taste of nutritional supplementation is not appealing. Which of the following would be an appropriate pharmaceutical agent for this patient?

    a. Megestrol acetate
    b. Estrogen
    c. Medroxyprogesterone acetate
    d. Depo-medroxyprogesterone acetate

14. An older adult female patient is brought to the ED because of worsening lethargy and somnolence. Medical history is significant for hypertension, hyperlipidemia, obesity, CHF, and hypothyroidism. The patient's husband reports she has had frequent exacerbations of her CHF requiring hospitalization due to inability to pay for her medications. The presence of which of these additional findings in this patient is most likely to suggest myxedema coma?

    a. Hyperventilation
    b. Hypertension
    c. Hypothermia
    d. Tachycardia

15. A patient is evaluated prior to undergoing subtotal thyroidectomy for Graves' disease. Which of these is most likely to increase this patient's risk for subsequent hypothyroidism?

    a. Large thyroid remnant
    b. Absence of subsequent iodine exposure
    c. Lymphocytic infiltration
    d. Protracted medical management for Graves' prior to surgery

16. An 85 year-old woman with minimal medical history presents to the ED with syncope and acute change in mental status. VS are: T 97.4F, HR irregular at 143 bpm, BP 98/50, O2 saturation 88% on RA. Per the nursing home, she has been increasingly lethargic over the last few days. Given this information, the AG-ACNP expects her thyroid function lab values to show:

    a. Normal free T4 and TSH levels
    b. Low free T4 and low TSH levels
    c. High free T4 and low TSH levels
    d. It is not necessary to check thyroid function in this patient

17. A young adult presents with nausea, vomiting, and abdominal pain a day after a party on the beach. He reports having drunk 12 to 16 beers yesterday. Vital signs include: temperature 37.5°C, heart rate 110, blood pressure 110/60, unlabored respirations of 24/min. Laboratory values include: white blood cells 16,000, hemoglobin and hematocrit (H/H) = 14/45. Basic metabolic panel reveals: sodium 148; potassium 3.4; chloride 102; carbon dioxide 14; blood urea nitrogen 30; creatinine 1.3; glucose 680. The most likely diagnosis is:

    a. Gastroenteritis
    b. Alcohol intoxication
    c. DKA
    d. HHS

18. A patient presents in DKA with the following laboratory values: white blood cells 16,000, hemoglobin and hematocrit (H/H) = 14/45; basic metabolic panel: sodium 148; potassium 3.2; chloride 102; carbon dioxide 14; blood urea nitrogen 30; creatinine 1.3; glucose 680. The AG-ACNP directs which of the following orders to be completed first:

    a. KCL 40 mEq IV over 1 hour
    b. NS @ 150 mL/hr
    c. Insulin 10 units IV bolus, followed by infusion at 10 unit/hr
    d. Blood cultures × 2 now

19. A patient presents in DKA with the following laboratory values: white blood cells 21,300, hemoglobin and hematocrit (H/H) = 16.2/51; ABG: pH 7.37/partial pressure of carbon dioxide in arterial blood (PaCO$_2$) 30/partial pressure of oxygen in arterial blood (PaO$_2$) 68/bicarbonate (Bicarb) 20/oxygen saturation (Sat) 92%/Base Excess-2; Basic metabolic panel reveals: sodium 153; potassium 4.3; chloride 102; carbon dioxide 17; blood urea nitrogen 68; creatinine 2.3; glucose 1,020. The AG-ACNP writes which of the following orders to be completed first:

    a. NS bolus 2 L IV now
    b. Insulin 0.1 unit/kg bolus, followed by infusion at 0.1 unit/hr
    c. Blood cultures × 2 now
    d. KCL 40 mEq IV over 1 hour

■ ENDOCRINE ANSWERS AND RATIONALES

1. **c) Begin normal saline and give furosemide 20 mg IV**. This patient has syndrome of inappropriate antidiuretic hormone (SIADH) with euvolemic hypotonic hyponatremia, a complication of the infectious bacterial pneumonia. If there were neurological symptoms, beginning hypertonic saline and increasing the sodium level by 1 to 2 mEq/L/hr would be appropriate. However, this patient is asymptomatic, therefore giving diuresis and sodium chloride (NaCl) is appropriate, increasing the sodium by 0.5 to 1 mEQ/hr. The current management is to correct the sodium level slowly. (b) is too rapid of a correction. Giving furosemide is incorrect, as the patient is euvolemic as demonstrated by the osmolarity values. The patient is symptomatic.

2. **a) Ischemia and infarction**. Caution should be used in older patients with underlying heart disease. Patients with a new diagnosis of hypothyroidism and known ischemic heart disease begin therapy following restoration of coronary perfusion by percutaneous coronary intervention (PCI) or coronary artery bypass graft (CABG) as the most serious side effect of treatment is ischemia and infarction. Pulmonary edema is not a concern, as the treatment does not interfere with fluid management, and the patient is already in atrial fibrillation. Deep vein thrombosis is also not a concern since thyroid disease does not have increased risk of clotting disorders.

3. **b) Thyroid studies**. This patient may be suffering from hypothyroidism. The appropriate test would be to obtain thyroid function tests. While electrocardiogram, echocardiogram and comprehensive metabolic profile, and hemoglobin A1c may be ordered as part of the work up, they will not come to a definitive diagnosis for this patient.

4. **d) 7 a.m. hyperglycemia**. Both the Somogyi effect and dawn phenomenon have 7 a.m. hyperglycemia, though the pathology of the two syndromes is different. Somogyi effect is a combination of hypoglycemia with rebound hyperglycemia, while the dawn phenomenon is the early rise in blood sugar secondary to elevation of a.m. hormones.

5. **b) Pituitary adenoma**. Acromegaly, as evidenced by the deepening of the voice, weight gain, and acne, are specific symptoms that should be evaluated. Most of the time, the cause of adult onset acromegaly is a pituitary adenoma. The other diseases do not have the symptomatology that was elicited from the patient.

6. **a) 0.1 to 0.15 unit/kg**. This patient is in DKA as evidenced by the laboratory and history. Regardless of the glucose level, fluid resuscitation and IV insulin are the mainstay, while looking of the underlying etiology of DKA. Infusions are started at 0.1 to 1.5 units/kg/hr and monitor glucose levels every hour. The other options are too high of an insulin loading dose.

7. **c) Administer an additional bolus dose of insulin and increase the drip**. The appropriate decrease in glucose on an infusion is 10% decrease after the first hour. Since this is not accomplished, an additional bolus of insulin with increase of the drip is recommended. No change in therapy is inappropriate, as the patient is still severely hyperglycemic. You cannot evaluate to increase the drip by 2 or 5 units since you have not been given information to evaluate that action.

8. **a) Closure of the anion gap**. In patients with DKA, discontinuation of the insulin drip is indicated when the anion gap is closed. Addition of dextrose in IV fluids occurs when the blood glucose levels are at or less than 250 mg/dL. Normal potassium and adequate hydration are not reasons for discontinuation of the drip.

9. **b) Cushing's syndrome**. Patients with Cushing's syndrome have nonspecific symptoms. However, they are high risk for pulmonary embolism, secondary to the hypercoagulable state. The constellation of symptoms of central obesity, DM, hypertension, and depression should lead the clinician to investigate for Cushing's syndrome. Conn's syndrome is primary hyperaldosteronism. Adrenal hyperplasia and syndrome of inappropriate antidiuretic

hormone (SIADH) do not present with the nonspecific symptoms that the patient has demonstrated.

10. **b) Glucocorticoids.** AIT has the classical laboratory value and presentation. There are two types of AIT. Type 2 is the result of a drug-related destructive thyroiditis, with no prior history of thyroid disease. Patients with type 2 AIT should receive a trial of glucocorticoids. Type 1 is associated with pre-existing nodular goiter or Graves' disease and should be treated with antithyroid therapy such as thionamide. For patients in whom the mechanism of the thyrotoxicosis is unclear, a combination of prednisone and antithyroid therapy may be considered.

11. **a) Thyroid storm.** Thyroid storm is manifested by an increase in the action of T4 and T3 that exceed the metabolic demands of the body. The classic symptoms are hyperthermia, atrial arrhythmias, high output cardiac failure, agitation and delirium, and gastrointestinal upsets. While sepsis can be considered, only the temperature would be part of the presenting symptoms. Cardiomyopathy does not present with fever and delirium. Hypothyroidism would present with hypothermia, lethargy, and so forth.

12. **c) Thyroid carcinoma.** Thyroid cancer is the most common endocrine malignancy in the United States. On presentation, the thyroid levels are normal, and therefore the patient is euthyroid. They will have small nodules and may also have regional lymph node invasion. The patient will typically complain of changes in the voice and swallowing. Myxedema coma will have more lethargy, high TSH, and low free T3, and T4 levels. Thyroid storm and hyperthyroidism will present with symptoms of tachycardia and high metabolism.

13. **a) Megestrol acetate.** Megestrol acetate would be most likely used to stimulate appetite, although it may cause potentially fatal secondary adrenal insufficiency and weight gain is mostly fat due to androgen deficiency. The remaining estrogens and progestins can cause secondary hypogonadism.

14. **c) Hypothermia.** Key diagnostic features of myxedema coma include altered mental status, hypothermia or absence of fever despite infectious disease, and a precipitating event such as this patient's CHF exacerbation. Hypoventilation, hypotension, bradycardia, and hyponatremia are also characteristic of myxedema coma.

15. **c) Lymphocytic infiltration.** Risk factors for hypothyroidism following subtotal thyroidectomy for Graves' hyperthyroidism include lymphocytic infiltration, small thyroid remnant, and subsequent exposure to iodine.

16. **c) High free T4 and low TSH levels.** The combination of lethargy and AF is a frequently cited presentation for apathetic thyrotoxicosis in the elderly. Lab values that suggest primary hyperthyroidism shows a reciprocal change in free T4 and TSH levels. Therefore, the NP would expect to see an opposite change. Because this is hyperthyroidism, there is an elevated free T4 level, and thus a reduced TSH level.

17. **c) DKA.** 80% of patients with DKA have a history of DM type 1, with 20% without the history of DM 1. Common complaints in DKA are nausea, vomiting, and severe abdominal pain. Kussmaul respirations and ketosis are also classic signs of DKA. Precipitating events of DKA include infection, trauma, myocardial infarction, drugs, alcohol, and inadequate insulin usage. HHS typically develops in older adults with DMII. HHS does not develop the same anion gap acidosis as DKA and does not have the same Kussmaul respirations. Gastroenteritis can cause DKA, but is not the cause of these laboratory values. Alcoholic ketoacidosis can resemble DKA, but there is not enough supporting evidence to state the patient is still intoxicated.

18. **a) KCL 40 mEq IV over 1 hour.** The therapeutic goals of DKA management include optimization of volume status; hyperglycemia and ketoacidosis; electrolyte abnormalities; and identifying and treating precipitating factors. Serum potassium should be closely monitored during DKA treatment. Insulin administration and correction of acidemia and hyperosmolality drive potassium intracellularly, resulting in hypokalemia that may lead to arrhythmias

and cardiac arrest. If serum potassium decreases to less than 3.3 mEq/L during DKA treatment, insulin should be stopped and potassium administered intravenously. Volume replacement of 150 mL/hr is not sufficient as DKA typically has a 6 L to 9 L water deficit; as such half should be replaced in the first few hours and the rest over the next 24 hours. Insulin bolus is based on 0.1 units/kg, followed by 0.1 unit/kg/hr. Blood cultures are important, but not the highest priority.

19. **a) NS bolus 2 L IV now**. The priority management strategy for HHS is volume repletion. It is important to start HHS therapy with a bolus of normal saline and monitor corrected serum sodium levels to determine appropriate timing to change to hypotonic fluids. Less insulin administration is required in HHS, as that insulin resistance is expected to improve with rehydration. Cultures are important, but are not the highest priority to stabilize this patient. There is less potassium shifts into the cell in HHS, compared to DKA.

■ BIBLIOGRAPHY

DiPiro, J., Talbert, T. L., Yee, G. C., Wells, B. G., & Posey, L. M. (2014). *Pharmacotherapy: A pathophysiologic approach* (9th ed.). New York, NY: McGraw-Hill.

Godara, H., Heirbe, A., Nassif, M., Otepka, H., & Rosenstock, A. (2014). *The Washington manual of medical therapeutics* (34th ed.). Philadelphia, PA: Wolters Kluwer-Lippincott Williams & Wilkins.

Gosmanov, A. R., Gosmanova, E. O., & Dillard-Cannon, E. (2014). Management of adult diabetic ketoacidosis. Diabetes, metabolic syndrome and obesity: Targets and therapy. *Dove Press, 7*, 255–264. doi: 10.2147/DMSO.S50516

Jameson, J. L DeGroot, L. J. (2016). *Endocrinology: Adult and pediatric* (7th ed.). Philadelphia, PA: Elsevier.

Kasper, D., Hauser, S., Jameson, J., Fauci, A., Longo, D., & Loscalzo, J. (2015). *Harrison's principles of internal medicine* (19th ed.). New York, NY: McGraw-Hill.

Marino, P. (2014). *Marino's the ICU book* (4th ed.). Philadelphia, PA: Wolters Kluwer Health I Lippincott Williams & Wilkins.

McCance, K. L. H. S. E. (2014). *Pathophysiology: The biologic basis for disease in adults and children* (7th ed.). St. Louis, MO: Elsevier.

Melmed, S. P. K., Larsen, P. R., & Kronenberg, H. (2011). *Williams textbook of endocrinology* (12th ed.). Philadelphia, PA: Saunders.

Papadakis, M. A., McPhee, S. J., & Rabow, M. W. (2017). *Current medical diagnosis & treatment 2017*. New York, NY: McGraw-Hill Education.

Parrillo, J., & Dellinger, R. (2013). *Critical care medicine: Principles of diagnosis and management in the adult* (4th ed.). Philadelphia, PA: Elsevier.

Tsang, W., & Houlden, R. L. (2009). Amiodarone-induced thyrotoxicosis: A review. *Canadian Journal of Cardiology, 25*(7), 421–424. doi:10.1016/S0828-282X(09)70512-4

14 Musculoskeletal

DONNA GULLETTE

MUSCULOSKELETAL QUESTIONS

1. A 25-year-old woman presents with complaint of acute onset of unilateral elbow swelling, warmth and tenderness, and cervical discharge for 1 week. She reports having two different sexual partners in the past month. Based upon these physical findings the AG-ACNP suspects she has?

   a. Gout
   b. Osteoarthritis
   c. Tennis elbow
   d. Gonococcal arthritis

2. A 40-year-old woman was diagnosed with rheumatoid arthritis and has been taking acetaminophen (Tylenol). Which of the following treatments will reduce joint inflammation and slow progression of the disease?

   a. Nonsteroidal anti-inflammatory drugs
   b. Joint aspiration
   c. Methotrexate
   d. Systemic corticosteroids

3. A 63-year-old woman presents with complaints of acute low back pain and loss of bowel function. She has a history of multiple myeloma and has been receiving chemotherapy. Physical examination reveals saddle anesthesia, decreased sphincter tone, and bilateral lower extremity weakness. The next step in management for this patient is:

   a. Consult neurosurgery
   b. CT of lower abdomen
   c. AP and lateral x-ray of lumbar spine
   d. Electromyography

4. A 66-year-old woman presents with results from her dual-energy x-ray absorptiometry (DEXA) scan. She has a T-score of a -1.5 SD at the hip and a -2.5 at the spine. Which of the following is the most accurate interpretation of these results?

    a. Osteoporosis at the spine and osteopenia at the hip
    b. Osteopenia of both areas
    c. A normal examination
    d. The Z score must be known to interpret the results

5. A 38-year-old obese waitress presents with 1 week of lower back pain, which she noted when lifting a pan full of dishes. She denies numbness, tingling, weakness, and bowel or bladder incontinence. Upon exam, deep tendon reflexes are intact, straight leg raise is normal, and patient is able to sit comfortably with legs crossed. Which of the following is the best next step?

    a. Regular doses of nonnarcotic analgesic
    b. Six days of bed rest
    c. MRI of the spine
    d. Plain film x-ray of lumbosacral spine

6. A 24-year-old man is transported to the ED in stable condition after a motor vehicle crash. His left leg was trapped under the car for several hours before he was freed. Upon examination of his left lower leg, there is ecchymosis with swelling, tenderness, severe pain, paresthesia, and pallor. The x-ray of his left leg is negative. The next step in the management of this patient is to:

    a. Apply a pressure dressing and ice to lower extremity.
    b. Consult surgery for evaluation of leg.
    c. Elevate leg above the level of the heart.
    d. Increase dosage of hydromorphone (Dilaudid).

7. A 54-year-old man was on a ladder painting the side of his house and fell, sustaining a compound fracture of his left tibia. He had an ORIF of the left tibia 3 weeks ago. He presents complaining of ongoing pain, tenderness, and nonhealing surgical site. An x-ray reveals osteomyelitis of the tibia. Which of the following antibiotic would be most appropriate to prescribe for him?

    a. Levofloxacin (Levoquin)
    b. Vancomycin (Vancocin)
    c. Cefepime (Maxipime)
    d. Ciprofloxacin (Cipro)

8. A 74-year-old woman fell on ice, landing on her buttocks. She presents with complaints of "tailbone" pain. An x-ray confirms the diagnosis of nondisplaced coccyx fracture. The best treatment of this patient is:

    a. Admit to orthopedic service for evaluation and treatment
    b. Discharge home with analgesic and bed rest for 3 to 4 weeks with hips flexed and abducted
    c. Orthopedic consultation with Hare splint application
    d. Admit for emergent ORIF to orthopedic service

9. A 60-year-old man with a history of diabetes and hypertension presents with complaint of left shoulder pain for 2 months. The pain is worse at night. He has limited range of motion in the shoulder. The AG-ACNP diagnoses the patient with adhesive capsulitis. What is the best treatment for him for immediate pain relief?

    a. Oral nonsteroidal anti-inflammatory drugs
    b. Oral prednisone
    c. Oral opioids
    d. Joint injection of lidocaine and cortisone

10. A 31-year-old female presents with complaint of severe right knee pain and swelling that began suddenly 3 hours ago. Vital signs are blood pressure 128/88 mmHg, heart rate 110, respiration

rate 18, and temperature 38.6°C. Vesiculopustular lesions are present on distal extremities. Past medical history is significant for IV drug use and 15-pack-year history of cigarette smoking. What would the AG-ACNP order to help confirm this diagnosis?

a. Bilateral ankle x-rays
b. Urine cultures
c. Blood cultures and synovial fluid aspirated
d. MRI of knee

11. A 33-year-old woman is admitted to the hospital with a diagnosis of gonococcal arthritis of her right ankle. Synovial fluid aspirate revealed a WBC count of 48,000 cells/mcL. Urine and blood cultures were positive for *Neisseria gonorrhoeae*. What antibiotics would the AG-ACNP order to treat this infection?

a. Azithromycin (Zithromax) 1 g orally now and ceftriaxone (Rocephin) 1 g IV q 12 hours
b. Amoxicillin 1 g orally now and levafloxacin (Levaquin) 750 mg q 24 hours
c. Cephalexin (Keflex) 1 g orally now and doripenem (Doribax) 500 mg IV q 8 hours
d. Procaine penicillin 1 million units intramuscularly now and ciprofloxacin (Cipro) 400 mg IV every 8 hours

12. A 41-year-old man presents with complaints of upper extremity weakness, pain, numbness, and swelling. Pain radiates from his neck down his arms, forearms, and hands. He complains of paresthesias of the volar distribution of his fourth and fifth digits of both hands. He reports his hands "feel" cold. The AG-ACNP asks him to raise his arms above his head and his hands become pallor. The AG-ACNP suspects he has?

a. Degenerative disk disease
b. Fibromyalgia
c. Thoracic outlet syndrome
d. Complex regional pain syndrome

■ MUSCULOSKELETAL ANSWERS AND RATIONALES

1. **d) Gonococcal arthritis**. She has gonococcal arthritis also known as migratory arthritis. Gonococcal arthritis presents as unilateral joint swelling, warmth, and tenderness. Even though gout causes painful inflammation in a single joint, it does not fit with the clinical presentation of cervical discharge and multiple sexual partners. Tennis elbow will cause inflammation and swelling but is related to tendonitis from overuse.

2. **c) Methotrexate**. Both NSAIDs and corticosteroids help to reduce inflammation, but neither will alter the progression of rheumatoid arthritis. DMARDs such as hydroxychloroquine, sulfasalazine, oral and parenteral gold, penicillamine, and methotrexate are most effective and methotrexate is considered the first-line treatment.

3. **a) Consult neurosurgery**. This patient has emergency situation of cauda equina syndrome requiring neurosurgery to evaluate and do the surgery. CT of the abdomen is not appropriate since it would not provide any information of the spinal cord. An MRI is the imaging that should be done. AP and lateral x-ray of the lumbar spine would show space narrowing but would not identify a lesion in the spinal cord. Electromyography (nerve conduction study) would be helpful in patients who have pain longer than 6 months.

4. **a) Osteoporosis at the spine and osteopenia at the hip**. The T-score is the number of standard deviations of a patient's bone mineral density from the mean of young adult white women. It is the standard measurement used by the World Health Organization. A score of (-2.5) standard deviation (SD) is the definition for osteoporosis. A Z-score is the number of standard deviations from the mean bone mineral density of women in the same age group.

5. **a) Regular doses of nonnarcotic analgesic**. The use of NSAIDs is best for acute pain. Bed rest has not been shown to improve low back pain. She should continue to be active as long as the activities do not make the pain worse. Imaging in not necessary with uncomplicated low back pain.

6. **b) Consult surgery for evaluation of leg**. He has likely developed compartment syndrome which requires surgery consult. Most surgeons prefer to check their own compartment pressure to determine if a fasciotomy is needed. Elevating the leg will help with swelling but not reduce the pressure from compartment syndrome. Applying a pressure dressing and ice would further compromise the extremity. Increasing dilaudid will mask symptoms and delay diagnosis and definitive intervention.

7. **b) Vancomycin (Vancocin)**. Vancomycin is the most appropriate and will cover MRSA. Fluoroquinolones may have a detrimental effect on the facture healing and may be associated with higher infection rates when used as a single agent. Other broad-spectrum coverage may be prescribed for Gram-negative coverage, but also needs MRSA coverage. If broad-spectrum coverage is started, de-escalate as soon as Gram stain and sensitivities result. Cefepime has greater coverage of Gram-negative organisms, whereas this is most likely a Gram-positive infection.

8. **b) Discharge home with analgesic and bed rest for 3 to 4 weeks with hips flexed and abducted**. There is not a treatment for fractured coccyx (unless fragments displaced) except bed rest and analgesics for pain. Schedule a follow-up with orthopedics in 2 to 3 weeks if pain continues. These fractures generally heal on their own.

9. **d) Joint injection of lidocaine and cortisone**. Adhesive capsulitis is very painful. Patients benefit most from lidocaine/cortisone injection in the shoulder. The patient will need to follow up with orthopedics for further evaluation. While oral NSAIDs, prednisone, and opioids would also provide pain relief, they would not take effect immediately.

10. **c) Blood cultures and synovial fluid aspirated**. This presentation is significant for nongonococcal acute bacterial arthritis. The synovial fluid aspirate would confirm the presences of elevated WBC count and low glucose level. The aspirate would also rule out gout, pseudogout, and gonococcal infections.

11. **a) Azithromycin (Zithromax) 1 g orally now and ceftriaxone (Rocephin) 1 g IV q 12 hours**. Azithromycin will also cover chlamydia if there is a coinfection and eradicates gonorrhea.

12. **c) Thoracic outlet syndrome**. The numbness, paresthesias, and pallor of the hands when raised above the head are consistent with thoracic outlet syndrome due to compression of the neurovascular structures in the upper extremities. MRI will confirm obstructed blood flow. Degenerative disk disease does not cause pallor of the hand but will cause numbness and paresthesias.

▪ BIBLIOGRAPHY

Halter, J. B., Oslander, J., Studenski, S., High, K. P., Asthana, S., Supiano, M. A., & Ritchie, C. (2017). *Hazzard's geriatric medicine and gerontology* (7th ed.). New York, NY: McGraw-Hill.

Hendrich, A. (2017). *Fall risk assessment for older adults: The Hendrich II fall risk model*. Retrieved from https://consultgeri.org/try-this/general-assessment/issue-8

Papadakis, M. A., McPhee, S. J., & Rabow, M. W. (2017). *Current medical diagnosis & treatment 2017*. New York, NY: McGraw-Hill.

Tintinalli, J. E. (2016). *Tintinalli's emergency medicine: A comprehensive study guide* (8th ed.). New York, NY: McGraw-Hill.

Workowski, K. A., & Berman, S. M. (2007). Centers for Disease Control and Prevention sexually transmitted diseases treatment guidelines. *Clinical Infectious Diseases, 44*(Suppl. 3), S73–S76. doi:10.1086/511430

15

Integumentary

GAIL LIS

INTEGUMENTARY QUESTIONS

1. The AG-ACNP is completing an assessment on a 78-year-old female who states she has had a painless area on her forehead for some time that she is concerned about. She is worried that she may have skin cancer. On exam the AG-ACNP notes an isolated papule that is rough, poorly circumscribed, and erythematous with white scaling. The AG-ACNP suspects the lesion to be:

   a. Actinic keratosis
   b. Basal cell carcinoma
   c. Squamous cell carcinoma
   d. Melanoma

2. The older adult patient is at increased risk for pressure ulcers secondary to which of the following integumentary changes associated with aging:

   a. Decreased threshold for pressure and touch
   b. Increased dermal thickness
   c. Decreased epidermal proliferation
   d. Decreased collagen cross-links

3. An 82-year-old female is being cared for on a medical unit for aspiration pneumonia. She is receiving broad-spectrum antibiotics and is primarily bedridden. The nurse caring for the patient tells the AG-ACNP that upon removing the patient's brief, she noticed redness to the lower back. Upon assessment the AG-ACNP notices diffuse erythematous patches to the lower back extending into the gluteal fold with small areas of pustules in a satellite pattern. The patient denies pain but states she can feel some irritation. Based upon this assessment, the AG-ACNP orders:

   a. Acyclovir
   b. Nystatin powder
   c. Transparent film
   d. Hydrocortisone 1% cream

4. Lesions associated with acne vulgaris are typically described as:

   a. Vesicular
   b. Pustular
   c. Bullous
   d. Papular

5. A 46-year-old male patient presents to the ED with a rash that is prominent over the trunk and proximal extremities. The patient states the rash started several days after completing a 7-day course of Bactrim for a mild skin infection. The patient is concerned because the rash seems to be getting worse and is now forming blisters. He even thinks they are inside his mouth on his lower lip. Upon exam, large vesicle target-like lesions are noted. The lesions are greater than 0.5 cm in diameter. Based upon this assessment, the AG-ACNP suspects:

   a. Allergic vasculitis
   b. Exfoliative dermatitis
   c. Drug exanthem
   d. SJS

6. The AG-ACNP is caring for an 82-year-old female with chronic aspiration pneumonia. Upon assessment the AG-ACNP notes an ulcer to the patient's left ischial tuberosity. The ulcer is noted to be partial thickness with a fluid-filled blister and the overall wound bed is red and moist. Based upon this assessment, the ulcer is staged at:

   a. Stage I
   b. Stage II
   c. Stage III
   d. Deep tissue injury

7. A 92-year-old patient is being cared for on the medical unit with sepsis secondary to infected decubitus ulcer. The ulcer is assessed to be stage IV with copious amounts of exudative drainage. The best treatment for this type of ulcer is:

   a. Foam island
   b. Hydrocolloids
   c. Alginate
   d. Hydrogel

8. A 24-year-old male with no past medical history and no known drug allergies presents with worsening redness, pain, and swelling to his right lower extremity. The symptoms started out as a small area of redness just below his knee where he wears his kneepads for protection while playing hockey, and increased in size to what appears to be a boil. Upon assessment, the AG-ACNP notes an erythematous, warm, raised lesion with mild fluctuance to the skin distal to the right patella. His vital signs are stable with the exception of a low-grade fever. Based upon this assessment, the AG-ACNP performs an incision and drainage and orders:

   a. Cephalexin (Keflex) 1 g oral every 8 hours for 7 days
   b. Ciprofloxacin (Cipro) 500 mg oral every 12 hours for 7 days
   c. Amoxicillin/clavulanate (Augmentin) 875 mg oral every 8 hours for 7 days
   d. Sulfamethoxazole/trimethoprim (Bactrim DS) 1 tablet oral, twice a day for 7 days

9. A 63-year-old patient is started on nafcillin IV every 4 hours for bacterial endocarditis. Shortly after starting the medication, the patient reports significant pruritus with raised lesions to his chest. Upon exam the AG-ACNP notes erythematous wheals to the patient's upper chest without respiratory compromise. This presentation is most likely associated with what type of drug reaction:

   a. Type I
   b. Type II
   c. Type III
   d. Type IV

10. A 45-year-old male was brought to the hospital via emergency medical services from his workplace following a chemical exposure with acid to his right upper extremity. Upon evaluation, a second-degree burn is suspected based upon which of the following assessment criteria:

   a. Mild pain, no blister formation
   b. Painless, no blister formation
   c. Painless, blister formation
   d. Moderate pain, blister formation

■ INTEGUMENTARY ANSWERS AND RATIONALES

1. **a) Actinic keratosis.** Actinic keratoses are benign precancerous lesions caused by chronic UV radiation and are characterized by tender, rough, poorly circumscribed, erythematous papules with white or yellow scaling. These lesions are typically found in older adults. They appear most often in areas with prolonged sun exposure. Basal cell carcinoma has three common appearances: (a) waxy translucent papule with overlying telangiectasias with central ulceration, (b) scar like, (c) erythematous macule or papule with fine scale or superficial erosion often surrounded by telangiectasia. Squamous cell carcinoma presents as occasional tender, erythematous papule, plaque, or nodule with keratotic scale. Melanoma is typically irregularly shaped with variations in tan, brown, and gray discoloration.

2. **c) Decreased epidermal proliferation.** Physiologic changes that occur with aging include thinning of the dermis and epidermis, decreased epidermal proliferation, and increased collagen cross links. These changes cause increased skin fragility and cell irregularity contributing to increased vulnerability to trauma and irritant dermatitis. Older adults have an increased threshold for pressure and touch thereby increasing the risk injury.

3. **b) Nystatin powder.** This patient is at risk for fungal skin infection related to administration of broad-spectrum antibiotics and bedridden status wearing a brief. Candidiasis is most common fungal skin organism. Candida pustules can develop on the backs of bedridden patients and appear as red patches, sometimes with erosion, and peripheral satellite pustules. Nystatin powder is a topical polyene that is used to treat fungal skin infections. Acyclovir is prescribed for herpes zoster and these lesions are typically grouped vesicles on an erythematous base along a dermatome. Transparent film will protect the area from friction but will not decrease the fungal load. Topical steroids are used to decrease inflammation and itching but will not inhibit the synthesis of ergosterol (an essential component of the fungal cytoplasmic membrane).

4. **b) Pustular.** Acne vulgaris is associated with pustular lesions. These lesions are filled with yellow proteinaceous fluid. Herpes zoster lesions are vesicular (palpable elevations with fluid-filled cavities). Impetigo and pemphigoid are associated with bullous lesions; these lesions are 1.0 cm or larger and fluid filled. Papular lesions are slightly raised; nonfluid filled are associated with basal cell carcinoma, hyperkeratotic lesions.

5. **d) SJS.** Target-like lesions with bulla beginning with the trunk and spreading to the proximal extremities with mucosal involvement are reflective of SJS. SJS is often associated with sulfonamides. Drug exanthema is typically morbilliform and maculopapular in appearance and does not involve the mucus membranes. Allergic vasculitis presents as a small (2 mm) purpuric papule on the lower extremity. Exfoliative dermatitis is red and scaly involving the entire skin surface and occurs 2 to 6 weeks after first dose of medication. All of the skin eruptions noted can be caused by sulfonamides.

6. **b) Stage II.** Stage I ulcers are intact with blanchable erythema. Stage II ulcers are partial thickness, loss of skin with exposed dermis. The wound bed is visible, pink, red, and moist, and may present as an intact or ruptured blister. Adipose fat or deeper tissues are not visible. Stage III ulcers are full thickness, adipose fat is visible in addition to slough and/or eschar. Deep tissue injury is assessed by intact or nonintact skin with nonblanchable, deep red or purple discoloration.

7. **c) Alginate.** Alginate is a silver-impregnated dressing that works to decrease the bioburden and is used for Stage III/IV ulcer with excessive drainage and infection. Foam island and hydrocolloids are used for Stage II/III ulcers with low to moderate exudate. Hydrogels alone are contraindicated in wounds with excess exudate and, if used, should be combined with a gauze dressing.

8. **d) Sulfamethoxazole/trimethoprim (Bactrim DS) 1 tablet oral, twice a day for 7 days**. Community-acquired MRSA (CAMRSA) is the suspected organism causing the symptoms. The patient's risk factor is sports-related use of equipment with close skin contact. Bactrim, doxycycline and clindamycin all have good sensitivity to CAMRSA bacteria and are first-line treatment for such a diagnosis. The patient would not meet admission criteria and it is feasible to begin oral antimicrobial after the incision and drainage. The remaining antibiotics would provide adequate coverage for streptococcus- and methicillin-sensitive staphylococcal organisms.

9. **a) Type I**. The patient is experiencing a Type I immediate immunologic reaction that is manifested by urticarial and angioedema of the skin (wheals). Type II is initiated by the interaction of drugs plus cytotoxic antibodies causing lysis of cells (platelets and leukocytes), leading to petechial rash. Type III is more delayed, with the development of immune complexes; this reaction may cause urticaria and vasculitis. Type IV is cell-mediated immune reaction that releases cytokines and cause morbilliform exanthematous reactions associated with SJS.

10. **d) Moderate pain, blister formation**. Second-degree or partial-thickness burns involve all of the epidermis and parts of the dermis. These burns are characterized by blister formation and moderate to severe pain. First-degree burns involve the epidermis only and are characterized by erythema but no blister formation. The site is painful. Third-degree burns are typically painless and have a white dry waxy appearance without blister formation.

■ BIBLIOGRAPHY

Benjamin, I. J., Griggs, R. C. Wing, E. J., & Fitz, J. G. (2010). *Andreoli and Carpenter's Cecil essentials of medicine* (8th ed.). Philadelphia, PA: Elsevier Saunders.

Bickley, L., & Szilagyi, P. (2013). *Bates' guide to physical examination and history taking*. Philadelphia, PA: Lippincott.

Doherty, G. (2015). *Current diagnosis and treatment: Surgery*. New York, NY: McGraw-Hill Education.

Flaherty, E. R. B (2014). *Geriatric nursing review syllabus: A core curriculum in advanced practice geriatric nursing*. New York, NY: American Geriatrics Society.

Goolsby, M. J. G. L. (2015). Advanced assessment interpreting findings and formulating differential diagnoses (2th ed.). Philadelphia, PA: F.A. Davis.

Halter, J. B., Oslander, J., Studenski, S., High, K. P., Asthana, S., Supiano, M. A., & Ritchie, C. (2017). *Hazzard's geriatric medicine and gerontology* (7th ed.). New York, NY: McGraw-Hill.

Kasper, D., Hauser, S., Jameson, J., Fauci, A., Longo, D., & Loscalzo, J. (2015). *Harrison's principles of internal medicine* (19th ed.). New York, NY: McGraw-Hill.

Liu, C., Bayer, A., Cosgrove, S. E., Daum, R. S., Fridkin, S. K., Gorwitz, R. J., & Murray, B. E. (2011). Clinical practice guidelines by the Infectious Diseases Society of America for the treatment of methicillin-resistant Staphylococcus aureus infections in adults and children. *Clinical Infectious Diseases, 52*(3), e18–e55. doi:10.1093/cid/ciq146

McKean, S. C., Ross, J. J., Dressler, D. D., & Scheurer, D. B. (2017). *Principles and practice of hospital medicine* (2nd ed.). New York, NY: McGraw-Hill.

Papadakis, M. A., McPhee, S. J., & Rabow, M. W. (2017). *Current medical diagnosis & treatment 2017*. New York, NY: McGraw-Hill Education.

Rosenthal, L. B. J. (2018). *Lehne's pharmacotherapeutics for advanced practice providers*. St. Louis, MO: Elsevier.

Soutor, C. H. M. (2013). *Clinical dermatology* (1st ed.). New York, NY: McGraw-Hill Education.

Stevens, D. L., Bisno, A. L., Chambers, H. F., Dellinger, E. P., Goldstein, E. J., Gorbach, S. L., & Wade, J. C. (2014). Practice guidelines for the diagnosis and management of skin and soft tissue infections: 2014 update by the Infectious Diseases Society of America. *Clinical Infectious Diseases, 59*(2), e10–e52. doi: 10.1093/cid/ciu444

Williams, B. A., Chang, A., Ahalt, C., Chen, H., Conant, R., Landefeld, C. S., Richie, C., . . . Yukawa, M. (2014). *Current diagnosis and treatment geriatrics* (2nd ed.). New York, NY: McGraw-Hill.

16

Psychosocial, Behavioral, and Cognitive Health

ANTHONY McGUIRE AND VICTORIA CREEDON

PSYCHOSOCIAL, BEHAVIORAL, AND COGNITIVE HEALTH QUESTIONS

1. A 19-year-old male presents with complaints of "heart racing." The ECG demonstrates a normal sinus rhythm with a rate of 96 and occasional premature atrial contraction (PAC) and no ST-segment changes. His troponin is 0.01 ng/mL (normal <0.05 ng/mL). On examination, the patient is noticeably nervous. He is sweating, and his skin is warm. He describes symptoms suddenly began as he started an oral presentation in one of his college classes. There is a history of three prior episodes like this in which he feels like he is "going to die." He states that he has been overwhelmed with school lately. What is the most appropriate management for this patient?

   a. Call a psychiatry consult for potential outpatient therapy.
   b. Admit the patient to the cardiology service for further workup.
   c. Give the patient haloperidol (Haldol) 5 mg IV ×1.
   d. Discharge the patient on lorazepam (Ativan) 1 mg orally as needed with instructions to follow up with his PCP.

2. A 31-year-old female who has been healthy is admitted to a medical–surgical floor for postoperative monitoring after an appendectomy. She is sitting up, alert and oriented, and sipping on some juice. She asks the AG-ACNP to order alprazolam 0.5 mg every night at bedtime and sertraline 100 mg orally daily because she takes them at home for her generalized anxiety disorder. The two medications are recorded on the reconciliation form that was completed during her admission assessment. What is the appropriate action for the AG-ACNP?

   a. Offer the patient trazodone 50 mg BID every night at bedtime instead.
   b. Do not restart either medication.
   c. Restart the sertraline only.
   d. Restart both medications.

3. A 76-year-old male has been in the ICU for 10 days recovering from CAP. He was transferred today to a bed on the floor where he has two roommates. The night nurse calls the AG-ACNP to report that the patient has been awake all night and is now very agitated and will not take his medications. Upon examination, the patient is noticeably confused and does not remember

why he is in the hospital. He is yelling and combative with the staff as they struggle to keep him from hurting himself. Which of the following is an appropriate step in managing this patient?

a. Move the patient down the hall to a quieter room.
b. Call the patient's family and ask if someone can speak to him to help him to reorient.
c. Prescribe lorazepam (Ativan) 0.5 mg IV every 2 hours as needed for agitation.
d. Check a corrected QT interval (QTc) and prescribe haloperidol (Haldol) 2.5 mg V ×1 now for agitation.

4. The AG-ACNP is asked to see an 88-year-old male with new onset disorientation and issues with attention. No other abnormalities are noted. These changes occurred over the past 24 hours and are a significant change in the patient's baseline. The AG-ACNP suspects delirium based on which of the following:

a. An additional cognitive disturbance (memory deficit, visuospatial or language-ability deficit)
b. Worry and fear with withdrawn behavior
c. A direct physiological consequence of another medical condition
d. The condition does not fluctuate over the course of the day

5. The AG-ACNP calls a neuropsychiatric consult for evaluation and management of a patient with Alzheimer's dementia. What pharmacologic management should be anticipated?

a. Carvidopa-levidopa (Sinemet)
b. Donepezil (Aricept) and memantine (Namenda)
c. Aspirin
d. Lorazepam and amitriptyline

6. Socioeconomic and cultural variations can make the diagnosis of major or minor neurocognitive changes due to Alzheimer's disease difficult. Which of the following statement is true?

a. It is easy to conduct objective cognitive assessments on those with low education.
b. Memory loss is always considered a natural part of aging in some cultures.
c. Individuals who face fewer cognitive demands in everyday life are more challenging to assess for functional decline.
d. Highly educated and financially well-off individuals are less likely to notice changes in cognitive function and do not access care.

7. Which of the following is a prognostic and/or risk factor for major or mild neurocognitive disorder due to Alzheimer's disease:

a. Traumatic brain injury
b. Klinefelter syndrome
c. Exposure to pesticides and herbicides
d. Viral illness

8. A 59-year-old patient with history of hypertension, hyperlipidemia, and DMII presents to the clinic for a follow-up appointment, where he reported not taking all his medications as prescribed. He suffered an intracranial hemorrhage 2 years ago due to hypertension. His wife accompanies him and says that he has been increasingly forgetful over the past several months. In order to optimize his condition, the AG-ACNP recommends which of the following:

a. Treating his underlying hypertension, hyperlipidemia, and DM
b. Starting donepezil (Aricept) and memantine (Namenda)
c. Starting carvidopa-levidopa (Sinemet)
d. Starting quetiapine (Seroquel)

9. A 27-year-old female presents with signs and symptoms of dehydration. She is crying and does not want to discuss anything. Her husband reveals to the AG-ACNP that his wife has been staying in bed more and more over the past month. He has noticed her appetite has significantly decreased in the past week. She is running out of sick time at her job and he is worried they will fire her. During a structured interview to assess for depression, the patient states she had a miscarriage 6 months ago and has not felt like herself since and cannot seem to engage in her usual hobbies and visits with friends. A psychiatry consult is requested. Which therapy would be anticipated?

   a. Amitriptyline (Elavil) and a support group referral
   b. ECT
   c. Fluoxetine (Prozac) along with cognitive behavioral therapy
   d. Lithium (Lithobid) with weekly mental health visits

10. A 32-year-old male patient is brought into to the ED by emergency medical services after a 911 call from a convenience store clerk. The patient was very aggressive and yelling at another customer. The clerk worried that the patient was on illicit drugs. On exam, the patient is speaking very quickly and seems to be jumping from thought to thought. He does not really answer questions and instead continues to talk with an obvious mood elevation. He keeps leaving the stretcher to pace around the room. His drug screen comes back negative. What is the most likely diagnosis of this patient?

   a. Borderline personality disorder
   b. Bipolar disorder with manic episode
   c. Antisocial personality disorder
   d. Schizophrenia

11. A 43-year-old male is being discharged from the hospital after a major myocardial infarction that required coronary artery bypass surgery. Prior to discharge, the nurse used the PHQ to screen for depression and notified the AG-ACNP that the score on the PHQ 2-item screening tool is 3 and the 9-item screening tool is 16. Based on this information, the AG-ACNP would:

   a. Start an SSRI and cancel the discharge to do cardiac monitoring for the next 24 hours.
   b. Discharge the patient with a referral for further assessment by a mental health professional.
   c. Consider the PHQ screening invalid because the patient has somatic symptoms from the myocaridal infarction which explains the high score on the tool.
   d. Give the patient a prescription for bupropion (Wellbutrin) and ask the wife to arrange psychotherapy.

12. A 34-year-old female presents with complaints of abdominal pain. Her diagnostic evaluation is negative. She is very agitated and states that she needs to be discharged with pain medication. She received 4 mg of morphine IV 30 minutes ago with some pain relief but now she is complaining of pain again. Pertinent history is that she has been in this facility 13 times in the past 4 months with similar complaints of abdominal pain. What is the best action the AG-ACNP should take next?

   a. Discharge the patient with a short course of oxycodone until she sees her PCP.
   b. Admit the patient as she is having ongoing pain issues.
   c. Discharge the patient with a short course of oral morphine.
   d. Run a report on the state's prescription monitoring database.

13. A 45-year-old male patient is admitted after being in a motor vehicle crash that left him with bilateral rib and right humeral fractures. The patient has a history of opioid abuse and is in recovery after being treated in a drug addiction program over a year ago. A new colleague has just seen the patient and requests a consult regarding reported poor pain control. The patient

is fearful of taking opioids because of his history. Which of the following therapies should be suggested?

a. Do not prescribe anything as the patient has an addiction history.
b. Prescribe Tylenol and ibuprofen only.
c. Suggest that the patient be evaluated for an epidural or regional block.
d. Prescribe oxycodone as needed with morphine for breakthrough pain.

14. A 35-year-old female patient is admitted with CAP. While being interviewed, the patient confides that she drinks six to seven alcoholic beverages almost every day. Her last drink was earlier this morning. What should the AG-ACNP order for this patient?

a. CIWA
b. Disulfiram (Antabuse) on discharge
c. Periodic opioid therapy to prevent withdrawal
d. Phenytoin to be given in case the patient seizes

15. A 52-year-old female with a history of depression presents to the ED with a large laceration on her right forearm that requires 28 sutures to close. When asked about the incident she says she was packing up her home when a large mirror broke, and she cut her arm in the process. Upon discharge the patient states that the she is packing up a lot of things that she does not need and that she "is trying to get everything in order." What is the next best action for the AG-ACNP to take?

a. Assess the patient for suicidal ideation.
b. Discharge the patient home.
c. Increase the patient's home antidepressant.
d. Ask the patient if she has been abusing drugs or alcohol.

16. Which of the following symptoms is a sign of suicidal behavior?

a. Putting affairs in order
b. Talking about plans for next week
c. Becoming more involved with friends
d. Beginning a new exercise routine

17. A 42-year-old male patient presents to the ED from urgent care with a chief complaint of a headache and blood pressure of 184/98. He reports having a history of hypertension and is on three antihypertensive medications. Additional pertinent history includes his discontinuation of two of the three medications because he felt he did not need all of them. The AG-ACNP orders labetalol 10 mg IV to be given now and his blood pressure is stabilized. Which of the following would be appropriate next steps for this patient?

a. Motivational interviewing
b. Give him educational handouts about his medications
c. Discharge him home with instructions to follow up with his PCP
d. Tell him he could have a stroke if he does not take his medications

■ PSYCHOSOCIAL, BEHAVIORAL, AND COGNITIVE HEALTH ANSWERS AND RATIONALES

1. **a) Call a psychiatry consult for potential outpatient therapy**. This patient is suffering from a panic disorder. He has had repeat panic attacks. Palpitations, sweating, and feelings of impending doom are all symptoms of panic attacks. His ECG and cardiac enzymes are normal, and there is no indication for a further cardiac workup. The treatment of choice for panic and other anxiety disorders is cognitive behavioral therapy. Patients can also be prescribed antidepressants, anxiolytics, and beta-blockers. Haloperidol (Haldol) is not an appropriate drug for this patient. While lorazepam (Ativan) is an anxiolytic, it would not be appropriate to initiate this therapy without consultation to a psychiatrist or referral to a more specialized clinician to manage the patient's prescription and care.

2. **d) Restart both medications**. The patient should be restarted on both medications. She is tolerating orally and should be allowed to take her home medications as long as there is no contraindication, which there are none indicated in this question. Restarting her benzodiazepine is important as she has the potential to have withdrawals from this medication which could result in adverse side effects including seizures. She is alert, oriented, and at relatively low risk for delirium given her age and overall good health status. In older adults or patients with other risk factors for delirium, providers should be cautious with the use of benzodiazepines and the hospitalization would offer a good opportunity to assess the tolerance of the benzodiazepine or change the treatment plan if necessary.

3. **b) Check a QTc and prescribe haloperidol (Haldol) 2.5 mg V ×1 now for agitation**. The patient is suffering from delirium. Nonpharmacologic options are preferred in these patients. This patient is in danger of hurting himself and the staff in his current state of acute agitation, so a low-dose Haldol injection would be appropriate. The QTc interval should be monitored in patients given Haldol to monitor for prolongation. Use Haldol with caution in patients with a QTc interval greater than 400 mS or those on other medications that increase the QTc or those with electrolyte imbalance. Benzodiazepines can contribute to delirium, especially in the elderly.

4. **a) An additional cognitive disturbance (memory deficit, visuospatial or language-ability deficit)**. The *Diagnostic and Statistical Manual of Mental Disorders*, fifth edition diagnostic criterion includes "an additional disturbance in cognition" (i.e., memory deficit, disorientation, language, visuospatial ability, or perception). Worry, fear, and withdrawn behavior would indicate anxiety or depression and not delirium. Physiologic conditions from other medical conditions would be pertinent negative in the diagnosis of delirium. The changes in orientation and attention tend to fluctuate over the course of a day with delirium, therefore, the lack of fluctuation would be a pertinent negative.

5. **b) Lorazepam and amitriptyline**. Cholinesterase inhibitors (donepezil/Aricept) and NMDA antagonists (memantine/Namenda) are indicated for slowing of progression of Alzheimer's dementia. Carvidopa-levidopa (Sinemet) can be part of therapy for Lewy body dementia with Parkinson's disease. Aspirin is indicated along with medical management of underlying vascular issues, hypertension, hyperlipidemia, and diabetes in vascular dementia. Part of Alzheimer's treatment is symptom management which can include antidepressants and anxiolytics, although benzodiazepines and antipsychotics are not first-line therapy for these patients.

6. **c) Individuals who face fewer cognitive demands in everyday life are more challenging to assess for functional decline**. It is more difficult to conduct cognitive assessments on people with lower educational levels. Memory loss may be considered a natural part of aging in some cultures, but not always or in every culture. Highly educated and financially well-off individuals are more likely to notice changes in cognitive function and do have access to care.

7. **a) Traumatic brain injury**. Traumatic brain injury, individuals reaching midlife with Down syndrome (trisomy 21), and a genetic susceptibility polymorphism apolipoprotein E4 are all risk factors for neurocognitive disorders due to Alzheimer's disease and delirium. Exposure to pesticides and herbicides are precursors for Parkinson's disease. Klinefelter syndrome may feature learning disabilities and delayed speech and language development. Viral illness, including respiratory or gastrointestinal viruses, are often cited a precursor to GBS.

8. **a) Treating his underlying hypertension, hyperlipidemia, and diabetes**. This patient has several risk factors for vascular dementia, including hypertension, hyperlipidemia, diabetes, and a previous intracranial hemorrhage. Care for these patients focuses on prevention and optimizing the treatment of their underlying conditions. Starting aspirin has also been associated with improvement in this patient population.

9. **c) Fluoxetine (Prozac) along with cognitive behavioral therapy**. This patient is most likely suffering from MDD. It is unknown if the patient had symptoms prior to the miscarriage. However, she is exhibiting anhedonia, increased sleeping, and appetite loss for an extended period of time. A psychiatry consult is in order to establish the MDD. First-line therapy for MDD is an SSRI (fluoxetine), cognitive behavioral therapy, and social support. In addition, fluoxetine is an SSRI generally considered safe for pregnancy if the patient is still actively trying to conceive. Amitriptyline (a tricyclic antidepressant) is not a first-line agent. ECT is also not a first-line therapy for MDD, and is usually started as an adjunct after failing pharmacotherapy and psychotherapy. Lithium is used for bipolar disorder.

10. **b) Bipolar disorder with manic episode**. The patient has several hallmark symptoms of a manic episode (persistent increased activity and/or energy, irritability, excessive mood elevation easily recognized by others) consistent with bipolar disorder. Borderline personality disorder is a pervasive history of unstable self-image, affects, and interpersonal relationships, along with impulsivity starting in early adulthood. Antisocial personality disorder must include a long history of a pervasive disregard of the rights of others with violation of the rights of others that began before the age of 15. Schizophrenia disorder requires "two or more of the following, each present for a significant portion of time during a 1-month period (or less if successfully treated). At least one of these must be (1), (2), or (3): 1. Delusions 2. Hallucinations. 3. Disorganized speech (e.g., frequent derailment or incoherence). 4. Grossly disorganized or catatonic behavior. 5. Negative symptoms (i.e., diminished emotional expression or avolition)."

11. **b) Discharge the patient with a referral for further assessment by a mental health professional**. The PHQ is a screening tool and is validated to be reliable and sensitive for depression. The scores range from 0 to 27. The first two items on the tool constitute the PHQ-2. If there is a score of zero on the first two items, there is no need to continue as a diagnosis of depression cannot be made (anhedonia and blue mood must be present and these are the target symptoms of the two PHQ-2 questions). Once there is a score of 1 or more on the PHQ-2, the PHQ-9 (7 additional questions added to the PHQ-2) is completed. A score of 15 to 19 indicates moderate to major depression is likely present. There is no need to do cardiac monitoring when starting a SSRI. SSRIs are first-line therapy for depression but should only be ordered once a mental health professional has done an exam to diagnose the depression. The PHQ can then be used to monitor symptoms, but no recommendation exists to base treatment on a screening tool score. The tool is valid even with somatic symptoms. Wellbutrin is not a first-line therapy, especially without a mental health professional assessment, and the wife should not be asked to make a referral on her own.

12. **d) Run a report on the state's prescription monitoring database**. The patient's frequent visits are red flags for possible doctor shopping associated with narcotic abuse and/or addiction. It would be most appropriate to first look up the patient on the prescription monitoring database to see if she has recently received other narcotic prescriptions before prescribing anything further.

13. **c) Suggest that the patient be evaluated for an epidural or regional block**. If the patient is concerned about using opioids, other types of analgesia should be used first. A regional

block or epidural is appropriate in this patient because it would allow the patient to have better local pain control for his rib fractures without requiring opioids. This patient would also benefit from multimodal analgesia such as adding Tylenol and gabapentin to his current medication regimen. If the patient was in an ICU setting, ketamine could be a viable option for continuous analgesia. Undertreating pain in patients with addiction histories has not proven to be beneficial and can in fact be harmful and predispose them to abusing drugs again.

14. **a) CIWA.** This patient is at risk for alcohol withdrawal. CIWA would be appropriate for this patient with as-needed benzodiazepines or standing phenobarbital. It would not be appropriate to discharge the patient on a medication like disulfiram (Antabuse), as that therapy requires strict outpatient monitoring. Opioids are not indicated for alcohol withdrawal. Phenytoin is contraindicated in alcohol withdrawal.

15. **a) Assess the patient for suicidal ideation.** One of the signs of suicidal behavior is giving away one's possessions. This, along with the patient's injury and history of depression, should raise a red flag for providers. The patient should be asked about suicidal ideation. Her safety is the primary concern. The patient is likely not stable from a psychiatric standpoint to be discharged home alone. Simply increasing an antidepressant dose is not going to help with suicidal behavior. Finding out about substance abuse is not the most important thing to do to ensure patient safety.

16. **a) Putting affairs in order.** Patients who are suicidal are likely to put their affairs in order, talk about feeling hopeless, and have changes in eating and sleeping habits. Becoming more involved with friends is not a symptom, as people tend to withdraw from friends and family when exhibiting suicidal behavior or tendencies. People who are suicidal don't typically make future plans or begin a new exercise routine.

17. **a) Motivational interviewing.** The patient has intentional medication nonadherence. He has multiple risk factors for this, including polypharmacy and lack of health literacy. Motivational interviewing has been found to be beneficial in these types of patients.

■ BIBLIOGRAPHY

Ahmed, S., Leurent, B., & Sampson, E. L. (2014). Risk factors for incident delirium among older people in acute hospital medical units: A systematic review and meta-analysis. *Age and Ageing, 43*(3), 326–333. doi:10.1093/ageing/afu022

American Psychiatric Association. (2013). *Diagnostic and statistical manual of mental disorders* (5th ed.). Washington, DC: Author.

American Psychological Association. (2017). *Older adult.* Retrieved from http://www.apa.org/pi/aging/resources/guides/older.aspx

Bohem, L. (2016). Assessment and management of delirium across the life span. *Critical Care Nurse, 36*(5), e14–e19. doi:10.4037/ccn2016242

Collier, R. (2012). Hospital-induced delirium hits hard. *Canadian Medical Association Journal, 184*(1), 23–24. doi:10.1503/cmaj.109-4069

Foster, J. G., & Prevost, S. S. (2013). *Advanced practice nursing of adults in acute care* (1st ed.). Philadelphia, PA: F. A. Davis.

Hugtenburg, J. G., Timmers, L., Elders, P. J., Vervloet, M., & van Dijk, L. (2013). Definitions, variants, and causes of nonadherence with medication: A challenge for tailored interventions. *Patient Prefer Adherence, 7*, 675–682. doi:10.2147/PPA.S29549

Kennedy-Malone, L., Fletcher, L. R., & Martin-Plank, L. (2014). *Advance practice nursing in the care of older adults.* Philadelphia, PA: F. A. Davis.

McGuire, A. W., Eastwood, J., Macabasco-O'Connell, A., Hays, R. D., & Doering, L. V. (2013). Depression screening: Utility of the PHQ-2 when used by nurses in patients hospitalized for ACS. *American Journal of Critical Care, 22* (1), 12–19. doi:10.4037/ajcc2013899

McGuire, A. W., Eastwood, J., Macabasco-O'Connell, A., Hays, R. D., & Doering, L. V. (2014). Depressed or not depressed: Untangling the somatic symptom conundrum in hospitalized CHD patients. *American Journal of Critical Care, 23* (2), 106–115. doi:10.4037/ajcc2014146

McKenzie, K. J., Pierce, D., & Gunn, J. M. (2015). A systematic review of motivational interviewing in healthcare: The potential of motivational interviewing to address the lifestyle factors relevant to multimorbidity. *Journal of Comorbidity, 6* , 162–174. doi:10.15256/joc.2015.5.55

Mert, D. G., Turgut, N. H., Kelleci, M., & Semiz, M. (2015). Perspectives on reasons of medication nonadherence in psychiatric patients. *Patient Prefer Adherence, 9* , 87–93. doi:10.2147/PPA.S75013

National Institute of Mental Health. (2016a). *Bipolar disorder.* Retrieved from https://www.nimh.nih.gov/health/topics/bipolar-disorder/index.shtml

National Institute of Mental Health. (2016b). *Depression.* Retrieved from https://www.nimh.nih.gov/health/topics/depression/index.shtml

National Institute of Mental Health. (2016c). *Substance abuse and mental health.* Retrieved from https://www.nimh.nih.gov/health/topics/substance-use-and-mental-health/index.shtml

National Institute of Mental Health. (2017). *Suicide prevention.* Retrieved from https://www.nimh.nih.gov/health/topics/suicide-prevention/index.shtml

National Institute of Neurological Disorders and Stroke. (2017). *Dementia information page.* Retrieved from https://www.ninds.nih.gov/Disorders/All-Disorders/Dementia-Information-Page

Quinlan, J., & Cox, F. (2017). Acute pain management in patients with drug dependence syndrome. *Pain Reports, 2*(4), e611. doi:10.1097/PR9.0000000000000611

Rosen, H. J., & Cummings, J. (2007). A real reason for patient with pseudobulbar affect to smile. *Annals of Neurology, 61*(2), 92–96. doi:10.1002/ana.21056

Substance Abuse and Mental Health Services Administration. (2017). *Recovery and support.* Retrieved from https://www.samhsa.gov/recovery

17

Multisystem

AUDREY SNYDER, HELEN MILEY, AND
MAJOR DAMON TOCZYLOWSKI

■ MULTISYSTEM QUESTIONS

1. A 25-year-old male arrives to the ED with a complaint of right lower extremity deformity with swelling, pain, discoloration, and numbness, stating he fell 15 feet from a balcony and landed directly on his leg. Initial evaluation of his lower extremity reveals absent pulses, loss of color and sensation, and 4+ pitting edema. An initial radiograph of the extremity shows a compound fracture of the tibia and fibular distal heads with diffuse edema and soft tissue trauma. Compartment pressures below the fracture read to 40 mmHg. Based on these findings, what is the most appropriate first intervention?

   a. Reduction of fracture with surgical consult
   b. Casting of leg for immobilization of extremity
   c. Ultrasound of lower extremity to evaluate for DVT
   d. Administration of tetanus prophylaxis and first-generation cephalosporin

2. While assessing a 29-year-old female involved in a motor vehicle crash with coup/counter coup injuries, the patient becomes hypotensive to 70/40 mmHg and bradycardic to 40 beats per minute with worsening mentation and loss of sensation below her waist. Given the known mechanism of injury, what should the AG-ACNP expect to do next?

   a. Order 0.5 mg atropine and fluid bolus
   b. Initiate dopamine after fluid optimization with crystalloids
   c. Type and screen for transfusion of packed red blood cells
   d. Order 1 mL of 1:10,000 epinephrine followed by fluid bolus

3. A 55-year-old male presents to the ED with traumatic amputation of his right hand sustained during repair of a lawn mower. Physical assessment reveals a missing right hand with a jagged stump at the wrist. Vital signs include sinus tachycardia with heart rate of 122, blood pressure of 80/40 mmHg, tachypnea, and altered mental status. The AG-ACNP initiates intravenous fluids with isotonic crystalloids based on the following rationale. Isotonic crystalloids are:

   a. Best for fluid resuscitation because the low sodium value helps ensure optimal intravascular volume via an osmotic gradient
   b. Better than fluids rich in dextrose for resuscitation because high blood glucose can complicate critical illnesses and lower sodium

    c. The fluid of choice for resuscitation because they are better at maintaining intravascular osmotic pressure than hypertonic saline (3% normal saline) or other colloid-based solutions

    d. Best for maintaining a normal pH because they have an acid/base balance very similar to that of blood

4. A 45-year-old female trauma victim is undergoing resuscitation with blood products, isotonic crystalloids (normal saline), and vasoactive drips. The patient weighs 100 kg (220 lb). Which of the following values indicates the patient is properly resuscitated?

	Heart rate	Blood pressure	Urine output last hour	Lactate	ABG: pH/PaCO$_2$/PaO$_2$/Sat/ Bicarb/Base excess
a)	115	100/50	40 mL	4.5 mmol/L	7.25/33/90/16/−6
b)	110	88/55	30 mL	3.5 mmol/L	7.30/38/88/18/−4
c)	100	95/60	50 mL	2.0 mmol/L	7.40/41/94/24/−1
d)	105	90/60	15 mL	5.0 mmol/L	7.20/28/92/20/−8

5. In caring for an elderly male who has had a motor vehicle crash sustaining a suspected hypoxemic-ischemic brain injury, which supportive measure is the AG-ACNP likely to order?

    a. Therapeutic hypothermia to 32°C

    b. Anticonvulsive medications

    c. Analgesic and sedative medications

    d. Hypertensive agents to keep cerebral perfusion pressure less than 40 mmHg

6. When caring for a patient with a suspected C-spine injury with TBI, the AG-ACNP notices the patient has waxing/waning mentation with a Glasgow Coma Scale score reduction to 8. The patient also has irregular breathing, increased systolic blood pressure with a widening blood pressure, and bradycardia. The AG-ACNP understands the highest priority is to order:

    a. C-spine precautions

    b. Benzodiazepines

    c. BiPAP

    d. HOB at greater than 30 degrees

7. A postsurgical otolaryngology patient who had sustained facial trauma reports to the ED 14 days postoperative with complaints of dizziness, nausea, diarrhea, fever, chills, and night sweats for 4 days. Vital signs reveal blood pressure 80/60, heart rate 122 (sinus tachycardia), O$_2$ saturation 88%, respiratory rate 26, and temperature 103.0°F. Physical examination reveals paranasal sinus, purulent nasal discharge, and altered mental status. CT of the head reveals paranasal sinus mass thought to be retained surgical packing. The AG-ACNP should anticipate the following antimicrobial after cultures and resuscitation has begun:

    a. Clindamycin (Cleocin) 900 mg IV every 8 hours

    b. Levofloxacin (Levoquin) 750 mg IV daily

    c. Metronidazole (Flagyl) 500 mg IV BID

    d. Fluconazole (Diflucan) 200 mg IV daily

8. An elderly patient from an assisted living facility presents to the ED in January, following a fall. The patient complains of fever, malaise, cough, nausea, and vomiting for 2 days. She is found to be febrile to 101.5°F, blood pressure to 85/40, and heart rate to 120, and a fluid bolus is given. Which of the following should the AG-ACNP do first?

   a. Place the patient in droplet precautions with influenza testing.
   b. Order metronidazole (Flagyl) 500 mg IV TID due to concern for bowel perforation.
   c. Place a central line and order norepinepherine (Levophed) due to concern for septic shock.
   d. Order loperamide (Immodium) 2 mg by mouth to treat acute viral gastroenteritis.

9. A 60-year-old female motor vehicle crash victim presented to the ED with a fractured humorous and evisceration of the small bowel. Vitals were stable upon arrival and she had immediate restorative surgery to correct her injuries. Preoperatively she was placed on empiric antibiotic coverage, had a urinary catheter placed, and was intubated. While conducting rounds on postoperative day 2, the AG-ACNP notices the patient has developed mild hypotension, fever, and leukocytosis. Understanding the patient is at risk for hospital-acquired infections, what is the best way to prevent development of an iatrogenic infection for this patient?

   a. Daily cultures while IV antibiotics are escalated to treat suspected infections
   b. Adhere to evidence-based care bundles and review daily in multidisciplinary rounds
   c. Replace invasive lines every 7 days
   d. Adopt policies from larger institutions to help reduce rates of infection because they have reduced their hospital acquired infection rate

10. A patient presents to the ED with complaint of trauma to the right foot after dropping a 15-lb bowling ball on his foot. He has a past medical history significant for chronic pain syndrome and is on high-dose narcotics/atypical medications (with a known pain contract per his pain manager). Other past medical history includes insulin dependent diabetes, CHF, and chronic kidney disease Stage III with a baseline Cr 2.05. X-ray of the foot reveals soft tissue damage to the ankle with a partial fracture to the lateral malleolus. The AG-ACNP implements the following pain management strategy:

   a. Order IV acetaminophen (Ofirmev) 1 g IV every 8 hours, orthopedic consult for reduction and splinting, and consult to pain specialist for further evaluation.
   b. Order ketoralac (Toradol) 60 mg IV every 6 hours for pain, hydromorphone (Dialudid) IV as needed for pain, with consult to pain specialist.
   c. Order a PCA of hydromorphone (Dilaudid) in addition to the patient's home medications and consult neurology.
   d. Consult pain management team for nerve block to lower extremity and consult to internal medicine/endocrinology to evaluate for neuropathy.

11. A patient with septic shock is on multiple vasoactive medications, intubated on mechanical ventilation, and on IV antibiotics, an insulin drip, sedation, and analgesia. After the insulin drip was discontinued, the glucose level continued to decline. The AG-ACNP understands:

   a. The antibiotics are likely causing a rebound hypoglycemic effect in the setting of septic shock.
   b. The patient likely has diabetes at baseline and is not getting enough feeds to compensate for the high dose of insulin they are on.
   c. The patient likely has ischemic liver (shock liver), with gluconeogenesis failing to respond to the stressors on the body.
   d. The insulin drip is taking too long to clear out of the patient's system, causing a downward trend in the patient's blood sugars.

12. While rounding in the ICU, an AG-ACNP correctly differentiates a patient who is at risk for developing sepsis and identifies which of the following patients requiring early goal-directed sepsis therapies: A patient

   a. Who is tachycardic and tachypneic with a history of anxiety
   b. Who is tachypneic, hypothermic, and tachycardic but just arrived from the OR
   c. With leukocytosis, fever, and tachycardia with a known bloodstream infection
   d. With hypothermia and tachycardia post-cardiac arrest

13. When writing admission orders for a 65-year-old female patient with septic shock from a urinary source, which of the following actions and rationale are part of the surviving sepsis campaign?

   a. Serum lactate levels every 12 hours while blood pressure is unstable to evaluate for adequate fluid resuscitation
   b. Sliding scale insulin if the patient has DMII, knowing that hyperglycemia has a higher risk for mortality than hypoglycemia in the ICU
   c. Blood cultures are drawn after antibiotics are started, but both are done in the first 3 hours of sepsis or septic shock recognition
   d. Two large-bore IVs are placed and possible placement of a central catheter if vasoactive agents are required

14. An elderly woman arrives to the ED confused, lethargic, and coughing after being rescued from an apartment fire by a neighbor. The AG-ACNP completes a physical examination and notices the patient continues to exhibit confusion and lethargy for the next hour despite having started O_2 at 4 L/min via nasal cannula and IV fluids (normal saline [NS] at 75 cc/hr). The AG-ACNPs next immediate order is:

   a. Order CT head to evaluate for an acute cerebral hemorrhage, as an altered mental status can be a sign of a CVA.
   b. Increase oxygen to high flow/non-rebreather mask (NRB) 100%, as this patient is likely suffering from CO toxicity.
   c. Order a STAT blood glucose to evaluate for hypoglycemia, as this could be the source of her confusion and lethargy.
   d. Order a urine culture and start empiric community-acquired UTI monotherapy.

15. A 27-year-old male self-presented to the ED with a report of an SSRI overdose (sertraline suspected). He states he took a handful of pills (number unknown) and continues to feel suicidal. After placing the patient on a 1:1 watch and obtaining (complete blood count and basic metabolic profile), he is admitted to the ICU for monitoring. When reviewing the admission orders, an AG-ACNP notices the inclusion of an antiemetic odansetron (Zofran). What should the AG-ACNP do when discovering this medication?

   a. Nothing, as this is routine supportive care for these patients; serotonin syndrome can present, which is an uncomfortable state often accompanied by nausea.
   b. Ask the patient if he is allergic to odansetron (Zofran), and if he indicates no, then plan to continue the medication and update the medication reconciliation form.
   c. Discontinue the medication odansetron (Zofran), as a known side effect of the medication can lead to a fatal arrhythmia.
   d. Look at the dosing of the medication, and if the medication dosing or frequency is incorrect, make any corrections needed.

16. An anxious and tachycardic patient who sustained blunt chest trauma presents with JVD, narrowing pulse pressure and distant heart tones. Immediate intervention for this patient would include:

    a. Chest tube insertion
    b. Needle decompression
    c. Pericardiocentesis
    d. Intubation

17. In a patient with inability to move his lower extremities and no sensation below the nipple line, the AG-ACNP suspects a spinal lesion at or above which of the following levels:

    a. Cervical 7
    b. Thoracic 4
    c. Thoracic 10
    d. Sacral 1

18. An elderly man fell 15 feet off a ladder, landing on his right side. He has fractures of rib 4 and rib 5, which are fractured both laterally and anteriorly. When he takes a deep breath, the injured area of his lung moves inward. The AG-ACNP diagnoses this as a/an:

    a. Tension pneumothorax
    b. Hemothorax
    c. Open pneumothorax
    d. Flail chest

19. What diagnostic/physical exam findings support an aortic injury?

    a. Widened mediastinum
    b. Distinct aortic knob
    c. Fractures of rib 3 and rib 4
    d. Transverse process fractures of the thoracic spine

20. A trauma patient with a grade III splenic laceration complains of acute pain in the tip of the shoulder when he is lying down with legs elevated. The AG-ACNP knows this as which of the following signs:

    a. Cullen sign
    b. Kehr's sign
    c. Rovsing's sign
    d. Psoas sign

21. A patient sustains a penetrating injury to the right eye when a pellet from a pellet gun entered the right orbit. The AG-ACNP is relieved when the ophthalmologist informs her the intraocular pressure is:

    a. 30 to 40 mmHg
    b. 15 to 25 mmHg
    c. 20 to 30 mmHg
    d. 10 to 20 mmHg

22. Using the rule of nines, calculate the percentage of TBSA burned in a 60 kg male with burns covering his entire right leg, anterior thorax including the abdomen, and entire surface of both arms.

    a. 18%
    b. 35%
    c. 54%
    d. 44%

23. Which of the following is part of the primary survey in a trauma patient?

    a. Head-to-toe exam
    b. Airway assessment
    c. Laboratory data
    d. GI exam

24. Which of the following types of thoracic trauma requires a #36 French pleural chest tube to be placed:

    A. Flail chest
    B. Cardiac tamponade
    C. Hemothorax
    D. Pneumothorax 40%

25. In an unstable trauma victim following a motor vehicle crash, a chest x-ray demonstrates a widened mediastinum, left second rib fracture, and deviation of the trachea to the right. The AG-ACNP is most concerned for a/an:

    a. Tension pneumothorax
    b. Aortic rupture
    c. Hemothorax
    d. Flail chest

26. An AG-ACNP assesses a trauma during the secondary survey and notes the patient has right flank bruising and pain with inspiration. The AG-ACNP recognizes this is most commonly associated with injury to which organ?

    a. Kidney
    b. Spleen
    c. Liver
    d. Gallbladder

27. Which of the following burn patients can be safely managed outside a level I trauma center?

    a. 44-year-old male diabetic with second-degree burn to his leg
    b. 35-year-old with inhalation injury
    c. 29-year-old with 15% third-degree burns
    d. 25-year-old with 30% first-degree burns

28. Which of the following is most consistent with high-grade splenic trauma?

    a. Kernig's sign
    b. Vomiting blood
    c. Decreased WBC count
    d. Positive focused assessment with sonography

29. A patient has been admitted from home with a peripherally inserted central catheter line for parenteral nutrition. She is lethargic, febrile, tachycardic, and hypotensive, requiring fluid resuscitation and vasopressor support. Blood cultures revealed heavy growth of Gram-positive cocci at 10 hours and the PICC line was immediately removed. This is an example of:

    a. Resuscitation therapy
    b. Source control
    c. Early goal-directed therapy
    d. Inotrope therapy

30. Which of the following parameter(s) is an endpoint in the resuscitation of a patient in septic shock?

    a. Central venous pressure 4 to 8 mmHg
    b. Lactate less than 2
    c. Urine output less than 0.5 mL/kg/hr
    d. Oxygen saturation greater than or equal to 95%

31. A 28-year-old patient is admitted to the ICU after being found in a motel room slumped over in a chair and unresponsive. He is intubated and now is being evaluated by the AG-ACNP. Laboratory evaluation shows a pH of 7.14, potassium 7.2 mEq/L, and a creatinine phosphokinase (CPK) of 40,000 U/L. He is producing little urine, which is dark and concentrated. Initial treatment includes:

    a. Aggressive volume resuscitation
    b. Hemodialysis
    c. Alkalization of urine
    d. Diuretics

32. Upon completing a focused assessment with sonography for trauma examination in a multi-trauma patient it is discovered that she has an acute splenic laceration with active bleeding. The patient's vital signs continue to downtrend despite administration of warmed 2 liters of lactated ringers and her blood pressure is now 70/50, heart rate 120 sinus tachycardia, and Glasgow Coma Scale score 12. Laboratory analysis reveals CBC of hemoglobin 6.0, hematocrit (HCT) 18.0, platelet count (PLT) 100k, international normalized ratio (INR) 3.0; chemistries reveal potassium 3.4, creatinine 2.0, lactate 3.0, calcium 8.5. A type and cross match was obtained for this patient. What is the best intervention for the AG-ACNP to take?

    a. Initiate the massive transfusion protocol and consult surgery.
    b. Order 2 units of packed red blood cells and 1 unit FFP to supplement the active bleed.
    c. Order 40 mEq of potassium and an ABG to assess for an anion-gap metabolic acidosis.
    d. Attempt to contact the patient's family members to ascertain code status.

33. A 37-year-old male was brought to the ED. It was reported that he was a street performer who was seen on a street hunched over after he inhaled a large amount of fire. Upon arrival to the scene paramedics assessed his airway as intact, found second- and third-degree burns to his face, and noticed burn marks to his mouth and nares. His vital signs on initial assessment were stable with an SPO_2 to 95% on room air. Upon arrival the ED he is found to have increasing oxygen demands, decreased breath sounds with wheezing bilaterally, and a hoarse voice that started upon arrival to the ED. What is the best initial intervention the AG-ACNP should complete?

    a. Obtain chest x-ray to assess for acute intrapulmonary findings.
    b. Administer nebulized albuterol via cool mist nebulizer.
    c. Prepare for rapid sequence intubation.
    d. Request a bronchoscopy to evaluate for trauma to tracheobronchial tree.

34. The AG-ACNP is working at an urgent care clinic at a ski resort. She receives a report from the ski patrol that a 26-year-old snowboarder was found off the ski trail next to a tree. He was alert and oriented sitting next to the tree when the ski patrol arrived. He appeared to have lost control, flew off the trail, striking the tree. As the snowboarder appeared to be stable, he was requested to walk up the hill to the ski trail, which he did. This demonstrates:

    a. Assessment based on appearance rather than mechanism of injury
    b. Appropriate request of the ski patrol, as using a toboggan to pull the patient up the hill would put their safety at risk
    c. Standard protocol for emergency services
    d. Assessment based on mechanism of injury rather than appearance

35. A 36-year-old female is transported to the ED by the ambulance. The ambulance crew states that the patient was reported to have been skiing at a nearby ski resort when she fell and slid down the ski slope into a tree, striking the left side of her chest. She has been complaining of shortness of breath and left-sided chest wall and abdominal pain since the accident. She was wearing a helmet, denies head trauma or loss of consciousness, and has been hemodynamically stable during transport. Upon arrival, she is awake, alert, and oriented × 4. She is holding the left side of her chest and appears to be in mild respiratory distress. She is able to talk and states, "I just had the wind knocked out of me," and continues to complain of difficulty breathing and extreme lateral chest wall and abdominal pain. What injuries would the AG-ACNP expect when evaluating this patient?

a. Cardiac contusion
b. Liver laceration
c. Pneumothorax
d. Aortic injury

36. The AG-ACNP is caring for an older adult trauma patient who just arrived in the ED. She has the following injuries: left anterior/lateral rib fractures 1–7, left pulmonary contusion, small left pneumothorax, grade I splenic laceration. What is the best plan of care for this patient?

a. Discharge home with Vicodin, rest, and follow-up in 24 hours.
b. Admit to ICU for monitoring and consider invasive pain management.
c. Admit to the inpatient acute care floor.
d. Observe in the ED for 6 hours and discharge home if stable.

■ MULTISYSTEM ANSWERS AND RATIONALES

1. **a) Reduction of fracture with surgical consult**. The patient has compartment syndrome below the level of the complex fracture and needs immediate reduction to allow for appropriate blood flow to the area along with surgical consultation for repair. Pain relief is important but is not the initial therapy, nor is tetanus/IV administration. Although a DVT can present with decreased blood flow/pallor, the patient presented with symptoms to suggest compartment syndrome.

2. **b) Initiate dopamine after fluid optimization with crystalloids**. This patient is suffering from vasomotor deficits with lowering vascular tone that necessitates need for fluid optimization and subsequent addition of vasoactive agents (phenylephrine, dopamine, norepinephrine) or inotropes (dobutamine). Atropine is appropriate for symptomatic bradycardia but not for neurogenic shock. The administration of blood products is not appropriate since as this is not hemorrhagic shock. Although anaphylactic shock is a variation of distributive shock; epinephrine is not indicated in this given instance known mechanism of injury.

3. **b) Better than fluids rich in dextrose for resuscitation because high blood glucose can complicate critical illnesses and lower sodium**. Isotonic crystalloids are more acidic that blood (pH of lactated ringers (LR) is close to 7.0 and pH of normal saline (NS) is close to 5.5). Isotonic crystalloids are not better at osmotic regulation as they do not cause as much of an osmotic shift as hypertonic saline, and isotonic crystalloids do not cause hyponatremia.

4. **c)**

Heart rate	Blood pressure	Urine output last hour	Lactate	ABG: pH/PaCO$_2$/PaO$_2$/Sat/ Bicarb/Base excess
100	95/60	50 mL	2.0 mmol/L	7.40/41/94/24/−1

Good end points of resuscitation include closing of a metabolic acidosis via lactic acidosis, good urine output (reduction of a prerenal state) and stable hemodynamics. Trauma patients in the ED frequently present with a lactate greater than 4.0 accompanied by a metabolic acidosis on ABG and poor urine output, which may be in the setting of stable or unstable vital signs.

5. **b) Anticonvulsive medications**. Anticonvulsive medications are indicated to prevent and treat seizures which helps prevent secondary brain injuries, which can exacerbate primary injuries and increase mortality. Analgesics and sedatives can mask reduce the best neurological examination. The goal is to keep cerebral perfusion pressure greater than 40. Therapeutic hypothermia is not indicated; however, the literature remains controversial regarding targeted temperature management.

6. **d) HOB at greater than 30 degrees**. This patient is having increased intracranial pressure, thus raising the head of bed to greater than 30 degrees allows for drainage of the third and fourth ventricles which is necessary to allow adequate cerebral perfusion pressures (this is in reference to the Monro-Kellie Doctrine). BiPAP is insufficient to manage this patient's airway. Intubation is indicated. Failure to establish a permanent airway can exacerbate secondary brain injuries due to hypoxemia/hypercapnia. Maintaining c-spine precautions is appropriate but will not treat the life-threatening condition of increased intracranial pressure. Benzodiazepines can further depress mental status and are not indicated. They are also known for causing ICU delirium, but are essential if seizure activity is present.

7. **a) Clindamycin (Cleocin) 900 mg IV every 8 hours**. The most likely diagnosis given the patient's known history of otolayngology surgery with likely retained packing is toxic shock Syndrome (strep/staph serving as the most likely organism). Beta lactams were historically

used (PCNases); however, clindamycin is more in favor given increased coverage (Gram positive/aerobic). Levofloxacin is appropriate for CAP monotherapy. Flagyl and fluconazole are not indicated for sinusitis.

8. **a) Place the patient in droplet precautions with influenza testing.** Knowing elderly populations in long-term facilities (skilled nursing facility [SNF]/long term acute care hospital [LTAC]/nursing homes) are at an increased risk for exposure to communicable disease, the AG-ACNP chooses correctly to place the patient in droplet precautions to limit the risk of transmission of influenza and sends for a screening test. Bowel perforation is on the differential, but there is no described history to support this. While a central line and norepinepherine is the correct for use in the setting of septic shock, this question does not indicate if the patient received sufficient fluids of if she responded to the fluids, thus this may be premature. Immodium is the correct dose for suspected gastroenteritis from an unknown etiology; however, acute gastroenteritis does not normally present with respiratory components.

9. **b) Adhere to evidence-based care bundles and are reviewed daily in multidisciplinary rounds.** Use of the A, B, C, D, E care bundles in an interdisciplinary manner has shown decreases in length of stay, complications, infections, and mortality. Daily cultures and escalation of antibiotics can have adverse outcomes. The goal is to deescalate antibiotics as soon as possible. Changing lines after an established time is not appropriate; lines do not need to be changed unless a cause is identified. Adapting a policy from a larger facility that has not been vetted appropriately through your institution can have adverse effects as different hospitals have differing populations and sizes.

10. **a) Order IV acetaminophen (Ofirmev) 1 g IV every 8 hours, orthopedic consult for reduction and splinting, and consult to pain specialist for further evaluation.** Given the patient's medical history use of IV Tylenol may offer reduction of immediate pain with consult to orthopedic specialist to reduce/repair fracture if needed and pain specialist to help with the plan moving forward. Patient will likely not tolerate IV ketoralac or hydromorphone given renal failure and already saturated opioid receptors. Consult to pain management is appropriate; however, anticipation of lower extremity block may be excessive and internal medicine/endocrine consult for neuropathy may be worked up as an outpatient.

11. **c) The patient likely has ischemic liver (shock liver) with gluconeogenesis failing to respond to the stressors on the body.** The identification of shock liver here is imperative as liver synthesis dysfunction is an ominous sign of liver failure. Supportive measures are needed to ensure fulminant liver failure is not allowed to occur. Antibiotics can be mixed in a dextrose solution, thus causing glucose levels to rise. Assuming a patient has diabetes is not accurate. Insulin does not accumulate in body tissues as other agents such as (i.e., benzodiazepines) and is cleared after the drip is discontinued.

12. **c) With leukocytosis, fever, and tachycardia with a known bloodstream infection.** It is important for an AG-ACNP to recognize that other etiologies can cause SIRS criteria; however, it is necessary to differentiate between patients with SIRS and sepsis.

13. **d) Two large bore IVs are placed and possible placement of a central catheter if vasoactive agents are required.** Per the surviving sepsis campaign directive: a patient should have two large bore IVs and placement of central catheter if vasoactive agents are required. Serum lactate should be drawn every 6 to 8 hours. There is a 50% risk of mortality associated with hypoglycemia in the setting of septic shock. Permissive hyperglycemia (140–180 mg/dl) is allowed. Blood cultures ideally should be drawn before antibiotics are started, not after.

14. **b) Increase oxygen to high flow/non-rebreather mask (NRB) 100% as this patient is likely suffering from CO toxicity.** All of the aforementioned answers can cause an altered mental status; however, given the fact that the patient was rescued from an apartment fire, she is suspected to have CO poisoning. A head CT and blood glucose are appropriate in the right clinical scenario. CO has a higher affinity for binding to the blood, therefore, it will take 250 to 320 minutes to clear, thus making ventilating with 100% oxygen the best clinical choice for this patient.

15. **c) Discontinue the medication odansetron (Zofran) as a known side effect of the medication can lead to a fatal arrhythmia**. SSRIs cause QTc prolongation, a common side effect in Zofran (a commonly prescribed medication in ICU settings). Recognition of this early on is an important finding that needs to be immediately addressed. Continuing this medication in any dose can cause harm and is not the safest action. Serotonin syndrome may present with nausea.

16. **c) Pericardiocentesis**. JVD, narrowing pulse pressure, and distant heart tones are signs of pericardial tamponade, a complication of blunt trauma and a true cardiac emergency. The immediate intervention is pericardiocentesis. The patient may need surgical intervention. Needle decompression or chest tube would treat a pneumothorax. A chest tube can also treat a hemothorax. Intubation may be needed later but the immediate life-saving intervention is a pericardiocentesis.

17. **b) Thoracic 4**. Sensation at the level of the nipple line is indicative of Thoracic 4 or above injury. The middle finger is Cervical 7, the level of the umbilicus is Thoracic 10, and sensation at the back of the leg is indicative of Sacral 1 or above spinal trauma lesion.

18. **d) Flail chest**. A flail chest occurs with two or more ribs fractured in two places and results in a floating rib section that moves paradoxically to normal inspiration and expiration. Tension pneumothorax is life threatening and occurs when air enters but does not exit the pleural space and puts pressure on the mediastinal structures. A hemothorax is a collection of blood in the pleural space, and with an open pneumothorax air enters and exits the chest cavity through the chest wound.

19. **a) Widened mediastinum**. A widened mediastinum is a hallmark of aortic injury. Obliteration of the aortic knob, fracture of the first or second rib and/or scapula as well as circulatory collapse are all findings associated with aortic injury. Transverse process fractures are too far away to cause injury to the aorta.

20. **b) Kehr's sign**. Cullen sign is periumbilical ecchymosis indicative of retroperiotoneal bleeding. Palpation of the left lower quadrant causing increased pain in the right lower quadrant is Rovsing's sign and may indicate appendicitis. Psoas sign, also called ilio-psoas sign, occurs when passive extension of the right hip causes pain in the right iliac fossa.

21. **d) 10 to 20 mmHg**. Normal intraocular pressure in penetrating ocular injury is 10–20 mmHg.

22. **c) 54%**. In the rule of nines calculation, a leg is 18%, anterior thorax is 18%, and each arm is 9%, for a total of 54% TBSA burn.

23. **b) Airway assessment**. The primary survey focuses on airway, breathing, circulation, disability (neurologic exam), and exposure and environmental control. The head to toe exam, laboratory data, and gastrointestinal assessment are part of the secondary survey.

24. **c) Hemothorax**. A hemothorax, tension pneumothorax, and pneumothorax of 40% or more require a chest tube. A flail chest may require internal stabilization with intubation and positive pressure ventilation. Cardiac tamponade requires a peridiaocentsis or pericardial window.

25. **b) Aortic rupture**. All of these signs on chest x-ray are suggestive of aortic rupture. A tension pneumothorax, hemothorax, and flail chest would not have a widened mediastinum.

26. **a) Kidney**. Bruising of the flank is referred to as Grey Turner's sign and is indicative of a potential kidney injury.

27. **d) 25-year-old with 30% first-degree burns**. The patient with first-degree burns can be managed and discharged from a nonburn center. The American Burn Association criteria for transfer to a burn center includes 10% partial thickness burns; any full thickness burn; electrical, chemical, or inhalation injuries; burn of the hands, feet, perineum, face, or major joints; and when there is increased risk for mortality including preexisting medical conditions. Patients with diabetes, inhalation injury, and third-degree burns would require transport to a burn center.

28. **d) Positive focused assessment with sonography**. A positive focused assessment with sonography for trauma exam will be positive when the splenic capsule is disrupted. An elevated, not decreased, WBC count is associated with splenic injury. A decrease in hemoglobin and hematocrit are expected findings form blood loss associated with splenic injury. Kehr's sign is considered a classic sign of ruptured spleen; pain in the shoulder from irritation of the diaphragm. Kernig's sign is seen in meningitis.

29. **b) Source control**. This is an example of source control, which is one of the tenets in the treatment of sepsis. Will resuscitation therapy, early goal direct therapy, and inotrope therapy are part of the bundle for sepsis, it is important to look at source control, which is the removal of the catheter.

30. **b) Lactate less than 2**. The endpoints of resuscitation include lactate clearance, CVP 8 to12, urine output (UOP) greater than 0.5 mL/kg/hr, mixed venous oxygenation 70% to 85%.

31. **a) Aggressive volume resuscitation**. Volume expansion regardless of the type of agent is the most important treatment modality. Hemodialysis is not indicated yet. Diuretics and hemodialysis may be of help once the patient has been adequately fluid resuscitated. Alkalization of urine has not proven to be beneficial.

32. **a) Initiate the massive transfusion protocol and consult surgery**. Although it is important to recognize that the patient likely has a metabolic acidosis (likely secondary to lactic acidosis resulting from hypoperfusion) and the patient has mild hypokalemia, this is not the initial area of concern. Ordering 2 units of PRBC and 1 FFP may help initially to control bleeding, but the exact degree of resuscitation cannot be predicted and it is imperative to order more products for the patient as she is likely going to need a surgical intervention with more anticipated blood loss. It is extremely important to attain the code status of the patient; however, the initial action of the NP is to ensure an appropriate resuscitation is transpiring.

33. **c) Prepare for rapid sequence intubation**. Immediate placement of a definitive airway is required in this patient given his declining respiratory status and changes to phonation after witnessed inhalation of an open flame. Consulting pulmonary medicine and chest radiography are likely secondary medical treatments; however, the initial treatment is to secure his airway. Nebulized albuterol is the treatment of choice for wheezing associated with asthma but should not be initially considered for this patient.

34. **a) Assessment based on appearance rather than mechanism of injury**. This patient was assessed based on appearance rather than mechanism of injury. The patient appeared to be a young healthy adult and requesting him to walk up the hill, rather than perform a primary survey of the patient, indicated mechanism of injury was not considered.

35. **c) Pneumothorax**. Blunt chest trauma can cause severe injuries. Rib fractures are the most common injury sustained following blunt chest trauma and the significance of rib injuries should never be underestimated. Upper ribs (1–3) may indicate a high magnitude of injury, placing the head, spine, and great vessels at risk. The majority of blunt trauma tend to affect the middle ribs (4–9) forcing the ends of the bones into the thorax, which may cause a pneumothorax. Splenic injury may occur with blunt trauma to the left side of the chest wall. A cardiac contusion and aortic injury are possible, they are not the most likely injuries given the mechanism and hemodynamic stability.

36. **b) Admit to ICU for monitoring and consider invasive pain management**. A common pitfall with rib fractures is underestimating the severe pathophysiology that can occur, especially in older adults and the elderly. Rib fractures are common and fractures can be significant in a patient with trauma to the thoracic cage. Rib fractures are painful and for those individuals who have suffered blunt trauma to the chest wall with several rib fractures, pain control is essential in order to prevent splinting that can lead to atelectasis and pneumonia. Continuous epidural infusion has been found to be helpful with these patients. Pulmonary contusions following rib fractures can be lethal. Patients need to be observed closely for 24 to 48 hours as respiratory failure can occur.

■ BIBLIOGRAPHY

Agnihotri, N., & Agnihotri, A. (2014). Transfusion associated circulatory overload. *Indian Journal of Critical Care Medicine, 18*(6), 396–398. doi:10.4103/0972-5229.133938

American College of Surgeons Committee on Trauma. (2012). *Advanced trauma life support* (9th ed.). Chicago, IL: American College of Surgeons.

ARDS Network. (2017). *Mechanical ventilation protocol summary.* Retrieved from http://www.ardsnet.org/files/ventilator_protocol_2008-07.pdf

Bauer, S. (2015). *Using teamwork to improve patient outcomes.* Society of Critical Care Medicine. Retrieved from http://www.sccm.org/Communications/Critical-Connections/Archives/Pages/Using-Teamwork-to-Improve-Patient-Outcomes.aspx

Bickley, L., & Szilagyi, P. (2013). *Bates' guide to physical examination and history taking.* Philadelphia, PA: Lippincott.

Buckley, N. A., Dawson, A. H., & Isbister, G. K. (2014). Serotonin syndrome. *British Medical Journal, 348,* g1626. doi:10.1136/bmj.g1626

Centers for Disease Control and Prevention. (2018). *Influenza.* Retrieved from https://www.cdc.gov/flu/index.htm

Dellinger, R. P., Levy, M. M., Rhodes, A., Annane, D., Gerlach, H., Opal, S. M., & Jaeschke, R. (2013). Surviving sepsis campaign: International guidelines for management of severe sepsis and septic shock, 2012. *Intensive Care Medicine, 39*(2), 165–228. doi:10.1097/CCM.0b013e31827e83af

Emergency Nursing Association. (2014). *TNCC: Trauma nursing core course provider* (7th ed.). Des Plaines, IL: Emergency Nurses Association.

Ethgen, O., Schneider, A. G., Bagshaw, S. M., Bellomo, R., & Kellum, J. A. (2015). Economics of dialysis dependence following renal replacement therapy for critically ill acute kidney injury patients. *Nephrology, Dialysis, Transplantation, 30*(1), 54–61. doi:10.1093/ndt/gfu314

Gerlach, A. T., & Dasta, J. F. (2007). Dexmedetomidine: An updated review. *Annals of Pharmacotherapy, 41*(2), 245–254. doi:10.1345/aph.1H314

Holcomb, J. B., Wade, C. E., Michalek, J. E., Chisholm, G. B., Zarzabal, L. A., Schreiber, M. A., & Park, M. S. (2008). Increased plasma and platelet to red blood cell ratios improves outcome in 466 massively transfused civilian trauma patients. *Annals of Surgery, 248*(3), 447–458. doi:10.1097/SLA.0b013e318185a9ad

Kasper, D., Hauser, S., Jameson, J., Fauci, A., Longo, D., & Loscalzo, J. (2015). *Harrison's principles of internal medicine* (19th ed.). New York, NY: McGraw-Hill.

Kunisawa, T. (2011). Dexmedetomidine hydrochloride as a long-term sedative. *Therapeutics and Clinical Risk Management, 7,* 291. doi:10.2147/TCRM.S14581

Madden, L. K., Hill, M., May, T. L., Human, T., Guanci, M. M., Jacobi, J., & Badjatia, N. (2017). The implementation of targeted temperature management: An evidence-based guideline from the neurocritical care society. *Neurocritical Care, 27*(3), 468–487. doi:10.1007/s12028-017-0469-5

Marx, J. A., Hocksberger, R. S., Walls, R. M., Biros, M. H., Ling, L. J., Danzl, D. F., & Jagoda, A. (2014). *Rosen's emergency medicine concepts and clinical practice* (8th ed.). Philadelphia, PA: Saunders.

Office on Women's Health U.S. Department of Health and Human Services. (2015). *Sexually transmitted infections, pregnancy, and breastfeeding.* Retrieved from https://www.womenshealth.gov/a-z-topics/stis-pregnancy-and-breastfeeding

Parrillo, J., & Dellinger, R. (2013). *Critical care medicine: Principles of diagnosis and management in the adult* (4th ed.). Philadelphia, PA: Elsevier.

Singer, M., Deutschman, C. S., Seymour, C. W., Shankar-Hari, M., Annane, D., Bauer, M., & Angus, D. C. (2016). The third international consensus definitions for sepsis and septic shock (Sepsis-3). *JAMA, 315*(8), 801–810. doi:10.1001/jama.2016.0287

Walker, P. F., Buehner, M. F., Wood, L. A., Boyer, N. L., Driscoll, I. R., Lundy, J. B., & Chung, K. K. (2015). Diagnosis and management of inhalation injury: An updated review. *Critical Care (London, England), 19*(1), 351. doi:10.1186/s13054-015-1077-4

Wyckoff, M., Houghton, D., & LePage, C. (2009). *Critical care concepts, role, and practice for the acute care nurse practitioner.* New York, NY: Springer Publishing Company.

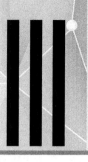

Practice Questions—Role, Professional Responsibility, and Healthcare Systems

18

Scope and Standards of Practice

DONNA GULLETTE AND MARY ANNE MᴄCOY

▣ SCOPE AND STANDARDS OF PRACTICE QUESTIONS

1. A patient involved in a drive-by shooting with a gunshot wound to the chest was transported to the ED. The AG-ACNP evaluates the patient and determines he needs a chest tube. The AG-ACNP asks the nurse to set up for chest tube insertion. She responds by asking, "Are you qualified to insert a chest tube?" The AG-ACNPs best response would be:

    a. "I don't have time to argue with you; get me the chest tube."
    b. "I have been approved by the hospital's credentialing committee to insert the chest tube."
    c. "If you have a problem, ask the ED physician to insert the chest tube."
    d. "I am certified to put in the chest tube because of my APRN license."

2. An AG-ACNP is treating a patient who has been recently diagnosed with hypertension and hyperlipidemia. A cost-effective, quality plan of care that involves monitoring patient progress is developed for the patient. The AG-ACNP educates the patient regarding management of the conditions prior to implementing the plan. Which process of healthcare does this scenario most closely resemble?

    a. Quality assurance
    b. Collaborative practice
    c. Continuous quality improvement
    d. Case management

3. AG-ACNPs should be aware of their role in mandatory reporting of rape to the proper authorities. Which of the following cases requires reporting to the authorities based on statutes found in most states?

    a. A 54-year-old female reporting rape by her son-in-law 2 weeks ago
    b. A 15-year-old female reporting rape by her 14-year-old boyfriend
    c. An 18-year-old high school student whose mother is reporting her daughter was raped
    d. An 82-year-old female who drove herself to the hospital after her neighbor raped her last night

4. Which of the following allows a patient the ability to decline life-saving interventions?

a. Patient Protection and Affordable Care Act
b. Patient Self-Determination Act
c. PSQIA
d. HIPAA

5. Which of the following statements is correct regarding prescriptive authority for AG-ACNPs?

a. They are granted after meeting educational requirements and obtaining national certification.
b. They are obtained through collaborative practice with a physician and the hospital credentialing board.
c. They are granted based upon state practice acts or statutes, which may restrict the prescription of certain categories of drugs.
d. They are granted by the state medical board where the AG-ACNP is practicing.

6. A 24-year-old female was admitted for 23-hour observation after presenting to the ED after being incapacitated from illegal-substance ingestion. Upon entering the patient's room, she tells you that she is going to kill herself and has a sheet wrapped around her neck. To keep her from harming herself, the AG-ACNP's best action to take first is:

a. Call for assistance and have the patient immediately restrained.
b. Call a psychiatric consult to assess for competency.
c. Order medication to prevent her from harming herself.
d. Remove any items she could use to harm herself and assess the patient.

7. A 66-year-old woman with terminal pancreatic cancer is considering her options and wants to pursue hospice. She is afraid she cannot afford it. The AG-ACNP advises her that she has several options but the Medicare Part A does not cover:

a. Short-term skilled nursing facility care
b. Hospice
c. Home health agency visits
d. Outpatient hospital care

8. An AG-ACNP has been hired to work with a group of pulmonologists. This role will incorporate unique differences in both the inpatient and outpatient clinic responsibilities. This position:

a. Will require him to obtain credentialing privileges for hospital practice
b. Will encompass substitutive care traditionally provided by physicians
c. Is considered to be a fee-for-service-based practice model
d. Must be supervised by a physician while in the inpatient setting

9. An AG-ACNP is interviewing for a new position. While interviewing at a major tertiary care facility, she was informed that claims-made malpractice insurance coverage is included as part of her compensation package. This means that she:

a. Would be protected from any claim made related to an incident while she was working there
b. Will be covered for any claim made from the date of her hire
c. Will need to consider purchasing tail coverage at some time
d. Should request a copy of the policy showing her name was added to list of insured providers

10. The AG-ACNP is rounding in the ICU on a patient with a TBI who has a Glasgow Coma Score of 12. The nurse asked the AG-ACNP to write an order for restraints to keep the patient from trying to get out of bed. Which of the following must be present to prevent the AG-ACNP from being held liable?

   a. An AG-ACNP is not allowed to order restraints on patients.
   b. AG-ACNP must document the exact reason and rationale for use of restraints, and safety checks.
   c. AG-ACNP must notify the medical director of the unit and obtain permission for the order.
   d. AG-ACNP must notify the family members and obtain their permission for restraints.

11. An AG-ACNP working in a specialty pulmonary clinic, which manages pulmonary hypertension, sees a 24-year-old woman who came to the clinic to establish care. Before the end of the long intake and physical exam, the patient requests the AG-ACNP to insert an IUD for conceptive prevention. The best response would be:

   a. "I will need to obtain a pregnancy test prior to insertion."
   b. "I will need to schedule you back when you are having your period for insertion of the IUD."
   c. "I will need to refer you to an OB/GYN NP, who can insert the IUD for you."
   d. "I will need you to obtain a consent form prior to the procedure."

12. The AG-ACNP is working in a very busy ED on the night shift. A 42-year-old Spanish-speaking patient is brought by his friends after he fell and broke his right arm. The patient does not speak English. What is the next action in caring for this patient?

   a. Since his friend speaks English, have his friend interpret for him.
   b. Call for a certified medical interpreter to be present or by phone.
   c. Have one of the medical assistants who speaks Spanish interpret for him.
   d. Refer him to another facility where there is someone who can speak Spanish.

13. An AG-ACNP is working in an ICU overnight and a critically ill patient is admitted in septic shock, requiring a CVC be placed urgently. The AG-ACNP has completed the required training and has submitted paperwork to add this procedure to his institutional credentialing, but has not yet received notification of approval. The AG-ACNP's best action is to:

   a. Proceed with the CVC placement.
   b. Obtain supervision for CVC placement.
   c. Manage the patient with peripheral vasopressors until day shift arrives.
   d. Obtain approval from the ICU attending to proceed with CVC placement.

14. What agency or organization enforces the protections safeguarded by the HIPPA?

   a. The OCR
   b. HHS
   c. AMA
   d. AHRQ

15. An AG-ACNP is managing a panel of patients with heart failure. She has implemented a new group-teaching program. She has made a series of modifications to the teaching plan based on the patient and provider feedback. She is evaluating the data at 6 months to see if the number of exacerbations and admissions has decreased. What process of healthcare does this most closely resemble?

   a. Quality assurance
   b. Collaborative practice
   c. CQI
   d. Case management

■ SCOPE AND STANDARDS OF PRACTICE ANSWERS AND RATIONALES

1. **b) "I have been approved by the hospital's credentialing committee to insert the chest tube."** It is the credentialing committee of the hospital that approves specific procedures that can be performed by the APRN. Being certified as an AG-ACNP does not provide you an automatic approval for invasive procedures. Being disrespectful to the nurse does not promote effective communication and a professional relationship. Neither is abdicating your role to the ED physician when faced with a concern from any healthcare provider advocating for the patient. This question is determining if you understand scope of practice and the credentialing process. Your APRN license in the state validates that you have met minimum education standards, but what you were credentialed to do may vary by specific service and by each institution where you may work.

2. **d) Case management.** This is an example of case management that uses a comprehensive, systematic approach to provide quality care by mobilizing, monitoring, and controlling patient resources during illness while balancing the quality of costs of these resources. The quality assurance process typically involves evaluating patient care according to established standards of care. Collaborative practice exists to enhance the quality of care and improve patient outcomes and would enhance efficiency in the case management process. The process of quality improvement often involves an environment in which management and staff strives to improve quality healthcare outcomes.

3. **b) A 15-year-old female reporting rape by her 14-year-old boyfriend.** In most states the AG-ACNP is not required to report the allegation of rape to the police when the individual is a competent adult. In those cases, the patient must report the rape to the police. However, the AG-ACNP can support the patient and assist in connecting the individual with a sexual assault nurse for rape evidence processing; evidence needs to be collected within 72 hours. The case of the 18-year-old whose mother reports her daughter's rape would require corroboration of the allegation by the daughter. The 15-year-old, even if the perpetrator is younger, is not considered a competent adult. Many states require medical personnel to make a report to law enforcement and/or social services following their treatment of a child, elderly person, or vulnerable adult who was the victim of a crime, including rape.

4. **a) Patient Self-Determination Act.** The Patient Self-Determination Act requires that all patients entering the hospital be given information of their right to execute advanced directives. PSQIA provides federal privilege and confidentiality protections for patient safety information, called the patient safety work product, to encourage reporting and analysis of medical errors. HIPAA covers the privacy of individually identifiable health information. The ACA expanded and reformed health insurance coverage for the underinsured or uninsured.

5. **c) They are granted based upon state practice acts or statutes, which may restrict the prescription of certain categories of drugs.** Prescriptive authority is granted by the state practice acts or state statutes and may have restrictions on what substances can be prescribed; the most common being controlled substances. A credentialing board and/or a state board of medicine in most cases do not grant prescriptive authority. A requirement to prescribe is to have completed the educational program requirements which individual states can set. Not all states require national board certification.

6. **d) Remove any items she could use to harm herself and assess the patient.** The AG-ACNP has the duty to protect someone from harming herself or others because of mental illness and may be found liable if the patient is discharged. However, the AG-ACNP should maintain the patient–provider relationship at all times. If the patient is combative or violent, use of restraints may be warranted and under most circumstances an AG-ACNP may legally subdue a patient who is danger of harming herself, with proper restraints or pharmaceutical agents. However, there is a common assumption that if someone seeks to attempt suicide has a method of choice blocked, she will simply find another method. Evidence in the literature disputed this assumption. A probable explanation is that suicidal crises are motivated by extreme pain or hopelessness; evidence suggests that removal of agents, equipment, etc.,

which a person may use to harm themselves,would be the most appropriate, along with a patient assessment. A psychiatric consult most likely will be required but it does not solve the immediate issue. The patient may need a temporary commitment to a psychiatric facility, but the immediate concern is patient safety.

7. **d) Outpatient hospital care**. Medicare Part A covers inpatient hospital care, skilled nursing facilities, hospice, in-patient rehab, home healthcare, and obesity bariatric surgery. The Medicare Part B supplement covers outpatient hospital care, physician visits, home care, radiology, laboratory, and other related services. In this case the patient can chose from in-patient or outpatient hospice care.

8. **a) Will require him to obtain credentialing privileges for hospital practice**. Credentialing privileges are only required to practice in the acute care setting. Credentialing demonstrates the AG-ACNP has the required education, licensure, and certification to practice. Care provided by an AG-ACNP may or may not always substitute care provided by a physician, be a fee for service or require physician supervision.

9. **c) Will need to consider purchasing tail coverage at some time**. Claim-made coverage only protects if the practitioner has the policy when the claim is made, which could be made after she leaves her current employer. Therefore, the practitioner will need to consider the purchase of tail insurance to cover claims that may occur after she leaves the facility. If the practitioner has occurrence policy form of insurance she would be covered for a claim made during and after her employment ends as long as the incident occurred during her covered policy.

10. **b) AG-ACNP must document the exact reason and rationale for use of restraints, and safety checks**. The AG-ACNP, to avoid being held liable in a state of law, must document the reason for the restraints, the rationale, the appropriate safety checks, and neuro checks, and must notify the attending physician. It is part of the scope of practice for AG-ACNP to order restraints, but restraints should be used only as last resort. The medical director or patient's primary care provider should be notified of the need for patient restraints. The family should also be notified of restraint use, particularly if it involved a change in condition, but they do not need to give permission.

11. **c) "I will need to refer you to an OB/GYN NP, who can insert the IUD for you."** This patient would need to be referred to a woman's health NP, family NP, or OB/GYN for insertion of the IUD. This procedure is out of the scope of practice for AG-ACNP and not part of the clinic care, which is for her pulmonary disease. Obtaining a pregnancy test and consent form, and a patient being on her period, are required as part of the process but not in this setting.

12. **b) Call for a certified medical interpreter to be present or by phone**. The legal foundation for language access lies in Title VI of the 1964 Civil Rights Act, which states: *"No person in the United States shall, on the ground of race, color, or national origin, be excluded from participation in, be denied the benefits of, or be subjected to discrimination under any program or activity receiving federal financial assistance."* Healthcare organizations must assure the competency of interpreters and bilingual staff to provide language assistance to patients and consumers of limited English proficiency.

13. **b) Obtain supervision for CVC placement**. The AG-ACNP still requires supervision with procedures until the proper credentialing process is completed and the AG-ACNP has documentation that the additional procedure has been approved and added to his institutional credentials. The attending physician does not have the authority to override the credentialing process. This patient may have untoward outcomes by managing the patient with peripheral vasopressors.

14. **a) The OCR**. The OCR enforces the protections safeguarded by HIPPA. The HHS is the administrative agency that developed the regulations for HIPPA. The AMA has nothing to do from an enforcement perspective. AHRQ is an independent organization concerned with reporting research of quality measures.

15. c) CQI. Quality assurance is the maintenance of a desired level of quality in a service or product, which is good, but this is a situation that has been modified. Collaborative practice is usually a relationship with a physician, which in some states, for an AG-ACNP to practice, a formal written agreement is required. CQI is the systematic process of identifying and analyzing problems and then testing, implementing, learning from, and revising solutions, which is exactly what this scenario is describing. Case management is a process of assessment, planning, facilitation, care coordination, evaluation, and advocacy for options and services to meet an individual's and family's comprehensive health needs.

■ BIBLIOGRAPHY

Agency for Healthcare Research and Quality. (2014). *The Patient Safety and Improvement Act of* 2005. Retrieved from https://www.ahrq.gov/policymakers/psoact.html

American Association of Critical-Care Nurses. (2017). *AACN scope and standards for acute care nurse practitioner practice 2017* (L. Bell Ed.). Aliso Viejo, CA: American Association of Critical Care Nurses.

Buppert, C. (2018). *Nurse practitioner's business practice and legal guide* (6th ed.). Boulder, CO: Jones & Bartlett.

Centers for Medicare and Medicaid Services. (2018). *Medicare part A: Hospice & respite care.* Retrieved from https://www.medicare.gov/coverage/hospice-and-respite-care.html

Dorman, T., Britten, F., Brown, D., & Munro, N. (2014). *Coding and billing for critical care: A practice tool.* Mount Prospect, IL: Society of Critical Care Medicine.

Hudon, C., Chouinard, M. C., Lambert, M., Dufour, I., & Krieg, C. (2016). Effectiveness of case management interventions for frequent users of healthcare services: A scoping review. *British Medical Journal Open, 6*(9), e012353. doi:10.1136/bmjopen-2016-012353

Hunt, D. (2016). *New 2016 ACA rules significantly affect the law of language access.* Retrieved from https://www.cmelearning.com/new-2016-aca-rules-significantly-affect-the-law-of-language-access

Kleinpell, R. M., Hravnak, M., Hinch, B., & Llewellyn, J. (2008). Developing an advanced practice nursing credentialing model for acute care facilities. *Nursing Administration Quarterly, 32*(4), 279–287. doi: 10.1097/01.NAQ.0000336724.95440

Larsen, P. D. (2018). *Lubkin's chronic illness impact and intervention* (10th ed.). Burlington, MA: Jones & Barlett Learning.

Linden, J. A. (2011). Care of the adult patient after sexual assault. *New England Journal of Medicine, 365*(9), 834–841. doi:10.1056/NEJMcp1102869

May, A. M., & Klonsky, E. D. (2013). Assessing motivations for suicide attempts: Development and psychometric properties of the inventory of motivations for suicide attempts. *Suicide and Life-Threatening Behavior, 43*(5), 532–546. doi:10.1111/sltb.12037

Nursing Service Organization. (2010). *Nurse practitioners and malpractice insurance: Frequently asked questions.* Retrieved from https://www.napnap.org/sites/default/files/userfiles/for_providers/NP_Malpractice_FAQ_NSO.pdf

O'Doherty, L., Hegarty, K., Ramsay, J., Davidson, L. L., Feder, G., & Taft, A. (2015). Screening women for intimate partner violence in healthcare settings. *Cochrane Database of Systematic Reviews, 30*(4), CD007007. doi: 10.1002/14651858.CD007007.pub3

Papadakis, M. A., McPhee, S. J., & Rabow, M. W. (2017). *Current medical diagnosis & treatment 2017.* New York, NY: McGraw-Hill Education.

Rape and sexual assault, 10 U.S. Code § 920 - Art. 120 C.F.R. (2018). Retrieved from https://www.law.cornell.edu/uscode/text/10/920

Reuben, D. B., Herr, K. A., Pacala, J. T, Pollock, B. G., Potter, J. F, & Selma, T. P. (2017). *Geriatrics at your fingertips* (19th ed.). New York, NY: American Geriatrics Society.

Safriet, B. J. (2011). Federal options for maximizing the value of advanced practice nurses in providing quality, cost-effective health care. In Committee on the Robert Wood Johnson Foundation Initiative on the Future of Nursing, at the Institute of Medicine, (Ed.), *The future of nursing: Leading change, advancing health* (pp. 443–475). Washington, DC: Institute of Medicine.

Sexual Assault Prevention and Response. (2010). *Rape reporting requirements for competent adult victims.* Retrieved from http://www.sapr.mil/public/docs/laws/arkansas.pdf

Springer, G.(2015). When and how to use restraints. *American Nurse Today, 10*(1), 26–27.

The Joint Commission Division of Health Care Improvement. (2016). Hospital accreditation standards: Provision of care treatment and services. In *standard P.C03.05.01 through P. C03.05.19.*

U.S. Department of Health and Human Services. (2013). *Summary of the HIPAA security rule.* Retrieved from https://www.hhs.gov/hipaa/for-professionals/security/laws-regulations/index.html

19

Research and Evidence-Based Practice

*HOPE MOSER, DAWN CARPENTER,
AND JAMES FAIN*

RESEARCH AND EVIDENCE-BASED PRACTICE QUESTIONS

1. A confidence interval for a mean is:

   a. The interval containing the unknown population mean
   b. A point in time estimate of a population mean
   c. A fixed parameter (interval)
   d. A discrete variable (parameter)

2. The FDA-approval process for drugs to get to market includes and utilizes multiple study phases I, II, III, IIIA, and IIIB. Phase IV studies are performed after the drug is approved for marketing and are used in market comparison. The AG-ACNP understands that phase II studies are:

   a. Used to determine toxicity and safety
   b. Large prospective studies to evaluate clinical efficacy
   c. The first controlled clinical studies of the drug involving a small group of patients
   d. Performed after preliminary evidence regarding the effectiveness of the drug has been demonstrated

3. Appraisal of clinical trials includes assessment for systematic errors. Reasons for systematic errors include:

   a. Multiple measurements
   b. Random chance
   c. Study design flaws
   d. Increased sample size

4. Ethnography is:

   a. The study of the nature or meaning of everyday experiences through the lived experience of subjects
   b. The study of discovering theory from data systematically obtained through research

    c. The study of philosophy focusing on exploration of the inner world of individuals

    d. The study of and description of a culture of a particular group of individuals

5. EBP is the conscious use of current best evidence to facilitate decision-making about patient care. It is grounded in:

    a. Information found in textbooks

    b. Best evidence and clinical expertise

    c. Systematically conducted research studies

    d. Expert opinion

6. Clinical practice guidelines:

    a. Are widely agreed upon between professional organizations

    b. Provide a strict legal protocol for AG-ACNPs to follow

    c. Contain best evidence, include cost-effective approaches to patient care

    d. Do not provide clinicians any protection from malpractice

7. A well-developed PICOT question helps the AG-ACNP:

    a. Find the largest amount of information.

    b. Search for focused evidence.

    c. Critically appraise the literature.

    d. Cultivate a spirit of inquiry.

8. Which of the following databases would the AG-ACNP use to find the most rigorous systematic reviews?

    a. PubMed

    b. CINAHL

    c. *ACP Journal Club*

    d. Cochrane Library

9. What is the correct order of hierarchy of evidence, from highest to lowest, on which to base treatment decisions?

    a. Meta-analyses, RCTs, case–control/cohort studies, descriptive studies

    b. Meta-analyses, case–control/cohort studies, RCTs, descriptive studies

    c. Systematic reviews, case–control/cohort studies, RCTs, expert opinion

    d. Systematic reviews, case–control/cohort studies, RCTs, descriptive studies

10. The AG-ACNP completes a literature search and identifies 30 potential articles on a particular topic of interest. To determine which of the 30 articles are appropriate, the AG-ACNP should first read the:

    a. Methods section of each article

    b. Discussion section of each article

    c. Abstract of each article

    d. Literature review of each article

11. The ability to generalize findings from a study's sample to the larger population is known as:

    a. Internal validity

    b. External validity

    c. Internal evidence

    d. External evidence

12. Which of the following is a limitation to EBP?

    a. Absence of research that explains practice
    b. Establishing linkages between academic and practice
    c. Access to evidence, time, money, and clinical resources
    d. Attending conferences where research is presented outside your institution

13. Test-retest reliability measures:

    a. Consistency of scores over time
    b. Consistency of scores obtained from two equivalent halves of the same exam
    c. Consistency with which a test measures a single construct/concept
    d. Degree of agreement between two or more scores

14. An AG-ACNP reads a research report that indicates the p value is $<.05$. The AG-ACNP concludes there was:

    a. Not a significant result and this would have only arose 5/10 times through chance
    b. Not a significant result and this would have only arose 5/100 times through chance
    c. A significant result and this would have only arose 5/10 times through chance
    d. A significant result and this would have only arose 5/100 times through chance

15. Which of the following is considered a scientific method used in action-oriented learning that impacts change and a desired outcome?

    a. PDSA
    b. NQF
    c. NDNQI
    d. PICOT

■ RESEARCH AND EVIDENCE-BASED PRACTICE ANSWERS AND RATIONALES

1. **a) The interval containing the unknown population mean.** The confidence level is the degree of certainty that the interval actually contains the unknown population parameter value. It provides the degree of assurance or confidence that the statement regarding the population parameter is correct. The more certainty we want, the wider the interval will have to be.

2. **c) The first controlled clinical studies of the drug involving a small group of patients.** Phase II studies are the first controlled clinical studies of the drug involving no more than several hundred patients. The primary objectives of phase II studies are to explore efficacy and less-common side effects. Phase I studies determine toxicity and safety. Phase III studies are larger prospective studies of clinical efficacy.

3. **b) Random chance.** Random errors can be introduced by chance. Variations due to chance can occur in most situations. Multiple measurements and larger sample sizes minimize chance of systematic errors.

4. **d) The study of and description of a culture of a particular group of individuals.** Ethnographic research studies describe a culture of a particular group of individuals. Grounded theory is the qualitative method discovering a theory from data systematically obtained through research. Phenomenology is the study of the nature or meaning of everyday experiences through the lived experience of subjects.

5. **b) Best evidence and clinical expertise.** EBP refers to the concept that clinical decisions should be supported by the strongest evidence, one's own clinical expertise, and patient preferences and values.

6. **c) Contain best evidence, include cost-effective approaches to patient care.** Practice guidelines have been developed by many professional organizations and agencies as a decision-making aid to caregivers. Most organizations attempt to incorporate the most recent available evidence and concerns of cost-effectiveness into their guideline formulations. Despite increasing levels of nuance in current guidelines, they cannot be expected to account for the uniqueness of each individual and his or her illness. Furthermore, many discrepancies exist in guidelines from major organizations. By setting a standard of reasonable care in most cases, clinical guidelines provide protection to both clinicians (from inappropriate charges of malpractice) and to patients, particularly those with inadequate healthcare resources. Even though guidelines do provide this protection, they do not provide a rigid legal constraint for the conscientious physician. The physician's challenge is to incorporate the useful recommendations provided by the experts in guidelines and incorporate them into the care of each individual patient.

7. **b) Search for focused evidence.** The PICOT question is used to identify the search terms for a successful and efficient focused search and begin the evidence-based process. Focused searches will identify studies that will efficiently answer the clinical question.

8. **d) Cochrane Library.** Cochrane Library contains the most rigorous systematic reviews. While PubMed contains many systematic reviews, the quality metrics of how the systematic reviews are performed may vary. CINAHL provides journal, primary studies, and reviews specific to nursing, but may miss key evidence from other professions. *ACP Journal Club* contains summaries of studies and expert clinical commentary.

9. **a) Meta-analyses, RCTs, case-control/cohort studies, descriptive studies.** Meta-analyses and systematic reviews of RCTs are the two highest levels of evidence, followed by RCTs, then controlled trials without randomization, case–control and cohort studies, systematic reviews of descriptive and qualitative studies, single descriptive or qualitative studies, and finally expert committees.

10. **c) Abstract of each article.** Reading the abstract will provide an initial screen for potential inclusion. The initial screen will include review of level of evidence, population, intervention,

and comparison groups as well as outcomes. Reading the methods sections of each article are parts of the rapid critical appraisal process to determine if the study results are valid, reliable, and applicable. Reading the literature review and discussion sections can help identify further articles that may also answer the PICOT question.

11. **b) External validity**. External validity refers to the generalizability to larger population. Internal validity refers to the independent variable having caused the change in the outcome. External evidence is generated through research processes and is intended to be used outside of one's own clinical practice setting.

12. **c) Access to evidence, time, money, and clinical resources**. Common limitations of EBP include possessing skill in searching and appraising the literature, time to master these skills, time to implement EBP scarce resources, and access to evidence.

13. **a) Consistency of scores over time**. Test-retest reliability is consistency of scores over time. Consistency of scores obtained from two equivalent halves of the same exam is split/half reliability. Consistency with which a test measures a single construct/concept is construct reliability. Degree of agreement between two or more scores is inter-rater reliability.

14. **d) A significant result and this would have only arose 5/100 times through chance**. Researchers use .05 as the standard level of significance, that is, researchers are willing to accept statistical significance occurring by chance five times out of 100.

15. **a) PDSA**. PDSA cycle is a widely adopted and effective model to test change on a small scale and evaluate impact on outcomes. PICOT components are the elements of a clinical question to be answered. These elements are used to create a search strategy for databases. NDNQI is a database that gathers data to understand factors influencing the quality of nursing care and outcomes at the unit level. NQF is a set of quality indicators to develop and implement a national strategy for healthcare quality measures and reporting.

■ BIBLIOGRAPHY

Chow, S. C. (2014). *Design and analysis of clinical trials: Concepts and methodologies* (3rd ed.). Hoboken, NJ: John Wiley & Sons.

Fain, J. (2017). *Reading, understanding and applying nursing research* (5th ed.). Philadelphia, PA: F.A. Davis.

Greenberg, R. S. (2015). *Medical epidemiology: Population health and effective health care* (5th ed.). New York, NY: McGraw-Hill.

Kasper, D., Hauser, S., Jameson, J., Fauci, A., Longo, D., & Loscalzo, J. (2015). *Harrison's principles of internal medicine* (19th ed.). New York, NY: McGraw-Hill.

Mazurek-Melnyk, B., & Fineout-Overhold, E. F. (2015). *Evidence-based practice in nursing & healthcare: A guide to best practice* (3rd ed.). Philadelphia, PA: Wolter Kluwer Health.

McKean, S. C. R. J., Dressler, D. D., & Scheurer, D. B. (2017). *Principles and practice of hospital medicine* (2nd ed.). New York, NY: McGraw-Hill.

Sharp, V. J., Kieran, K., & Arlen, A. M. (2013). Testicular torsion: Diagnosis, evaluation, and management. *American Family Physician, 88*(12), 835–840.

Van Norman, G. A. (2016). Drugs, devices, and the FDA: Part 1: An overview of approval processes for drugs. *JACC: Basic to Translational Science, 1*(3), 170–179. doi:10.1016/j.jacbts.2016.03.002

20 Education and Facilitation of Learning

LEANNE H. FOWLER

EDUCATION AND FACILITATION OF LEARNING QUESTIONS

1. A 45-year-old patient is admitted to the hospital for chest pain. The patient has no prior medical or surgical history and an unknown family history. The patient has a 40-pack-year tobacco history and social alcohol use. Cardiac workup revealed normal chest x-ray, 12-lead ECG with no ischemic changes, normal sinus rhythm, and LV hypertrophy. The patient is preparing for discharge home. What behavior coaching skill should the AG-ACNP use to help the patient make long-term changes to reduce the risk for chronic illness?

   a. Ask closed questions.
   b. Avoid paraphrasing patient responses.
   c. Use active listening.
   d. Avoid empathetic communication.

2. Which coaching skill, used by the AG-ACNP, will best assist the patient to generate strategies to overcome barriers related to lifestyle changes?

   a. Problem solving
   b. Goal setting
   c. Active listening
   d. Paraphrasing

3. What strategy is an interviewing approach performed by the AG-ACNP to understand and help the patient resolve ambivalence about a behavioral change by increasing the awareness for and building a desire to adopt new behaviors to improve health?

   a. Advanced communication
   b. Motivational interviewing
   c. Self-reflection
   d. Cultural competence

4. Which of the following is a health literacy strategy aimed to help reduce health disparities and improve the quality and safety of care?

   a. Providing patients with educational materials that were prepared utilizing complex detailed language
   b. Referring patients to health information on the Internet
   c. Documenting the years of education a patient has completed
   d. Advocating for programmatic approaches and policies for simpler education materials

5. According to the TTM for behavior change (Norcross, Krebs, & Prochaska, 2011), behavior change occurs through five stages. The AG-ACNP is assessing a patient with an 80-pack-year history of smoking. The AG-ACNP believes the patient is in the "preparation stage" to learn lifestyle changes when:

   a. The patient is not interested in learning about or thinking about his high-risk behaviors.
   b. The patient admits to knowing the hazards of tobacco abuse and benefits of cessation.
   c. The patient is still smoking occasionally but has a detailed plan to quit within a month.
   d. The patient has already quit and feels confident he can sustain tobacco abstinence.

6. A 55-year-old male has recently been diagnosed with DMII. The patient and his spouse have begun walking 1 hour, 5 days per week and adhering to strict dietary restrictions. The spouse reports the patient has been compliant with the metformin regimen prescribed for him. What factors or behaviors should the AG-ACNP recognize as a risk for the patient to relapse to high-risk behaviors?

   a. The patient reports new stressors of losing his job.
   b. The patient reports less desire for sugary foods and drinks.
   c. The patient reports losing weight and a reduction in finger-stick glucose levels.
   d. The patient reports looking forward to taking walks with his spouse.

7. Which systems-level process improvement strategy should the AG-ACNP acknowledge is a barrier to an optimal patient-learning environment:

   a. Identification of key stakeholders within the organization needed to support the patient-level change
   b. Engaging interprofessional collaboration to identify and discuss barriers to an optimal learning environment
   c. Identifying processes and procedures needed to support the patient-level change
   d. Limiting patient visitation or group settings during teaching moments

8. Identify the term that is defined as the approach to developing learning materials written and designed to be engaging, accessible, and easy to read:

   a. Health literacy
   b. Plain language
   c. Education level
   d. Functional literacy

9. Which term is defined as the skills patients use to communicate their needs and preferences; to understand the choices, consequences, and context of information; and to make sense of health information and services?:

   a. Health literacy
   b. Plain language
   c. Education level
   d. Competence

10. A 39-year-old patient diagnosed with late-stage, metastatic ovarian cancer is admitted to the hospital with acute pain and persistent nausea with vomiting. She reports having a living will and would like to formulate a plan of care that will help keep her out of the hospital and that will allow her to spend the rest of her time with her family "until I die." What action should the AG-ACNP take to facilitate patient-centered care?

    a. Discuss palliative and hospice treatment options with the patient and her oncologist.
    b. Order comfort measures, antiemetics, and analgesics routinely in preparation for discharge home.
    c. Consult the oncologist to address the patient's cancer management plan.
    d. Consult the social worker to have hospice or palliative-care agencies evaluate the patient.

11. The AG-ACNP spent approximately 15 minutes with a patient and family discussing therapeutic lifestyle changes the patient can make to improve cardiovascular health. What term should the AG-ACNP use in documentation for billable services that reflect the CPT coding system for patient evaluation and management services?

    a. Education
    b. Counseling
    c. Coaching
    d. Mentoring

12. A 35-year-old African American male patient is being treated in the observation unit for a lower extremity abscess. Upon review of medical records the AG-ACNP notes that the patient was most recently seen by his PCP and was diagnosed with Stage 1 essential hypertension with a low-risk atherosclerotic cardiovascular disease score. The patient's blood pressure is noted to be 136/88. The best action for the AG-ACNP to take at this time would be to:

    a. Reinforce education provided to the patient at PCP's office that includes disease and significance of initiating therapeutic lifestyle changes.
    b. Refer the patient to cardiology clinic for Stage B heart failure evaluation and treatment.
    c. Prescribe hydrochlorthiazide 25 mg daily with amlodipine 5 mg daily and ask him to follow up in 4 weeks with his PCP.
    d. Prescribe furosemide 10 mg daily as monotherapy and ask him to follow up in 4 to 6 weeks with his PCP.

13. An independent 71-year-old patient presents to the ED with a productive cough, subjective fever, and generalized weakness that has not gotten any better over the past week. The patient is alert and oriented and able to provide appropriate history. Chest radiograph reveals a left lower lobe infiltrate suspicious for pneumonia. The patient's vital signs include a temperature of 100.1°F, blood pressure of 145/85 mmHg, heart rate of 87, respiratory rate of 22, and a pulse oximeter reading of 96% on room air. All laboratory values are within normal limits except for a WBC of 12.4. The patient has a medical history of hypertension, for which he takes lisinopril 5 mg daily and a multivitamin. The AG-ACNP was consulted by emergency medicine for hospital admission. What is the next best action?

    a. Admit the patient to the medical-surgical unit for intravenous antibiotic therapy.
    b. Discharge the patient home with oral antibiotic therapy, patient/family education for CAP, and a follow-up referral with the PCP in 1 week.
    c. Admit the patient to the medical ICU for at least 24 hours and intravenous antibiotic therapy.
    d. Discharge the patient home with oral antiviral therapy, patient education for lower respiratory infections caused by viruses, and a follow-up referral with the PCP in 1 week.

14. A staff nurse asks the hospital medicine AG-ACNP rounding that day "why can't family members just use the alcohol-based hand-hygiene products after visiting" a patient diagnosed with history of (HO) CDI. Which statement is the best response to the nurse?

   a. "Family members who are not involved in the direct care of the patients with a CDI can follow universal precautions."
   b. "Hand hygiene with alcohol-based products before contact and after glove removal is adequate if there has been no direct contact with the patient's feces or perineal region."
   c. "When family members don all personal protective equipment for CDI contact precautions, alcohol-based hand-hygiene products can be used immediately after glove removal."
   d. "Visitors can refrain from contact precautions and CDI-recommended hand hygiene if they are not visiting other patients in the hospital."

15. A 36-year-old female presents to the ED complaining of "another urinary tract infection." The patient has been followed and treated by a PCP for uncomplicated cystitis over the past month. The patient completed two courses of ciprofloxacin and states the last urinalysis continues to show bacteria. She denies fever, dysuria, vaginal discharge, cloudy urine, hematuria, and incontinence. The patient would like a second opinion and a prescription for a different antibiotic. A urine pregnancy test is negative and a repeat urinalysis revealed some bacteriuria, no pyuria, and no leukocyte esterase. Using evidence-based guidelines, the AG-ACNP should:

   a. Request the urinalysis, culture, and sensitivity results from the lab to identify a susceptible drug for treatment.
   b. Refer the patient to infectious diseases for drug-resistant infection evaluation and referral to a new PCP.
   c. Provide patient education for the urinalysis findings and the risk for CDI with overuse of fluoroquinolones.
   d. Consult hospital medicine for admission and initiate orders for indwelling catheter placement and intravenous antibiotic therapy.

■ EDUCATION AND FACILITATION OF LEARNING ANSWERS AND RATIONALES

1. **c) Use active listening**. Active listening nonverbally communicates to patients they have your full attention and care about their issues that may be related to the behavior needing modification. Other behavior-changing skills include asking open-ended questions to help explore the patient's thoughts about a topic; paraphrasing patient responses to demonstrate you were listening and understand the patient's issue; and using empathetic communication to demonstrate the AG-ACNP understands the meaning of that issue to the patient. These are skills of successful coaching sessions with patients aimed to facilitate long-term behavioral changes.

2. **a) Problem solving**. Problem solving is a behavior coaching skill the AG-ACNP can use to engage patient-centered care and patient/family participation with finding solutions for difficult but necessary lifestyle modifications. The other responses are coaching skills that do not directly engage the patient's perspective of how to overcome limitations or barriers.

3. **b) Motivational interviewing**. Motivational interviewing has proven to improve patient health by facilitating change in the patient's thoughts and behaviors. The AG-ACNP actively listens during the interview and engages the patient through situated/strategic questions aimed to elicit self-reflection about the patient's motivations surrounding barriers to change. The other responses are skills and components of motivational interviewing.

4. **d) Advocating for programmatic approaches and policies for simpler education materials**. AG-ACNP's need to advocate for programmatic approaches and policies for simpler education materials. Language in educational materials should be in plain language. Before referring patients and families to the Internet for information, the AG-ACNP should evaluate the material for appropriate level of plain language. The number of years of education a patient has completed is not an adequate indicator of the patient's reading level or computational literacy. Also, patients with higher levels of education completed can still have difficulty processing complex information about new diagnoses or illnesses due to situational stressors.

5. **c) The patient is still smoking occasionally but has a detailed plan to quit within a month**. Patients are more open to the AG-ACNP's advice during the preparation stage of the TTM framework for behavior change. Because of this learning readiness, the AG-ACNP can collaboratively work with the patient to identify and anticipate barriers for cessation and develop specific strategies to overcome them. In the precontemplative stage, the patient is not ready to acknowledge the need to learn behavior changes. In the contemplation stage the patient demonstrates ambivalence and uncertainty. In the action stage, the patient is beyond learning readiness and has already changed the behavior.

6. **a) The patient reports new stressors of losing his job**. The patient who has undergone a recent behavior change can indicate the risk for relapse when new stressors occur that may interfere with the patient's new behavioral routine and tempt him to revert to former, high-risk coping strategies. The AG-ACNP can assess the patient's risk for relapse by reviewing the patient's plan to overcome and manage the new stress without reverting back to prior high-risk and unhealthy behaviors.

7. **d) Limiting patient visitation or group settings during teaching moments**. Promoting a learning environment within a healthcare setting requires a coordinated and collaborative approach. An optimal learning environment should also include and encourage appropriate social support for the patient and family. Limiting visitation can inhibit patient engagement and become a barrier to the patient's motivation to participate in the learning process of behavior change.

8. **b) Plain language**. Patient education materials should use "plain language" to facilitate clear communication and reader-friendliness. Plain language principles are used to address and improve the patient's health literacy aiming to reduce health disparities and improve the quality and safety of care.

9. **a) Health literacy**. The AG-ACNP must understand the terminology used for adequate patient education. By understanding the meaning of health literacy, the AG-ACNP can appreciate the significance a patient's health literacy capacity has upon the patient's health. The patient's health literacy capacity can also impact medical adherence and readmission rates. Plain language is writing designed to ensure the reader understands as quickly, easily, and completely as possible.

10. **a) Discuss palliative and hospice treatment options with the patient and her oncologist**. This patient realizes she is at the end of her life due to progressive and late-stage cancer. Ensuring the patient's care preferences are included in the collaborative management of her illness with the oncologist facilitates shared decision making and informed decisions about her options. The AG-ACNP collaborating with the patient's oncologist facilitates optimal coordination of care and communication between all medical providers and the patient. Including the patient in the decision-making process will allow her to understand and determine comfort-care options. The social worker can contact the appropriate agency after an initial discussion with the patient has occurred.

11. **b) Counseling**. The AG-ACNP should capture time spent on patient education as counseling services to demonstrate the impact upon the patient's health. Coaching and mentoring are AG-ACNP competencies involved in patient education but are not terms used in the CPT coding system of billable services.

12. **a) Reinforce education provided to the patient at PCP's office that includes disease and significance of initiating therapeutic lifestyle changes**. The best action would be to educate the patient on his disease and advised management. Stage 1 essential hypertension in a patient with a low-risk atherosclerotic cardiovascular disease score can be managed by therapeutic lifestyle changes without pharmacotherapeutic interventions. This patient's disease state does not warrant cardiology consultation and is not indicative of Stage B heart failure.

13. **b) Discharge the patient home with oral antibiotic therapy, patient/family education for CAP, and a follow-up referral with the PCP in 1 week**. The AG-ACNP should use an evidence-based tool to facilitate clinical decision making related to the admission or discharge of an older adult. Admission to the hospital is not warranted for this patient using the CURB-65 tool. Considering this patient is independent, does not live alone, and reports having adequate follow-up care, discharging the patient home with adequate instructions for care is reasonable. Patient education for CAP would include an explanation of the disease process, signs and symptoms of decline, treatment options, and when to seek urgent/emergent medical attention.

14. **b) "Hand hygiene with alcohol-based products before contact and after glove removal is adequate if there has been no direct contact with the patient's feces or perineal region."** According to 2018 CDI guidelines for infection control, hand hygiene before contact and after glove removal with either soap and water or an alcohol-based hand-hygiene product is strongly recommended. Contact precautions should be used for all patients diagnosed or suspected to have a CDI. If the hospital is experiencing a CDI outbreak or has sustained high rates of CDIs, hand hygiene with soap and water to more effectively remove spores is weakly recommended by the guidelines and has low quality of supporting evidence.

15. **c) Provide patient education for the urinalysis findings and the risk for CDI with overuse of fluoroquinolones**. Treatment with antibiotics is not recommended for asymptomatic bacteriuria in nonpregnant, premenopausal females. Treatment of asymptomatic bacteriuria is associated with untoward outcomes including antimicrobial resistance, adverse effects, and increased cost.

■ REFERENCE

Norcross, J. C., Krebs, P. M., & Prochaska, J. O. (2011). Stages of change. *Journal of Clinical Psychology, 67*(2), 143–154. doi:10.1002/jclp.20758

■ BIBLIOGRAPHY

Adult-Gerontology Nurse Practitioner Competencies Work Group. (2016). *Adult-gerontology acute care and primary care NP competencies.* Retrieved from http://c.ymcdn.com/sites/www.nonpf.org/resource/resmgr/competencies/NP_Adult_Geri_competencies_4.pdf

Agency for Healthcare Research and Quality. (2014). *Behavior coaching.* Retrieved from https://www.ahrq.gov/professionals/education/curriculum-tools/stepmanual/step8.html

Centers for Disease Control and Prevention. (2016a). *Everyday words for public health communication.* Retrieved from https://www.cdc.gov/other/pdf/everydaywords-060216-final.pdf

Centers for Disease Control and Prevention. (2016b). *What is health literacy?* Retrieved from https://www.cdc.gov/healthliteracy/learn/index.html

Eckel, R. H., Jakicic, J. M., Ard, J. D., De Jesus, J. M., Miller, N. H., Hubbard, V. S., . . . Yanovski, S. Z. (2014). 2013 AHA/ACC guideline on lifestyle management to reduce cardiovascular risk: A report of the American College of Cardiology/American Heart Association task force on practice guidelines. *Journal of the American College of Cardiology, 63*(25, Pt. B), 2960–2984. doi:10.1161/01.cir.0000437740.48606

Hamric, A., Hanson, C., Tracy, M. F., & O'Grady, E. T. (2014). *Advanced practice nursing: An integrative approach* (5th ed.). St. Louis, MO: Elsevier Saunders.

Institute for Healthcare Improvement. (2018). *Person- and family-centered-care: Overview.* Retrieved from http://www.ihi.org/Topics/PFCC/Pages/Overview.aspx

Mandell, L. A., Wunderink, R. G., Anzueto, A., Bartlett, J. G., Campbell, G. D., Dean, N. C., . . . American Thoracic Society. (2007). Infectious Diseases Society of America/American Thoracic Society consensus guidelines on the management of community-acquired pneumonia in adults. *Clinical Infectious Diseases, 44*(Suppl. 2), S27–72. doi:10.1086/511159

McDonald, L. C., Gerding, D. N., Johnson, S., Bakken, J. S., Carroll, K. C., Coffin, S. E., . . . Wilcox, M. H. (2018). Clinical practice guidelines for clostridium difficile infection in adults and children: 2017 update by the Infectious Diseases Society of America and Society for Healthcare Epidemiology of America. *Clinical Infectious Diseases, 66*(7):e1–e48.doi:10.1093/cid/cix1085

Moyers, T. B. (2014). The relationship in motivational interviewing. *Psychotherapy (Chic), 51*(3), 358–363. doi:10.1037/a0036910

Nicolle, L. E., Bradley, S., Colgan, R., Rice, J. C., Schaeffer, A., Hooton, T. M., . . . American Geriatrics Society. (2005). Infectious Diseases Society of America guidelines for the diagnosis and treatment of asymptomatic bacteriuria in adults. *Clinical Infectious Diseases, 40*(5), 643–654. doi:10.1086/427507

Whelton, P. K., Carey, R. M., Aronow, W. S., Casey, D. E., Collins, K. J., Himmelfarb, C. D., & Jones, D. W. (2017). 2017 ACC/AHA/AAPA/ABC/ACPM/AGS/APhA/ASH/ASPC/NMA/PCNA guideline for the prevention, detection, evaluation, and management of high blood pressure in adults: A report of the American College of Cardiology/American Heart Association task force on clinical practice guidelines. *Journal of the American College of Cardiology, 71*(6):1269-1324.

21

AG-ACNP–Patient Relationship

LEANNE H. FOWLER

AG-ACNP–PATIENT RELATIONSHIP QUESTIONS

1. The AG-ACNP is caring for a comatose patient in the critical care unit. What strategy can be used to maintain communication and a therapeutic relationship with this patient?

   a. Utilize appropriate touch and reassuring tone of voice during care.
   b. Have the patient's family communicate to the patient what you as the AG-ACNP are doing.
   c. Avoid communicating with the patient as this may cause distress to the patient.
   d. Limit family interaction with the patient.

2. A 19-year-old patient is suspected to be injured secondary to intimate partner violence. The patient is evasive and withdrawn. Which communication skill should the AG-ACNP demonstrate to facilitate patient-centered therapeutic communication?

   a. Address the patient's complaints matter-of-factly, with an erect posture, and focused on the mechanism of injury.
   b. Use closed questioning to isolate extraneous details from relevant data.
   c. Inquire about the patient's thoughts, perspectives, expectations, and/or goals about her injuries.
   d. Counsel the patient about the epidemiology of intimate partner violence and risk for further injury.

3. What strategy can the AG-ACNP use to work toward resolution of situations causing his or her own moral distress?

   a. Reflective practice
   b. Coaching and guidance
   c. Evidence-guided practice
   d. Therapeutic communication

4. An AG-ACNP identifies inconsistent care of critically ill patients with traumatic brain injuries. The provider coordinates a staff meeting with hospital administrators and nursing, respiratory therapy, and medical staff to discuss the latest research supporting standardized approaches to care of this population of patients. The AG-ACNP obtains support to implement a standardized approach to care, coordinates clinician training, and develops algorithms with information technology to support computerized order-entry and documentation efforts of this practice change. According to the AACN Synergy Model for Patient Care (2003), what professional competency is the AG-ACNP demonstrating the most with this initiative?

   a. Clinical judgment
   b. Interprofessional collaboration
   c. Clinical inquiry
   d. Professional and patient advocacy

5. A 79-year-old patient recently experienced the loss of her spouse of 42 years who was the patient's primary caregiver financially and physically. The patient is losing sleep over this change and is considering moving into a long-term care facility for safety and assistance with activities of daily living. What intervention should the AG-ACNP utilize when initiating crisis prevention techniques?

   a. Prescribe an appropriate pharmacotherapeutic agent.
   b. Actively listen to the patient's concerns with minimal interruptions.
   c. Hand off this process to a social worker or case manager.
   d. Inquire about the family's thoughts and feelings surrounding this life change.

6. A 38-year-old patient with a significant family history for breast cancer is seeking genetic counseling at an oncology clinic under the duress of her mother, sister, and aunt. The AG-ACNP will provide posttest counseling to discuss the results and implications of the results. Which ethical concerns regarding the disclosure of test results should the AG-ACNP caution against during posttest counseling with the patient and other family members?

   a. Issues of justice
   b. Moral distress
   c. Beneficence
   d. Privacy and confidentiality

7. The AG-ACNP is caring for an older adult trauma patient with bilateral rib fractures. The patient developed acute respiratory failure for which he was intubated in the early morning hours. The AG-ACNP's next step is to:

   a. Call and notify family.
   b. Update note in medical record that describes patient's change in medical condition.
   c. Bill for services.
   d. Inform the charge nurse.

8. A young adult is in cardiac arrest. Family is in the waiting room and is demanding to come into the room. The AG-ACNP's best response is to:

   a. Allow the family to be in the room but stand in the corner.
   b. Allow the family to come to the doorway to observe.
   c. Allow the family to come in the room and ensure support is provided to the family.
   d. Not allow it as it is against hospital policy.

9. The AG-ACNP is obtaining consent from a patient for a CVC to be placed for vasopressor therapy. The consent form needs to include the benefits, risks, and:

   a. Consequences
   b. What device will be used
   c. Technique for insertion
   d. Alternatives

10. A new AG-ACNP, working in a tertiary care hospital, is obtaining consent from a patient to insert a CVC for management of septic shock. The patient asks the AG-ACNP how many catheters has she inserted, to which she responds five. The patient becomes upset and refuses to allow the AG-ACNP to insert the catheter. The best response by the AG-ACNP is to:

   a. Inform the patient that they are in a teaching hospital and critically ill, requiring this be done immediately.
   b. Acknowledge the patient's concerns, reassure him the AG-ACNP will be careful, and proceed to set up for the procedure.
   c. Acknowledge the patient's concerns and offer to find a more seasoned person to perform the procedure.
   d. Inform the attending physician of the patient's refusal to have the procedure.

■ AG-ACNP–PATIENT RELATIONSHIP ANSWERS AND RATIONALES

1. **a) Utilize appropriate touch and reassuring tone of voice during care.** Studies report patients who were unconscious were able to hear and sometimes respond emotionally to those speaking to them. Therefore, the AG-ACNP should still communicate to the patient and assess for patient response despite the patient's limited ability to interact. The family should not, however, interact with the patient on behalf of the nurse. It is imperative that the AG-ACNP state to the patient what he or she is doing. Avoidance of communication may cause more distress, especially if touch or some type of procedure is done without informing the patient that this is going to be done first.

2. **c) Inquire about the patient's thoughts, perspectives, expectations, and/or goals about her injuries.** Therapeutic communication should include open-ended questioning aimed to engage the patient's participation and facilitate open and honest communication between the patient and provider. The AG-ACNP should avoid matter-of-fact verbalization of information and unrelaxed postures in an effort to create an environment of social connectedness. Therapeutic communication should also include motivational interviewing techniques and principles such as assessing the patient's readiness to learn about high-risk behaviors or situations before providing counseling.

3. **a) Reflective practice.** Reflective practice is an AG-ACNP competency that can be used to demonstrate professional accountability for decisions made and lifelong learning from prior situations. When experiencing moral distress, the AG-ACNP can also utilize the skill of reflective practice along with the 4A framework aimed to address moral distress among nurses. Coaching and guidance are strategies used to facilitate patient education and strengthen the AG-ACNP–patient relationship. Evidence-guided practice is a competency the AG-ACNP uses prior to distressful situations with the intent to support his or /her medical decision making with the best evidence. Therapeutic communication is also a fundamental competency aimed to support the AG-ACNP–patient therapeutic relationship.

4. **d) Professional and patient advocacy.** Working on another's behalf and representing the best interest of the profession and/or patient are the tenets of advocacy. The scenario demonstrates the AG-ACNP serving as a moral agent in recognizing and helping to resolve a clinical problem. Clinical judgment involves the AG-ACNP's ability or capacity of clinical decision making, critical thinking, and an overall grasp of the clinical situation. Interprofessional collaboration does include the ability to work with other healthcare providers and fostering an interdisciplinary healthcare community. However, the scenario is not demonstrating collaboration more than it is advocacy. Clinical inquiry involves the ongoing process of questioning and evaluating practice aimed to ultimately create practice changes. Clinical inquiry in this scenario is necessary and serves as a means for advocacy.

5. **b) Actively listen to the patient's concerns with minimal interruptions.** Active listening is part of developing a therapeutic relationship. The patient has a relationship with the AG-ACNP and handing this off to another team member is not the best option. Working through this change as a team is a better option. Pharmacotherapeutic agents should not be used in patients unless effective screening and diagnosis is made. The patient's perceptions, thoughts, and feelings are more important than the family at this time.

6. **d) Privacy and confidentiality.** Disclosure of test results to other family members can raise ethical concerns because genetic information is crucially linked to privacy and confidentiality issues related to the continued use of that data beyond identification of the patient's risk for disease. Failure to obtain informed consent to include family members in posttest counseling can also raise patient privacy and confidentiality issues.

7. **a) Call and notify family**. The AG-ACNP is responsible for notifying the healthcare proxy or next of kin regarding this acute change in status. Families need timely communication and updates to help make sense of the changing conditions. Updating the medical record is important but can wait until the family is notified. The medical record can include documentation of the family communication, including who was called and what was communicated. Thus the note will be done after the call. The bill for services cannot be done until the note is written. Updating the list is an administrative function that is not the highest priority. Contacting the charge nurse can be done after the patient's family is contacted and the medical record has been updated.

8. **c) Allow the family to come in the room and ensure support is provided to the family**. Witnessing a code can be overwhelming for a family member, thus it's important to have someone with the family member explaining the events of the code. Family may want to touch the patient during the code, especially if survival is unlikely. Thus, it is important to make family part of the care team and make space at the bedside for the family.

9. **d) Alternatives**. Informed consent is an agreement or permission that is accompanied by full disclosure about the care, interventions, and/or services that are the subject of the consent. A patient must be fully apprised of the nature, risks, and alternatives for the medical procedure or treatment before the healthcare professional begins the procedure.

10. **c) Acknowledge the patient's concerns and offer to find a more seasoned person to perform the procedure**. Patients have a right to participate in shared decision making regarding their care. An ethical principle guiding this is the right to self-determination. Providers should be accepting that individual self-determination is a desirable goal, and that clinicians need to support patients to achieve this goal, wherever and whenever feasible. While this patient is critically ill, he is still able to talk, thus deeming this an emergent procedure is not correct. The patient did not refuse to have the procedure; rather, he wants someone with more experience.

■ REFERENCE

American Association of Critical-Care Nurses. (2003). *Synergy model: Basic information about the AACN synergy model for patient care*. Retrieved from https://www.aacn.org/nursing-excellence/aacn-standards/synergy-model

■ BIBLIOGRAPHY

American Association of Critical-Care Nurses. (2004). *The 4A's to rise above moral distress*. Retrieved from http://www.aacn.org/wd/practice/docs/4as_to_rise_above_moral_distress.pdf

Elwyn, G., Frosch, D., Thomson, R., Joseph-Williams, N., Lloyd, A., Kinnersley, P., . . . Barry, M. (2012). Shared decision making: A model for clinical practice. *Journal of General Internal Medicine, 27*(10), 1361–1367. doi:10.1007/s11606-012-2077-6

Flaherty, E. R. B. (2014). *Geriatric nursing review syllabus: A core curriculum in advanced practice geriatric nursing*. New York, NY: American Geriatrics Society.

Hamric, A., Hanson, C., Tracy, M. F., & O'Grady, E. T. (2014). *Advanced practice nursing: An integrative approach* (5th ed.). St. Louis, MO: Elsevier Saunders.

Iversson, K. (2016). Improvised medicine: Providing care in extreme environments (2nd ed.). New York, NY: McGraw_Hill.

Joint Commission Division of Health Care Improvement. (2016). *Informed consent: More than getting a signature, quick safety; An advisory on safety and quality issues*. Retrieved from https://www.jointcommission.org/assets/1/23/Quick_Safety_Issue_Twenty-One_February_2016.pdf

Rushton, C. H. (2006). Defining and addressing moral distress: Tools for critical care nursing leaders. *AACN Advanced Critical Care, 17*(2), 161–168. doi:10.1097/00044067-200604000-00011

Steinbock, B., Arras, J. D., & London, A. J. (2012). *Ethical issues in modern medicine: Contemporary readings in bioethics* (8th ed.). New York, NY: McGraw-Hill.

Tintinalli, J. E. (2016). *Tintinalli's emergency medicine: A comprehensive study guide* (8th ed.). New York, NY: McGraw_Hill.

Wallis, L. (2015). Moral distress in nursing. *American Journal of Nursing, 115*(3), 19–20. doi:10.1097/01.NAJ.0000461804.96483.ba

Wetzig, K., & Mitchell, M. (2017). The needs of families of ICU trauma patients: An integrative review. *Intensive and Critical Care Nursing, 41*, 63–70. doi:10.1016/j.iccn.2017.02.006

22
Diversity and Inclusion

*DIANE FULLER SWITZER, KENNETH PETERSON,
CARLA CARTEN, AND DAWN CARPENTER*

▨ DIVERSITY AND INCLUSION QUESTIONS

1. The AG-ACNP is working at a rural clinic and receives a call from the ambulance personnel at a ski resort. The EMT states, "We have a 27-year-old snowboarder who was found on the ground next to a tree approximately 15 feet below a ski trail. The patient states that he was heading to the lodge when he hit ice, lost control, slid down the ski trail, then flew backwards airborne 15 feet into a tree, striking the left side of his chest. There was no loss of consciousness, he was wearing a helmet, and is awake and alert, moving all extremities." The EMT states: "He appears to have been traveling too fast and was probably racing down the hill to the bar. You know how those snowboarders are." This statement demonstrates:

   a. Standard practice of emergency field care
   b. Cultural bias
   c. Appropriate management of trauma
   d. Poor communication by EMS

2. A 21-year-old female sex worker is seen in the emergency room by an AC-AGNP for a sexual assault by a known heroin user that occurred the day prior to this admission. The physical examination shows trauma to the anal area. The patient's history includes having been seen and treated 1 week prior for a chlamydial infection. Her HIV testing results from the prior visit was negative. The AC-AGNP recognizes the patient's HIV risk is very high. The best approach to decrease this patient's chances of HIV infection is to:

   a. Encourage use of condoms for oral, vaginal, and anal penetration.
   b. Repeat HIV testing now and again in 3 and 6 months.
   c. Prescribe postexposure prophylaxis immediately.
   d. Encourage regular sexually transmitted disease screenings every 6 months.

3. An AC-AGNP working in a hospitalist role is contacted by the nurse manager of an inpatient medical unit regarding the room assignment for a transgender female patient with no past surgical history. The patient is requesting a private room, but one is not available. There is a semi-private room available and the other bed is occupied by another female patient. The AC-AGNP advises the nurse manager to:

   a. Tell the admission's office to find a different floor for the patient.
   b. Admit the patient to the available room with the female patient.
   c. Admit, but switch the current female patient with a male patient.
   d. Encourage the transgender patient to consider a room with a male patient.

4. An AG-ACNP in the medical ICU is reviewing her patient assignment for her shift. She notices a discrepancy with names for one of her assigned patients. The daily census printout identifies the patient in room 3 as John Singleton, but the assignment board lists the patient in room 3 as Kaitlyn S. She asks the unit clerk if there was a mistake. The unit clerk responds with "No, that's correct. You have him or her. He refers to himself as she, but the medical record system has him listed as a 23-year-old male. I'm so confused about this whole gender identity thing, I'm not certain how to address him." Which response offered by the AC-AGNP regarding gender identity and pronouns would promote respect and dignity for this patient? The AG-ACNP should:

   a. Refer to a patient by the assigned name in the medical record.
   b. Ask the patient which name and pronouns are preferred.
   c. Refer to the patient with pronouns that match the patient's appearance.
   d. Refer to the patient by the assigned gender in the medical record.

5. An AG-ACNP who engages in a process of lifelong self-critique and self-awareness that identifies and examines personal patterns of unintentional and intentional racism, classism, ethnocentrism, and homophobia in response to lack of knowledge about a patient's health beliefs and life experiences would be demonstrating:

   a. Cultural competence
   b. Motivational interviewing
   c. Cultural humility
   d. Active listening

6. An AG-ACNP cares for underserved populations and desires to advocate for his/her diverse patient population. Which healthcare policy strategy has the best potential for positively influencing issues of health equity?

   a. Develop new funding opportunities to support simulation courses.
   b. Increase ethnic and racial diversity in the nursing workforce.
   c. Support legislation to mandate nursing unions in all healthcare settings.
   d. Recruit a lobbyist to work between the various nursing associations.

7. The lead AC-AGNP for the hospitalist service is notified about complaints received from three recently admitted patients. These complaints came from patients who reported feeling discriminated against because of: (1) their gender identity (transgender woman), (2) sexual identity (gay male), and (3) race (African American male). The AC-AGNP's next step includes leading a discussion with the provider group to help providers better understand the patients' experiences. Which of the following frameworks would best support that plan?

   a. Motivational interviewing
   b. Intersectionality
   c. Diffusion of innovation
   d. Health belief model

8. Which of the following patients is most likely to have an overall poor health status:

   a. African American man who is college educated who is currently laid off without insurance
   b. Caucasian American woman who does not eat a nutritious diet or exercise
   c. Caucasian American male with lower educational and income levels
   d. Hispanic man who follows an ethnic diet and earns $75,000 per year

9. A 30-year-old emigrant from Vietnam presents into the ED with a fever of 104.0°F with tachycardia and tachypnea. Upon exam, the AG-ACNP notes several symmetrical, striated, and abrasive marks on the patient's back. The nurse is concerned that she may be a victim of physical abuse, and that the break in skin integrity might be the source of infection. The AG-ACNP asks the patient about the marks on her back and she explains that her husband put the marks there on purpose. She explained he rubs a small coin down the middle of her back until he sees a little

blood under the skin and this takes away the wind that causes a fever. Which of the following is the best action for the AG-ACNP to take?

a. Call social services to assess for interpersonal violence.
b. Educate the patient about the ineffectiveness of coining and its potential for increasing infection.
c. Work with the patient to integrate coining into the treatment plan.
d. Offer contact information and resources for the interpersonal violence.

10. An AG-ACNP is co-managing a 22-year-old Puerto Rican woman, who is in the ICU for treatment of eclampsia. She is status-post cesarean section to a full-term baby girl 12 hours ago. The obstetrical nurse assesses, bathes, and changes the baby. While the nurse is attending to the baby, the AG-ACNP observes the mother leave the room. The nurse is surprised that the mother left but assumed all is well. She tells the AG-ACNP that she would be worried if this happened with another patient but not a Latina because they take good care of their newborns. What is the AG-ACNP's best response to the nurse?

a. Reassure her that there is nothing to worry about, she's right about Latinas.
b. Call social work services to monitor the mother for neglect.
c. Inquire with the mother about why she left the room.
d. Consult psychiatry to evaluate for postpartum depression.

11. A patient is in a private room in the ICU and has a large family, many of whom have been visiting throughout the day. It is late in the evening, but family members continue to arrive, bringing food and beverages to the patient's room. Everyone is happy as if celebrating at a party. The charge nurse tells the AG-ACNP she has politely informed the family that only two visitors should be in the room at a time and that visiting hours are ending shortly. The patient's son tells the AG-ACNP that in their culture, for a patient to heal properly, they must never be left alone in the hospital. He continues to say that the patient must have his family with them and that the family must eat. Which is the best response by the AG-ACNP?

a. Call the nursing supervisor to enforce the hospital visitation policy at the end of visiting hours.
b. Reinforce the hospital policies, but allow two family members to stay overnight.
c. Provide a separate location for family to congregate, allow family members to rotate visitation.
d. Consult clergy to explain the hospital regulations and negotiate a compromise.

12. A 45-year-old woman is admitted to the hospital complaining of having symptoms of a heart attack. She discloses that she suffers from anxiety and thought she was just anxious until her chest felt like it was being squeezed, her jaw and neck hurt, her arm was numb, and it was hard to breathe. While collecting her history, she laughs that her husband often makes her nervous so maybe this is just nerves. She then tells you that she wants to have a pelvic exam while she is there because she has been experiencing pain, especially during sex. She says that maybe she just isn't ready for sex sometimes, especially when her husband is in the mood and she isn't, and when she often wakes up because he is having sex with her. She used to tell him to stop, but he told her he has needs and is it better to let him do his thing. She says it is best to get it over with after all, her husband tells her it is her wifely duty. What is the AG-ACNP's best response?

a. Recommend her to use personal lubrication to ease the pain.
b. Inform her this is assault and provide resources.
c. Explain this is a primarily a cultural practice between husband and wife.
d. Request a GYN consult to identify the cause of the pain.

13. A mother brings her 18-year-old autistic son in to be checked for a head injury he self-inflicted at high school. The school insisted that she bring him in because he has been very agitated and hit his head multiple times, resulting in a very large hematoma near his scalp. The mother explains that he often gets upset and bangs his head, especially after he eats American food. She explains she plans to have an Ethiopian Orthodox Christian (Tewahedo) priest "call out the evils" that has existed in her family for generations. She assures you her son will be fine and only needs some ice for his head and assures the AG-ACNP there is no other action needed. What is the AG-ACNP's best response?

    a. Obtain consent to perform a CT scan of the brain.
    b. Ask the mother about the process of "calling out the evils."
    c. Apply ice to the scalp hematoma.
    d. Consult social services to intervene.

14. An AG-ACNP joined the ICU 3 weeks ago and has noticed that there is a group of nurses who have been together for over 15 years and another group that all went to the same school together. The AG-ACNP observes a new nurse who seems to be an outsider to the groups and seems to be ignored. The AG-ACNP observes the nurses invited people to a party right in front of the new nurse, who was not asked to attend. The same thing happened with another after-work event last week. The AG-ACNP notes the nurse is getting more upset about being excluded, and the nurse shared she feels she has been dismissed when she attempted to reach out to the other nurses. The AG-ACNP recognize the behaviors of the nurses represents:

    a. Normal behavior
    b. Vertical violence
    c. Lateral violence
    d. Social isolation

15. The AG-ACNP observed a new grad nurse on a busy medical/surgical unit, who asked a senior nurse for help with care of a patient. The AG-ACNP observed the senior nurse rolling her eyes as she turned to follow the nurse into the patient's room. Later the AG-ACNP walked into the break room and heard the senior nurse telling other senior nurses about the new nurse's request for help. They abruptly discontinued their conversation when the AG-ACNP entered the room. What action should the AG-ACNP take?

    a. Ignore the conversation as the AG-ACNP doesn't know the whole story.
    b. Report the encounter to the nursing manager.
    c. Report the lateral violence to human resources.
    d. Inform the nurses their behaviors represent workplace bullying.

■ DIVERSITY AND INCLUSION ANSWERS AND RATIONALES

1. **b) Cultural bias**. This is an example of cultural bias. The EMT is judging the patient based on his own cultural assumptions regarding snowboarders. Although we mostly think of cultural bias occurring when race, ethnicity, or religion is the difference present, it can occur with anyone who may have a distinct group identity, for example, social groups, sporting clubs, or members of a neighborhood.

2. **c) Prescribe postexposure prophylaxis immediately**. This patient has had a high-risk exposure. Postexposure prophylaxis is required within 72 hours for sexual assault and prevention of HIV transmission. Use of condoms will help prevent future exposures, but the question is asking how to prevent HIV infection after exposure. Repeat sexually transmitted disease and HIV testing will be performed to monitor for conversion, but not will not prevent infection.

3. **b) Admit the patient to the available room with the female patient**. Caring for transgendered patients is commonplace and room assignments can be challenging, especially during times of high census. When room assignments are gender-based, transgender patients should be assigned to rooms based on their self-identified gender, regardless of whether this self-identified gender aligns with their physical appearance, surgical history, genitalia, legal sex, sex assigned at birth, or name and sex as it appears in hospital records. If a transgender patient requests a private room and there is one available, it should be made available to the patient. Sufficient privacy can be ensured by use of curtains.

4. **b) Ask the patient which name and pronouns are preferred**. A person's gender identity is their own. Gender expression varies and is often on a continuum. A person's gender is not always a match to theassigned sex at birth. A patient-centered approach to care that takes into consideration the many variations of gender identification and expression would include asking the patient for the names and/or pronouns the patient prefers to use.

5. **c) Cultural humility**. Cultural humility involves a lifelong commitment to self-appraisal to balance the patient–provider relationship and develop a nonpaternalistic clinical partnership with patients and defined populations. Active listening is an element of cultural humility. Cultural competence encompasses an understanding and appropriate response to unique cultural and diversity variables that the AG-ACNP brings to interactions with patients. Cultural humility and/or cultural competence is needed for motivational interviewing. The provider recognizes and accepts the fact that clients who need to make changes in their lives approach these changes from different levels of readiness to change their behaviors.

6. **b) Increase ethnic and racial diversity in the nursing workforce**. The Institute of Medicine's report, *The Future of Nursing: Leading Change, Advancing Health*, recommends key interventions related to diversity. To improve access, care should be delivered in an appropriate manner that is culturally relevant so that patients can contribute and participate in their care. Strategies should focus on increasing the diversity of undergraduate and doctoral students, which will expand a workforce that is more prepared to deliver care to diverse populations. Diversity of the nursing profession should focus on diversification by race/ethnicity, gender, and geographic area.

7. **b) Intersectionality**. The intersectionality model identifies how interconnecting systems of power can impact and oppress marginalized groups. Intersectionality considers that class, race, sexual orientation, disability, and gender do not exist separately, but are complexly interwoven. Motivational interviewing is typically referred to when assessing a patient's readiness to implement change. Diffusion of innovation model explains how an idea gains momentum and or spreads through a specific population or social system. The health belief model explains and predicts health-related behaviors, predominantly in regard to the use of healthcare services.

8. **c) Caucasian American male with lower educational and income levels**. The two most common social determinants of health include education and income, which are the most frequently used socioeconomic measures in the U.S. Americans who are poor and have not graduated from high school report noticeably worse health status on average than more

wealthy or educated Americans. Diet, exercise, smoking and alcohol can all adversely affect overall health, but not to the same degree as education and income.

9. **c) Work with the patient to integrate coining into the treatment plan**. This helps build trust between the AG-ACNP and patient and increases the patient's adherence to the course of treatment. The desired intervention is a culturally competent and patient-centered approach to care. There are several mnemonic models that focus on delivering culturally competent and patient-centered care and incorporate the patient's values, beliefs, and practices into the treatment plan. Calling social services or offering information and resources for domestic violence indicates that the AG-ACNP is working from her assumption of mistreatment without trying to understand other possible causes for the striated and abrasive marks on the patient's back. Attempting to educate a patient that their approach is wrong or ineffective is placing a negative judgment on their belief or practice reducing the probability that an "educated" treatment is followed. In patient-centered and culturally competent care, the patient is more likely to follow a treatment plan presented by a caregiver who strives to understand the point of view of the other and thus responds with compassion rather than judgment.

10. **c) Inquire with the mother about why she left the room**. It is best to engage with the new mother to see why she left the room. Often people make assumptions based on perceived patterns; however, perceptions and patterns are not facts. The other answers are based on assumptions that can lead to an improper intervention and treatment. While some nurses may experience a certain group as having a particular pattern of behavior, such as taking good care of their newborns, this is an assumption. While patterns can give insight, care needs to be made on an individual basis. Evaluation for postpartum depression is premature. However, postpartum depression can present through many behaviors, including feeling overwhelmed, reduced concentration, and withdrawal. The other answers are also based on assumptions: contacting social work services for potential parental neglect and dismissing the behavior as normal because new mothers need a break and may quietly leave when they get a chance.

11. **c) Provide a separate location for family to congregate and allow family members to rotate visitation**. Nurses and AG-ACNPs should facilitate unrestricted access of hospitalized patients to their chosen support person(s) who can provide emotional and social support 24 hours a day in alignment with patient preference, unless the support person(s) infringe on the rights or safety of other patients, or is medically contraindicated.

12. **b) Inform her this is assault and provide resources**. Initial interventions should include: ensure consultation is conducted in private; ensure confidentiality, while informing the patient of the limits of confidentiality (e.g., when there is mandatory reporting); be nonjudgmental and supportive; validate what the patient is saying; provide care and support that responds to her concerns; ask about other history of violence; listen without pressuring her to talk; provide information about resources, including legal and other services; assist her to increase safety for herself and her children (if applicable); and provide or mobilize social support.

13. **b) Ask the mother about the process of "calling out the evils."** The autistic child is considered a vulnerable population. The AG-ANCP's role is to recognize vulnerable populations and extend protection from additional harm, when they may not be able to effectively advocate for themselves. Thus the AG-ACNP needs to gain additional information about the cultural practices of exorcism. Exorcisms are practiced in the Ethiopian Orthodox (Tewahdo) Church, as well as among other cultures. In this religion, exorcisms are performed to cure mental health conditions, which involve the application of holy water, holy oil, a small wooden cross, and holy ash. It is not typically physical in nature, but there are reports of exorcisms that have cause harm, and even death. CT scans do not require consent. Application of ice is not the best answer and there is no reason given in the scenario that warrants a social service consult, although it may be once further information is obtained.

14. **c) Lateral violence**. Lateral violence in nursing is a defined as an aggressive behavior directed by a nurse towards a nurse. The aggression can be verbal or nonverbal and can have psychological, emotional, and/or behavioral effects on nurses. Lateral violence can be in the form of gossiping, targeted personal jokes, ostracism, insults, unwarranted criticism, belittling, and verbal aggression. This humiliation and putting down of nursing colleagues including rudeness and aggressions will demoralize the sense of self-worth. AG-ACNPs are leaders within healthcare organizations and have an obligation to prevent and respond to lateral violence. Vertical violence occurs between two different levels of the hierarchical system. Social isolation is a lack of contact between an individual and society.

15. **d) Inform the nurses their behaviors represent workplace bullying**. Lateral violence in nursing is a defined as an aggressive behavior directed by a nurse towards a nurse. The aggression can be verbal or nonverbal and can have psychological, emotional, and/or behavioral effects on nurses. Lateral violence can be in the form of gossiping, targeted personal jokes, ostracism, insults, unwarranted criticism, belittling, and verbal aggression. This humiliation and putting down of nursing colleagues, including rudeness and aggression, will demoralize the sense of self-worth. AG-ACNPs are leaders within healthcare organizations and have an obligation to prevent and respond to lateral violence or workplace bullying. The AG-ACNP witnessed the events, and as such is in the best position to immediately address the situation. Reporting to the manager or human resources may also be performed, but are not the best options.

■ BIBLIOGRAPHY

AACN Practice Alerts. (2012). Family presence: Visitation in the adult ICU. *Critical Care Nurse, 32*(4), 76–78.

Asfaw, B. B. (2015). Demonic possession and healing of mental illness in the Ethiopian Orthodox Tewahdo church: The case of Entoto Kidane-Mihret monastery. *American Journal of Applied Psychology, 3*(4), 80–93. doi:10.12691/ajap-3-4-2

Berlin, E. A., & Fowkes Jr, W. C. (1983). A teaching framework for cross-cultural health care—application in family practice. *Western Journal of Medicine, 139*(6), 934.

Braveman, P. A., Egerter, S. A., & Mockenhaupt, R. E. (2011). Broadening the focus: The need to address the social determinants of health. *American Journal of Preventive Medicine, 40*(1 Suppl. 1), S4–S18. doi:10.1016/j.amepre.2010.10.002

Campinha-Bacote, J. (2011). Delivering patient-centered care in the midst of a cultural conflict: The role of cultural competence. *Online Journal of Issues in Nursing, 16*(2). doi:10.3912/OJIN.Vol16No02Man05

Chapman, E. N., Kaatz, A., & Carnes, M. (2013). Physicians and implicit bias: How doctors may unwittingly perpetuate health care disparities. *Journal of General Internal Medicine, 28*(11), 1504–1510. doi:10.1007/s11606-013-2441-1

Chu, R. Z., & Evans, M. M. (2016, November-December). Lateral violence in nursing. *Medsurg Nursing, 25*, S4+. doi:10.12968/bjon.2016.25.20.s4

DeNisco, S. M. (2018). *Role development for the nurse practitioner.* Burlington, MA: Jones & Bartlett Learning.

Gender Spectrum. (2017). *Understanding gender.* Retrieved from https://www.genderspectrum.org/quicklinks/understanding-gender/

Graham, E., & Chitnarong, J. (1997). Ethnographic study among Seattle Cambodians: Wind illness. Retrieved from https://ethnomed.org/clinical/culture-bound-syndromes/ethnographic-study-among-cambodians-in-seattle

Human Rights Campaign Foundation. (2016). *Creating equal access to quality health care for transgender patients: Transgender-affirming hospital policies.* Retrieved from https://assets2.hrc.org/files/assets/resources/TransAffirming-HospitalPolicies-2016.pdf?_ga=2.39461546.844116398.1521502413-701768635.1521321255

It's Prounounced Metrosexual. (2018). *The genderbread person v3.* Retrieved from http://itspronounced metrosexual.com/2015/03/the-genderbread-person-v3/

Levin, S., Like, R., & Gottlieb, J. (2000). ETHNIC: A framework for culturally competent clinical practice. *Appendix: Useful clinical interviewing mnemonics. Patient Care, 34*(9), 188–189.

Martinez, M., Prabhakar, N., Drake, K., Coull, B., Chong, J., Ritter, L., & Kidwell, C. (2015). Identification of barriers to stroke awareness and risk-factor management unique to Hispanics. *International Journal of Environmental Research and Public Health, 13*(1), 23. doi:10.3390/ijerph13010023

National LGBT Health Education Center: A Program of the Fenway Institute. (2015). *Taking routine histories of sexual health: A system-wide approach for health centers.* Retrieved from http://www.lgbthealtheducation.org/wp-content/uploads/COM-827-sexual-history_toolkit_2015.pdf

O'Doherty, L., Hegarty, K., Ramsay, J., Davidson, L. L., Feder, G., & Taft, A. (2015). Screening women for intimate partner violence in healthcare settings. *Cochrane Database of Systematic Reviews, 22*(7), CD007007. doi:10.1002/14651858.CD007007.pub3

Olaussen, A., Bade-Boon, J., Fitzgerald, M., & Mitra, B. (2018). Management of injured patients who were Jehovah's Witnesses, where blood transfusion may not be an option: A retrospective review. *Vox Sanguinis, 113*(3), 283–289. doi:10.1111/vox.12637

Paradies, Y. (2006). A systematic review of empirical research on self-reported racism and health. *International Journal of Epidemiology, 35*(4), 888–901. doi:10.1093/ije/dyl056

Rainford, W. C., Wood, S., McMullen, P. C., & Philipsen, N. D. (2015). The disruptive force of lateral violence in the health care setting. *The Journal for Nurse Practitioners, 11*(2), 157–164. doi:10.1016/j.nurpra.2014.10.010

Tervalon, M., & Murray-Garcia, J. (1998). Cultural humility versus cultural competence: A critical distinction in defining physician training outcomes in multicultural education. *Journal of Health Care for the Poor and Underserved, 9*(2), 117–125. doi:10.1353/hpu.2010.0233

The Future of Nursing: Campaign for Action. (2011). *Institute of Medicine: The future of nursing: Leading change, advancing health recommendations related to diversity.* Retrieved from https://campaignforaction.org/wp-content/uploads/2016/04/IOM-Diversity-Recommendations3.pdf

Workowski, K. A., & Berman, S. M. (2007). Centers for Disease Control and Prevention sexually transmitted diseases treatment guidelines. *Clinical Infectious Diseases, 44*(Suppl. 3), S73–S76. doi:10.1086/511430

World Health Organization. (2013). *Responding to intimate partner violence and sexual violence against women: WHO clinical and policy guidelines.* Retrieved from https://www.ncbi.nlm.nih.gov/books/NBK174251/

23 Ethics, Advocacy, and Moral Agency

MARY SULLIVAN AND MARY ANNE McCOY

ETHICS, ADVOCACY, AND MORAL AGENCY QUESTIONS

1. A 56-year-old patient presents for treatment of a local irritation on her breast. Upon taking her history the AG-ACNP discovers she has a diagnosis of breast cancer in situ, for which she has refused traditional treatment. She states that she believes applying a balm her aunt gave her will cure her. On physical exam the AG-ACNP determines that the irritation is a contact dermatitis from the balm. She refuses to discontinue the balm and requests to be discharged. The AG-ACNP feels conflicted and troubled about the patient's decision but determines that the patient has decision-making capacity and must respect her wishes to proceed in this manner. The AG-ACNP is experiencing?

    a. Moral obligation
    b. Moral distress
    c. Moral dilemma
    d. Moral resiliency

2. In caring for patients with chronic, life-limiting illnesses, the most important task of the AG-ACNP is to:

    a. Obtain advance directives with the patient.
    b. Write and order for DNR/DNI as indicated.
    c. Identify the healthcare proxy.
    d. Determine the family decision-maker.

3. Informed consent includes the ability to:

    a. Comprehend information, contemplate options, and evaluate risks and consequences.
    b. Make decisions based on written information that is provided about acceptable care.
    c. Answer questions about information that is provided.
    d. Perform a full competency evaluation on the patient.

4. When an AG-ACNP consults a patient's healthcare proxy for medical decision making, the expectation is that the proxy will be able to make decisions as nearly as possible as what the incapacitated individual would decide for themselves. The ethical principle describing this concept of a person and their self-determination is:

   a. Veracity
   b. Autonomy
   c. Beneficence
   d. Justice

5. The elements of decision making include being able to:

   a. Communicate verbally.
   b. Understand alternative approaches.
   c. Sign your name.
   d. State positive outcomes if treatment is refused.

6. The use of a decision tree in analyzing ethical dilemmas is helpful because constructing a decision tree:

   a. Delineates the legal parameters
   b. Shows the best solution
   c. Allows all the options to be considered
   d. Explains the ethical principles

7. The ethical conduct and responsibilities of the AG-ACNP are guided by:

   a. Religious preferences
   b. Social norms
   c. Collaborative practice agreements
   d. ANA Code of Ethics

8. A 72-year-old man is refusing transfer to rehab following a left-hip replacement, stating he is fine to go home. He lives alone and has little support. The AG-ACNP does not think this is a good discharge plan for him. His insistence on going directly home instead of rehab is an example of him employing his right to:

   a. Justice
   b. Self-determination
   c. Beneficence
   d. Informed consent

9. A patient is admitted to rehab after surgery for a bowel obstruction. At time of surgery it was discovered that she had metastatic ovarian cancer. She has two daughters who are under the age of 21. She tells the AG-ACNP that she does not want to tell her daughters of her diagnosis. The AG-ACNP knows that her decision to withhold this information is based upon the ethical principle of:

   a. Autonomy
   b. Veracity
   c. Informed consent
   d. Shared decision making

10. The decision to withhold or withdraw life-sustaining care can be an appropriate determination with the patient, surrogate. and/or an ethics committee. Opiates and benzodiazepines are often used to manage the analgesia and anxiety of the patient in this situation. If death is hastened by the use of these medications, this is ethically acceptable due to which concept?

   a. Double effect
   b. Self-determination
   c. Euthanasia
   d. Autonomy

11. The AG-ACNP is deciding whether to recommend that a patient follow a long-term medication regimen that will help control disease symptoms but may also create troublesome side effects. The decision involves consideration of which ethical principle?

   a. Fidelity
   b. Autonomy
   c. Beneficence
   d. Nonmaleficence

12. A referring physician tells you that he has not disclosed a new diagnosis of lung cancer to his patient, who told him he would commit suicide if he was ever diagnosed with cancer. This is an example of:

   a. Fidelity
   b. Utilitarianism
   c. Paternalism
   d. Justice

13. Who has the highest authority to make medical decisions when a patient does not have capacity?

   a. Legal guardian
   b. Legal next of kin
   c. Healthcare proxy
   d. Varies by state

14. AG-ACNP prescribing practices for controlled substances is regulated by:

   a. Collaborative practice agreements
   b. The DEA
   c. The practice protocols of the hospital
   d. The SBON

15. The definition of the ethical principle of justice is:

   a. The responsibility to promote the well-being of another
   b. The duty not to inflict harm or evil
   c. The duty to treat all fairly, equally
   d. The duty to respect another's personal liberty and the right to make choices

16. An 80-year-old man is brought in by his daughter, who has concerns about her father's daytime drowsiness. As a result of the AG-ACNP's interview, she discovers that he has three chronic conditions for which he takes seven different medications. Using a patient centered-approach to care, which should be the next step?

    a. Ask the patient and his daughter which medication they would like you to discontinue.
    b. Discuss his medication adherence and identify strategies to help him take his meds.
    c. Discuss goals of care with him and his daughter.
    d. Contact the pharmacist to identify which medication is most likely causing the drowsiness.

17. A frail elderly woman is being discharged after admission for a UTI. Her past medical history is significant for mild dementia, chronic pain secondary to arthritis, and poorly controlled DMII. She lives alone, but is able to get around with the use of a cane. She states that her main concern is preserving her mobility. She is fearful of breaking her hip. The various specialists consulted during this hospitalization have recommended adding tramadol (Ultram) and insulin, increasing her ACE inhibitor dose and adding a cholinesterase inhibitor. Based on the AG-ACNP's understanding of management strategies in caring for patients with multiple chronic conditions, which of the following is likely to occur:

    a. Changes in the patient's medication regimen may increase the patient's risk for falls.
    b. The patient's new medication regimen will result in better outcomes for her.
    c. Addition of tramadol may decrease her pain and thus decrease her risk of falling.
    d. Adding a cholinesterase inhibitor should help improve her memory and her ability to be compliant with medications.

18. The elements of beneficence include which of the following:

    a. Promote good for self.
    b. Prevent harm to self.
    c. Make the best choice for another.
    d. Prevent evil by acting in the best interest of others.

19. An AG-ACNP is responsible for billing codes submitted to insurance:

    a. For all activities on the unit when he/she is scheduled
    b. For all "incident to" events
    c. When the evaluation and management criteria have been met
    d. When the electronic medical record (EMR) flags incomplete charges for procedures

20. The group responsible for granting or suspending the license of an AG-ACNP regarding specific norms of practice is the:

    a. AG-ACNP's state licensing board
    b. Credentialing committee associated with the practice setting
    c. National credentialing organization
    d. Credentialing insurance companies

■ ETHICS, ADVOCACY, MORAL AGENCY ANSWERS AND RATIONALES

1. **b) Moral distress**. Ethical conflicts are evident daily in healthcare. The AG-ACNP must be aware that what they consider is their fiduciary relationship with the public, moral obligation is not the confusion with what they consider the correct decision in the situation. Moral distress is experienced by healthcare providers when they feel that they know the ethically or medically correct action to take in a given situation, but they are restricted by (in this case) the opinion of the designated decision maker. Moral dilemmas are situations, pressures, and obstacles that make healthcare such difficult work, but not what care providers may be feeling. Moral resiliency is the ability to manage moral distress and moral dilemmas.

2. **a) Obtain advance directives with the patient**. It is important to initiate conversations with patients with chronic and terminal illness regarding advance care planning before an emergency arises. Further, good AG-ACNP practice is to make a routine practice of discussing patient preferences at regular intervals and visits. You may write for a DNR/DNI if your state SOP allows. Furthermore, you may be involved or working with a patient's healthcare proxy or family decision maker in a situation where the patient is not competent to make a decision.

3. **a) The patient must be able to comprehend information, contemplate options, evaluate risks and consequences**. The patient needs a chance to ask questions, not rely solely on written materials. The patient does not need to be able to answer questions, but does need to be able to ask questions about the procedure. A full competency evaluation is not required.

4. **b) Autonomy**. Autonomy or self-determination states that patients have the moral and legal right to determine what will be done with their own person.

5. **b) Understand alternative approaches**. Patients need to be able to understand alternative approaches, communicate preferences, and state possible outcomes if treatment is refused. Patients do not need to be able to communicate verbally. Using adaptive devices can achieve the same goals. Patients do not need to be able to sign their name. Decision making does not require the physical ability to write or sign. Decision making requires only that the patient has the ability to express their choice in an understandable fashion.

6. **c) Allows all the options to be considered**. Decision-tree analysis allows for identification of options in a setting that involves complex or substantial risk of uncertainty and possible morbidity for patients in a prescriptive manner to determine an outcome.

7. **d) ANA Code of Ethics**. The ANA Code of Ethics is a statement of the ethical obligations and duties of every individual who enters into the nursing profession.

8. **b) Self-determination**. The patient is exertion his right to autonomy or self-determination, which is the principle of recognizing each individual's right to make his or her own decisions on healthcare. Justice is treating others fairly. Beneficence is doing good for the client and informed consent is the process of promoting self-determination.

9. **a) Autonomy**. Autonomy is the ethical principle recognizing an individual's right to make their own decisions about healthcare, including the right to refuse treatment even if it is not beneficial to the individual's health.

10. **a) Double effect**. The doctrine of double effect (DDE) is an ethical principle dating back to the 13th century that explains how the bad consequences of an action can be considered ethically justified if the original intent was for good intention. An example is the use of pain medication that may make one constipated. The unintended side effect does not make the use of pain medicine unethical. Self-determination and autonomy may be the doctrine used by the patient in the discussion, but it does not describe what the question asks. DDE in fact forbids euthanasia and the achievement of good ends by wrong means, and it is generally accepted that the DDE does not provide moral justification for euthanasia or physician-assisted death.

11. **d) Nonmaleficence**. Nonmaleficence means nonharming, or inflicting the least harm possible to reach a beneficial outcome. Harm and its effects are considerations and part of the ethical decision-making process in healthcare. Short-term and long-term harm, though

unintentional, often accompany life-saving treatment in the acute care even with side effects. Fidelity is keeping commitment to the patient, beneficence is to do well, and autonomy is the right of the patient to make decisions regarding his or her personal health.

12. **c) Paternalism.** Paternalism is making the choice for people, believing that the individual knows what is best for others. Utilitarianism is the doctrine that actions are right if they are useful or for the benefit of a majority; while fidelity is faithfulness to a person and justice quality of being fair and reasonable.

13. **d) Varies by state.** Medical ethics allows for several levels of decision making for patients who become incapacitated. State statutes define who has the greatest authority to make healthcare decisions when a patient does not have capacity, and these statutes vary from state to state. Many times it is the healthcare proxy, where a surrogate is selected as a decision maker for another when they are unable to do so. The principle is that the designated surrogate decision maker would respect the person's wishes and make decisions that most closely align with those wishes.

14. **b) The DEA.** The federal government oversees the prescribing of all controlled substances for AG-ACNPs and other healthcare providers.

15. **c) The duty to treat all fairly, equally.** Justice is the obligation to be fair and equitable in the distribution of benefits.

16. **c) Discuss goals of care with him and his daughter.** Clinical decision making with regard to elders with multiple chronic co-conditions must be based on the weighting of influential factors, including the patient's priorities and preferences, potential benefit and risk, as well as life expectancy and practical issues such as transportation and ability to comply with treatment.

17. **a) Changes in the patient's medication regimen may increase the patient's risk for falls.** Clinical decision making is difficult in the setting of multiple comorbidities and the effects of aging. The risk/benefit ratio may be decreased and the risks of adverse drug reactions and drug-drug interactions increase with the number of medications and the severity of frailty, increasing the risk of poor outcome. The patient has outlined her goals and ethically we are bound to respect them, taking all factors into consideration.

18. **d) Prevent evil by acting in the best interest of others.** Beneficence is the principle of doing good, preventing harm, and acting in the best interest of others. Making the choice for another would be paternalism.

19. **c) When the evaluation and management criteria have been met.** The evaluation and management codes have specific criteria that are required be met for reimbursement. Reimbursement is a high-stakes issue. AG-ACNPs are responsible for individual practice regarding the submission and authenticity of care delivered. AG-ACNPs are not responsible for all activity on a unit, they do not bill "incident to" in an inpatient setting, and electronic medical records (EMRs) are usually separate from the billing services, although the documentation is developed from content placed into the EMR or patient's chart.

20. **a) AG-ACNP's state licensing board.** Licensing for RNs, including APNs, is administered through SBON. SPAs assure that licenses are subject to disciplinary action when it is determined that a licensee has violated law or regulation.

■ BIBLIOGRAPHY

American Nurses Association. (2001). *Code of ethics for nurses with interpretive statements.* Nursesbooks.org. Silver Spring, MD: Author.

Austin, W. (2012). Moral distress and the contemporary plight of health professionals. *HEC Forum, 24*(1), 27–38. doi:10.1007/s10730-012-9179-8

Buppert, C. (2018). *Nurse practitioner's business practice and legal guide* (6th ed.). Boulder, CO: Jones & Bartlett.

DeNisco, S. M. (2018). *Role development for the nurse practitioner.* Burlington, MA: Jones & Bartlett Learning.

DeNisco, S. M., & Barker, A. M. (2016). *Advanced practice nursing: Essential knowledge for the profession* (3rd ed.). Burinington, MA: Jones & Bartlett Learning.

Fowler, M. D. M. (2008). *Guide to the code of ethics for nurses: Interpretation and application*. Silver Spring, MD: Nursesbooks.org.

Kasper, D., Hauser, S., Jameson, J., Fauci, A., Longo, D., & Loscalzo, J. (2015). *Harrison's principles of internal medicine* (19th ed.). New York, NY: McGraw-Hill.

Ruston, C. H., Schoonover-Shoffner, K. & Kennedy, M. (2017). Executive summary: Transforming moral distress into moral resilience in nursing. *American Journal of Nursing, 117*(2), 52–56. doi:10.1097/01.NAJ.0000512298.18641.31

Wholihan, D., & Olson, E. (2017). The doctrine of double effect: A review for the bedside nurse providing end-of-life care. *Journal of Hospice and Palliative Nursing, 19*(3), 205–211. doi:10.1097/NJH.0000000000000348

24 Health Policy

MARY ANNE McCOY AND DONNA GULLETTE

■ HEALTH POLICY QUESTIONS

1. The discharge of a patient with CHF requires that the AG-ACNP provider understands the MS-DRG-based prospective payment method penalizes the hospital for:

   a. Overspending the amount of the bundle payment for all services based on the original admission diagnosis
   b. Any 30-day readmission on select MS-DRG-based cases to the original hospital, even if the patient is admitted elsewhere
   c. Accepting a high-risk patient case-mix
   d. Not accepting the Medicare-calculated cost of the related DRG

2. There are a multitude of factors that influence health outcomes, but the most influential factor that influences health is:

   a. SES
   b. Racial and gender disparities
   c. Access to healthcare
   d. Lack of insurance

3. What should influence the discharge orders that an AG-ACNP is preparing for a 68-year-old male who has a complicated wound care treatment plan and no supplemental insurance plan?

   a. Part B coverage will cover 80% of the wound treatment pharmaceuticals, but the patient is responsible for 20% until their deductable is met.
   b. Part B coverage will cover 80% of the costs of the wound care dressings, but the patient is responsible for 20% until their deductable is met.
   c. The treatment plan for the wound care greatly influences the ability to discharge a patient to home care, depending on the frequency of care needed and/or the level of involvement the wound requires.
   d. A home care agency that accepts a patient with a requirement for wound care is responsible under its bundled payment to use the dressings and wound care agents ordered by the provider.

4. Free markets typically secure more economic prosperity than government, with its centralized planning, because:

   a. The price system utilizes more local knowledge of means and ends.
   b. Markets rely upon coercion, whereas government relies upon voluntary compliance with the law.
   c. More tax revenue can be generated from free enterprise.
   d. Government planners are too cautious in spending taxpayers' money.

5. The AG-ACNP has been concerned that there is a delay in initiation of tube feeding in the ICU primarily because the delay is getting small-bore feeding tube inserted in eligible patients. A policy exists that tube feedings cannot be given via nasogastric tubes. The continued practice and policy is related to the strong feelings of a now-retired intensivist that had proposed the policy years ago. What is the best potential approach for the AG-ACNP to change this practice?

   a. The AG-ACNP should conduct a needs assessment to see if the medical group would be interested supporting this practice change now that the intensivist is no longer there.
   b. The AG-ACNP should conduct a formal policy analysis.
   c. The AG-ACNP should do a retroactive data review of the time from admission to time of small-bore feeding tube placement to evaluate the problem.
   d. The AG-ACNP should bring this issue up to the Nursing Practice Council in the ICU to gain its support in the project.

6. There was an important change to the recent release of the 2017 rules on the MACRA. What effect does it have on AG-ACNPs for purposes of recognition and future growth of the profession?

   a. It recognized the importance of all providers, including AG-ACNPs, to participate in EHRs and requiring patient access to their medical records to improve communication.
   b. "Eligible professional" was replaced with the term "eligible clinician," expanding the population of individuals covered by MIPS, which now includes all four APRN groups.
   c. It specifically addresses the need to utilize electronic prescribing and sharing of records across institutions to control costs and waste.
   d. It exempted hospital-based professionals from penalties that could occur if their facilities did not meet quality standards.

7. The AG-ACNP is rounding on a patient scheduled for a cholecystectomy for persistent obstructive symptoms later today. The AG-ACNP confirms the consent for the procedure was signed by the patient last evening. However, the patient is now found to be confused to place and time. She states that she is not having surgery today. The best action for the AG-ACNP to take would be:

   a. Notify the surgeon, and determine if the patient had decisional capacity at the time she signed the consent form.
   b. Call the surgeon and cancel the surgery until the patient's confusion is evaluated.
   c. Notify the ethics committee of the hospital.
   d. Place an urgent consult to psychiatry for assessment of competency.

8. The AG-ACNP working in a specialty clinic is seeing a young adult man who is complaining of pain and demands a prescription for oxycodone and MS Contin. As the AG-ACNP begins to explain that she is not able to prescribe these medications, he begins to curse and threatens to sue the AG-ACNP and the clinic. What is your best action in this situation?

   a. Have one of the other physicians write for the medications.
   b. Have the nurse call hospital security.
   c. Have the nurse call the police.
   d. Make an appointment for him in the pain management clinic.

9. The AG-ACNP has been caring for a young adult diabetic patient for past 4 months. The patient has refused to take her insulin and other antidiabetic medications. The patient has been hospitalized three times for DKA in the past 3 months. What step would the AG-ACNP take for discharging this patient from the practice?

a. Refuse to schedule future appointments.
b. Call another AG-ACNP or physician to see if he would be willing to care for the patient.
c. Send a certified letter with return request receipt requested stating the reason for dismissal and continue to provide care for 30 days beyond termination.
d. Notify the Patient Safety Committee that the patient will no longer be seen at the clinic by you.

10. A 55-year-old woman has advanced metastatic breast cancer. Her pain is managed on long-acting opioids and she is able to participate in very limited ADL. Her husband is her primary caregiver and would like to discuss the code status of his wife. With respect to ethical principles that guides nursing practice, what is the best response?

a. The attending physician would need to be consulted.
b. The patient must be involved in the discussion.
c. This topic should be discussed during the palliative care consultation.
d. The patient can't consent to DNR while on hydromorphone.

11. For Medicare patients, which plan under Medicare offers coverage for prescriptions but also requires a co-pay and monthly premium?

a. Medicare A
b. Medicare B
c. Medicare C
d. Medicare D

12. A 77-year-old patient discharged from the hospital can expect that Medicare would pay how much of the hospital bill?

a. 75%
b. 80%
c. 85%
d. 100%

13. Which of the following is required for an AG-ACNP to have to become a Medicare provider?

a. DNP degree in nursing
b. Credential by the hospital
c. Certification as an AG-ACNP by a recognized national certifying body
d. Federal DEA and state prescribing licenses in the state in which he/she intends to practice

14. Which of the following laws require most hospitals to provide an examination and necessary stabilization treatment without consideration of insurance coverage or ability to pay?

a. EMTALA
b. HIPAA
c. ACA
d. Stark Law

15. The purpose of obtaining consent in a research study is to:

a. Follow IRB regulations and procedures.
b. Reduce study bias against alternative treatments.
c. Release legal liability from the sponsors of the research funding group.
d. Ensure the participant understands his/her rights and responsibilities.

■ HEALTH POLICY ANSWERS AND RATIONALES

1. **b) Any 30-day readmission on select MS-DRG-based cases to the original hospital, even if the patient is admitted elsewhere.** The MS-DRG-based bundle payment considers the principal admission diagnosis, the facilities case-mix and type of institution (teaching or nonteaching), along with the other weighting measures to calculate a prospective bundled payment (Shi & Singh, 2010). How the hospital manages the costs is then the hospital's responsibility, assuming that it is still meeting all core measures and prudent care. Therefore, overspending the amount of the bundle payment for all services based on the original diagnosis is not a penalty per se, as this is an inherent risk of inefficient care. A high-risk case mix is built into the system, and Medicare does not mandate the participation of a facility in Medicare. To prevent too early of a discharge for patients, a "penalty" can be placed on a hospital if there are excessive 30-day readmissions for the same medical condition whether they are readmitted to the first facility or to another hospital (Shi & Singh, 2010, p. 159).

2. **a) SES.** Although there are a multitude of factors that influence the health, such as racial and gender disparities and access to quality care, the single most influential factor is SES. SES is pervasive barrier to health insurance, under-insurance, healthcare access, ability to pay co-pays, adequate food and housing, and environmental stressors. Statistics support that SES is the predominant influence on health.

3. **c) The treatment plan for the wound care greatly influences the ability to discharge a patient to home care depending on the frequency of care needed and or the level of involvement the wound requires.** The AG-ACNP needs to know the discharge support agencies in the Medicare bundled-payment system to achieve a cost-effective quality discharge for his/her patients. Traditional Medicare does not cover any topical drugs/biologics, although it covers the dressings. Nontraditional Medicare "advantage plans" would cover the wound pharmaceuticals. In this case, the patient does not have Part D coverage. It is true that an 80-20 split is the percentage of payment for Part B coverage; however, that is not the best answer as the key to the treatment plan is to know how to order the dressing and topical agents which are most acceptable to a home care agency. Too complicated of a plan may lead to the risk of an increased length of stay or trying to find an agency that will accept your patient. Under the Medicare payment system called the Home Health Resource Group Prospective, Payment Service agencies would be responsible for the dressings and the wound care but are not obliged to include the topical agents or biologics.

4. **a) The price system utilizes more local knowledge of means and ends.** In a free market, market forces determine demand, with many individuals independently determining what to buy. In healthcare, local market needs are partially influenced by local knowledge, which is difficult to determine in large practice plans such as Medicare. That is one reason the Medicaid plans differ significantly, based on local knowledge and public opinion. Free markets require information to be shared with potential consumers, therefore coercion is not a good tactic. In the U.S., tax revenues are required to be taken out of monies earned from everyone for government-subsidized Medicare and Medicaid so they generate more tax revenue. In this day and age, it's hard to justify that Washington is too cautious in spending taxpayers' money.

5. **b) The AG-ACNP should conduct a formal policy analysis.** Faced with a strong institutional history regarding this policy, the AG-ACNP needs to approach this issue carefully. The AG-ACNP should know that not all policies or practices in healthcare are evidence-based, therefore using a systematic approach to the problem is best. The other three options may well need to be done, but the components of a formal, theoretically supported policy analysis allows the AG-ACNP to have a firm understanding of the issue and allows the AG-ACNP to set the agenda.

6. **b) "Eligible professional" was replaced with the term "eligible clinician," expanding the population of individuals covered by MIPS, which now includes all four APRN groups.** MACRA was introduced by the CMS in 2015 with rules promulgated in late 2017. MACRA replaced the former means of physician payment with a program of bonuses and penalties for not meeting quality measures that progressively increase. This question is specifically asking about what MACRA did which recognizes APRNs (including AG-ACNPs), which is particularly important for the future of the profession and recognition. Answers a, c, and d, although part of the many changes in MACRA, do not answer the question. Only answer b that changes the narrower "eligible professional" with "eligible clinician," which includes all four APRN groups, allows formal recognition of Medicare and Medicaid payments and payment incentives as potentially available for all APRN group members.

7. **a) Notify the surgeon, and determine if she had decisional capacity at the time she signed the consent form.** Part of informed consent is that the patient is able to make personal decision and able to understand, reason, differentiate between good and bad, and communicate. Therefore the best answer is to call the surgeon to determine her decisional capacity at the time she signed the consent form. Notifying the ethics committee is not appropriate, nor is canceling the surgery if the need is indeed the best option for this patient. A psychiatric consult would be acceptable only in the setting of possible dementia.

8. **c) Have the nurse call the police.** This level of activity is considered Type II by NIOSH/NORA Organization of Work team. Type II is the most common to the healthcare setting, and is defined as a situation in which the perpetrator has a legitimate relationship with the business and becomes violent while being served by the business. The criminal justice system believes the concept that ignoring or tolerating low-level crime creates an environment conducive to more serious crime. The example here of verbal abuse, threats of assault, and low-level daily violence, if tolerated in healthcare environments, may perpetuate more serious forms of violence. Recognize that this is an unsafe situation for you as a provider, and have the nurse call the police. You cannot assume that all institutions' security forces cover a clinic setting even if there is an affiliation. A referral to a pain management clinic may need to be done, but official counselling by a law enforcement officer is the safest route.

9. **c) Send a certified letter with return request receipt requested stating the reason for dismissal and continues to provide care for 30 days beyond termination.** The AG-ACNP cannot withdraw from caring for a patient without notification, and reasons for dismissal include refusal to pay, abuse from the patient, and persistent nonadherence to recommended care. A certified letter with return receipt requested must state the reason. You must continue to provide primary care 30 days beyond termination to allow time for the patient to find another provider.

10. **b) The patient must be involved in the discussion.** She can provide some care for herself, therefore she must be included in the discussion. This is part of the patient's autonomy. The attending physician may be involved at some point, but it is not necessary for the initial discussion. Palliative care would be available after she elects for DNR status.

11. **d) Medicare D.** Medicare Part D requires a co-pay and a monthly premium. Medicare Part A covers hospitalization and skilled nursing facilities for individuals 65 and older. Medicare Part B covers physician services, out-of-hospital services, and lab and diagnostic procedures. Medicare Part C or Medicare "advantage" patients enrolled in A and B are eligible to enroll in C to receive healthcare through health maintenance organizations (HMOs), preferred provider organizations (PPOs), and so on.

12. **b) 80%.** Medicare covers 80% of the hospital bill if the facility accepts Medicare. The facility can charge the patients the additional difference between the Medicare payment and the total remaining balance of the hospital stay. The patient is responsible for a minimum of 20%. The 85% of the calculated physician fee payment is what Medicare will pay for an AG-ACNP service.

13. **c) Certification as an AG-ACNP by a recognized national certifying body.** The AG-ACNP must have an MSN or higher. A DNP degree is not required. National certification and licensure in the state is required. Credentials from by the hospital and potential DEA/state prescribing is not required to be Medicare provider, but they may be needed to fulfill the role.

14. **a) EMTALA.** Federal law states the EMTALA requires hospitals to provide an assessment and emergency treatment and stabilization without consideration of ability to pay when a patient presents with a medical emergency or is in labor. This policy ensures access to healthcare and reduces financial barriers. The ACA does not include this requirement. Stark Laws apply to providers who have a financial stake in ancillary services.

15. **d) Ensure the participant understands his/her rights and responsibilities.** The primary purpose of the consent form is to provide key information essential for the subject candidate to make a decision that a reasonable person would want to have. The subject being recruited must know this agreement is voluntary and how long the participation is required in the study and procedures. All reasonable and foreseeable risks or discomforts, possible benefits, and if any alternative procedures might be advantageous to the subject need to be discussed.

■ REFERENCE

Shi, L., & Singh, D. (2010). *Essentials of the US health care system*. Burlington, MA: Jones & Bartlett Learning.

■ BIBLIOGRAPHY

Bodenheimer, T., & Grumbach, K. (2012). Understanding health policy. New York, NY: McGraw-Hill Professional.

Buppert, C. (2018). *Nurse practitioner's business practice and legal guide* (6th ed.). Boulder, CO: Jones & Bartlett.

Centers for Medicare and Medicaid Services. (2017). *MACRA: Delivery system reform, Medicare payment reform*. Retrieved from https://www.cms.gov/Medicare/Quality-Initiatives-Patient-Assessment-Instruments/Value-Based-Programs/MACRA-MIPS-and-APMs/MACRA-MIPS-and-APMs.html

Centers for Medicare and Medicaid Services. (2018). *Home health PPS*. Retrieved from https://www.cms.gov/Medicare/Medicare-Fee-for-Service-Payment/HomeHealthPPS/index.html

Chadwick, G. L. (2018). *Comprehensive guide to informed consent*. Retrieved from https://about.citiprogram.org/en/final-rule-resources/#consent

Lilly, C. M., McLaughlin, J. M., Zhao, H., Baker, S. P., Cody, S., Irwin, R. S., & UMass Memorial Critical Care Operations Group. (2014). A multicenter study of ICU telemedicine reengineering of adult critical care. *Chest*, 145(3), 500–507. doi:10.1378/chest.13-1973

McPhaul, K., & Lipscomb, J. (2004). Workplace violence in health care: Recognized but not regulated. *Online Journal of Issues in Nursing*, 9(3), 7.

Patton, R., Zalon, M., & Ludwick, R. (2014). *Nurses making policy: From bedside to boardroom*. New York, NY: Springer Publishing Company.

Phillips, J. P. (2016). Workplace violence against health care workers in the United States. *New England Journal of Medicine*, 374(17), 1661–1669. doi:10.1056/NEJMra1501998

Polit, D. F. B. C. T. (2012). *Nursing research: Generating and assessing evidence for nursing practice* (9th ed.). Philadelphia, PA: Wolters Kluwer Health/Lippincott, Williams & Wilkins.

Rudner, N. L. (2016). Full practice authority for advanced practice registered nurses is a gender issue. *Online Journal of Issues in Nursing*, 21(2), 6–6. doi:10.3912/OJIN.Vol21No02PPT54

Schaum, K. D. (2014). Medicare payment: Surgical dressings and topical wound care products. *Advances in Wound Care*, 3(8), 553–560. doi:10.1089/wound.2013.0434

Seavey, J. W., Aytur, S. A., & McGrath, R. J. (2014). *Health policy analysis*. New York, NY: Springer Publishing Company.

U.S. Health Policy Gateway. (2018). *Access to care*. Retrieved from http://ushealthpolicygateway.com/vi-key-health-policy-issues-financing-and-delivery/k-barriers-to-access/

25

Quality of Healthcare Practice

ALEXANDER MENARD

QUALITY OF HEALTHCARE PRACTICE QUESTIONS

1. QSEN has outlined six key topics that graduate-level nurses need to be competent in patient-centered care, teamwork and collaboration, EBP, quality improvement, safety, and Informatics. How does QSEN define safety?

   a. Minimizing harm to patients
   b. Minimizing risk of harm to patients and providers through both system effectiveness and individual performance
   c. Use data to monitor the outcomes of care processes and use improvement methods to design and test changes to continuously improve the quality and safety of healthcare systems
   d. Recognize the patient or designee as the source of control and full partner in providing compassionate and coordinated care based on respect for patient's preferences, values, and needs

2. In which clinical scenario would the AG-ACNP evaluate for a quality improvement policy?

   a. A recent case of *Clostridium difficile* in an immunocompromised patient with recent use of antibiotics
   b. An expected/projected increase in admissions for the flu
   c. A projected decrease in rhinovirus presentation to the ED
   d. A new onset of frequently diagnosed CAUTIs

3. The AG-ACNP is caring for an 85-year-old male who presents to the hospital with acute chronic heart failure. After initial workup the AG-ACNP consults the heart failure service for further management recommendations. What QSEN competency does this embrace?

   a. Patient-centered care
   b. Teamwork and collaboration
   c. Best patient care
   d. Healthcare resource management

4. There have been an increased number of complaints from patients regarding a medical–surgical floor's noise level at night. The AG-ACNP has been asked to be a member of a new interprofessional team to address this issue. At the first meeting, the AG-ACNP identifies this as the team's first task:

   a. Identify those night staff members causing the excess noise.
   b. Install noise meters to collect data.
   c. Identify the interprofessional team's project goals.
   d. Fire the nurse manager for not intervening on the noise complaints.

5. Prior to the AG-ACNP intubating a 96-year-old male patient who presented from the floor in acute respiratory distress and septic shock secondary to CAP, the AG-ACNP discusses with the patient's wife and healthcare proxy (HCP) the plan to intubate the patient. The HCP states that the patient would not want to be intubated. After discussing the alternatives of treatment with the HCP, the patient's goal of care was changed to comfort measures only. This is an example of what QSEN competency?

   a. EBP
   b. Patient-centered care
   c. Teamwork and collaboration
   d. Safety

6. A 28-year-old female patient was discharged home after a prolonged hospital stay secondary to a stroke. During this hospitalization the patient was diagnosed with a hypercoagulable disorder. It was determined she would require lifelong anti-coagulation. Prior to discharge home the patient was being given therapeutic doses of enoxaparin while she was transitioned to warfarin. The patient was subsequently sent home on warfarin after 10 days in the hospital with an international normalized ratio (INR) of 1.2, but without a prescription for enoxaparin. The patient subsequently was readmitted to the hospital 5 days later with a new ischemic stroke and was noted to have and INR of 1.3. The AG-ACNP identifies the lack of bridging therapy for the patient with enoxaparin as a medication error. What is the best way for an institution to understand this how this mistake occurred?

   a. Discipline the provider who discharged the patient.
   b. Write up the nurse who discharged the patient.
   c. Suggest completion of a RCA.
   d. Say nothing, as there are tremendous legal implications.

7. The AG-ACNP is developing a QI project for decreasing falls in patients 65 years of age or older admitted the medical–surgical floors of a large suburban hospital. When preparing for the project, the AG-ACNP knows the highest quality of evidence will be obtained from:

   a. RCT
   b. Expert opinion
   c. Cohort study
   d. Case series

8. After the initiation of a quality care improvement process to decrease the amount of CLABSI through educating staff members about proper application of sterile drapes, the AG-ACNP will evaluate its effectiveness by:

   a. Polling nurses to see if drapes are being applied properly
   b. Comparing pre-intervention CLABSI rates to postintervention CLABSI rates
   c. Counting the amount of sterile drapes used compared to the number of central lines placed
   d. Polling providers who insert central lines regarding proper sterile techniques

9. A family friend notices the AG-ACNP in the cafeteria during his/her lunch break and asks if he/she is caring for someone they know. The AG-ACNP knows the information the family friend is requesting is protected health information. How should the AG-ACNP respond to the request for information?

   a. Give the family friend the admitting diagnosis but no other information.
   b. Respectfully inform the family friend you are unable to share patient data.
   c. Share what you know regarding the patient.
   d. Call security.

10. The AG-ACNP recognizes which of the following as an example of EBP:

    a. Obtain daily chest x-rays on all intubated patients.
    b. Prescribe broad-spectrum antibiotics to patients who present in septic shock within 1 hour.
    c. Order stress ulcer prophylaxis for all elderly patients admitted to the hospital.
    d. Order blood, urine, and sputum cultures for all patients who spike a fever.

11. The Joint Commission certifies more than 21,000 healthcare organizations and programs in the United States. The AG-ACNP recognizes the mission of the Joint Commission is best addressed in which of the following statements:

    a. To reduce the amount of fraud throughout healthcare in the United States
    b. To continuously improve healthcare for the public by inspiring hospitals to excel in providing safe and effective care of the highest quality and value
    c. To reduce harm to patient and increase revenue for healthcare facilities by implementation of guideline-based interactions
    d. To address racial and ethnic disparities throughout healthcare

12. The CMS uses quality measures in its quality improvement, public reporting, and pay-for-reporting programs for specific healthcare providers. What set of goals does CMS intend these quality measures to address?

    a. Effective, safe, efficient, patient-centered, equitable, and timely care
    b. The CMS is not concerned with quality
    c. Safe, equitable, and efficient care
    d. Effective, evidence-based, and timely care

13. Which of the following best describes an accountable care organization:

    a. Any hospital in the United States that cares for patients is an accountable organization
    b. Groups of doctors, hospitals, and other healthcare providers that come together voluntarily to give coordinated high-quality care to their Medicare patients
    c. A group of facilities that specialize in minimizing expenses to care for their patient population
    d. Groups of doctors, hospitals, and other healthcare providers that come together voluntarily to give coordinated high-quality care primarily to wealthy patients

14. When evaluating the effectiveness of a new protocol related to reducing rates of newly documented pressure ulcers, the AG-ACNP expects which of the following outcomes to indicate the new protocol is effective:

    a. Increased patient satisfaction scores
    b. Reduction in staff injuries with repositioning patients
    c. Reduction in the rate of newly documented pressure ulcers
    d. Increased job satisfaction among new staff members

15. QSEN designates informatics as one of the six competencies to continuously improve the quality and safety of the healthcare systems within which they work. Which of the following best defines informatics?

    a. The use of information and technology to communicate, manage knowledge, mitigate error, and support decision-making
    b. Reducing harm to patients and families through automated text updates and best-practice alerts
    c. The use of databases and decision-making tools to aid in clinical decision making
    d. The use of information and technology to assess the readiness of the healthcare community to transition to an electronic medical record

■ QUALITY OF HEALTHCARE PRACTICE ANSWERS AND RATIONALES

1. **b) Minimizing risk of harm to patients and providers through both system effectiveness and individual performance**. While QSEN does minimize harm to patients it also minimizes risk of harm to providers, as such this answer is not the best answer. Using date to monitor the outcome of care processes and use improvement methods to design and test changes to continuously improve quality and safety is QSEN's definition of quality improvement processes. Recognizing the patient or designee as the source of control and full partner in providing compassionate and coordinated care based on respect for patient's preferences, values and needs is QSEN's definition of patient-centered care.

2. **d) A new onset of frequently diagnosed CAUTIs**. A new onset of frequent CAUTI warrants a QI process. CAUTI rates are used for quality markers. The new onset means there is something that has changed and can therefore be evaluated for a QI policy. A recent case of *C. difficile* in an immunocompromised patient is an isolated case and there is a high risk for developing the infection.The increase in flu admissions was expected/projected. A decrease in rhinovirus presentation to the ED was projected.

3. **b) Teamwork and collaboration**. QSEN defines this as the knowledge and skills to function effectively within nursing and interprofessional teams, fostering open communication, mutual respect, and shared decision making to achieve quality patient care. Healthcare resource management and best patient care are not among the six QSEN competencies for graduate-level nursing (patient-centered care, teamwork and collaboration, EBP, QI, safety, and informatics). Patient-centered care is defined as recognizing the patient or designee as the source of control and full partner in providing compassionate and coordinated care based on respect for the patient's preferences, values, and needs.

4. **c) Identify the interprofessional team's project goals**. The best answer is to identify the interprofessional team project goals. Anytime a team is developed it is crucial to identify and outline the project goals prior to starting to work on the problem. Identifying the night staff members causing the excess noise or installing noise meters may be effective interventions, but goals need to be defined to have a successful intervention. Firing the nurse manager is not a rationale intervention at this time; no data has been collected and no interventions have been attempted.

5. **b) Patient-centered care**. The best answer is patient-centered care. The AG-ACNP recognized the patient or designee as the source of control and full partner in providing compassionate and coordinated care based on respect for patient's preferences, values, and needs. EBP, safety, and teamwork and collaboration are all used to provide patient-centered care.

6. **c) Suggest completion of a RCA**. A RCA will help all parties involved discover the core reason(s) why this medication was not prescribed at discharge when the patient required anticoagulation and was not therapeutic on her enoxaparin. Understanding the core problem will prevent this from happening in the future. Disciplining the provider or writing up the nurse who discharged the patient is premature, as the core of the problem is not understood. Saying nothing is unethical.

7. **a) RCT**. Expert opinion, cohort study, and case reports fall below RCT when assessing levels of evidence. Systematic reviews and meta-analyses produce higher-quality evidence than RCTs, but are not option in this question.

8. **b) Comparing pre-intervention CLABSI rates to postintervention CLABSI rates**. Polling nurses and providers on proper draping as well as counting drapes and comparing to number of lines placed can provide data to assess effectiveness of the training, but will not directly measure the desired outcome which is to decrease the number of CLABSIs.

9. **b) Respectfully inform the family friend you are unable to share patient data**. The HIPAA of 1996 required the secretary of the U.S. Department of HHS to develop regulations protecting the privacy and security of certain health information (HHS, 2018). The admitting diagnosis and anything else you know regarding the patient is protected health information.

Calling security is not the best answer; many people are not aware of what constitutes protected health information.

10. **b) Prescribe broad-spectrum antibiotics to patients who present in septic shock within** 1 hour. Ordering and administering broad-spectrum antibiotics to a patient presenting in septic shock within 1 hour of presentation to the ED is EBP. Daily chest x-rays are not indicated on all intubated patients. Stress ulcer prophylaxis is not indicated for all admitted patients. Hospitalized patients have reasons to become febrile other than infection, and thus not all require an infectious workup.

11. **b) To continuously improve healthcare for the public, by inspiring them to excel in providing safe and effective care of the highest quality and value** (see the Joint Commission website, www.jointcommission.org). Reducing fraud, racial and ethnic disparities and increasing revenue are not part of the mission of the Joint Commission and are not inclusive of their mission. Therefore, these are not the best answers.

12. **a) Effective, safe, efficient, patient-centered, equitable, and timely care.** The CMS does have a large focus on quality care. Safe, equitable, and efficient care, and effective, evidence-based, timely care address only some of the goals CMS intends to address with quality measures.

13. **b) Groups of doctors, hospitals, and other healthcare providers that come together voluntarily to give coordinated high-quality care to their Medicare patients** (CMS.gov). Accountable care organizations (ACC) do not care just for wealthy patients. ACCs are not isolated hospitals, but include a comprehensive range of providers, hospitals and services. While minimizing expenses is a likely outcome, it is not the complete definition of ACCs.

14. **c) Reduction in the rate of newly documented pressure ulcers.** Data on a reduction in the rate of newly documented pressure ulcers directly assess the intervention's effectiveness. Increased patient satisfaction scores, a reduction in staff injuries with repositioning patients, and increased job satisfaction among new staff members may be results of the new protocol, but do not directly assess the effectiveness of the protocol and its ability to reduce newly documented pressure ulcers.

15. **a) The use of information and technology to communicate, manage knowledge, mitigate error, and support decision making.** These uses encompass all aspects of informatics as defined by QSEN. Use of information systems may reduce harm by automating best practices, using decision making tools and assessing healthcare communities are elements of informatics, by themselves are not the best definition of informatics.

■ REFERENCE

U.S. Department of Health & Human Services. (2018). Summary of the HIPAA privacy rule. Retrieved from https://www.hhs.gov/hipaa/for-professionals/privacy/laws-regulations/index.html

■ BIBLIOGRAPHY

Alhazzani, W., Alshahrani, M., Moayyedi, P., & Jaeschke, R. (2012). Stress ulcer prophylaxis in critically ill patients: Review of the evidence. *Polskie Archiwum Medycyny Wewnetrznej, 122*(3), 107–114. doi: 10.20452/pamw.1173

Centers for Disease Control and Prevention. (2012). *Central line-associated bloodstream infection.* Retrieved from http://www.cdc.gov/nhsn/PDFs/pscManual/4PSC_CLABScurrent.pdf

Center for Medicare and Medicaid Services. (2017). *Final policy, payment, and quality provisions in the Medicare physician fee schedule for calendar year 2018.* Retrieved from https://www.cms.gov/

Centers for Medicare and Medicaid Services. (2017a). *MACRA: Delivery system reform, Medicare payment reform.* Retrieved from https://www.cms.gov/Medicare/Quality-Initiatives-Patient-Assessment-Instruments/Value-Based-Programs/MACRA-MIPS-and-APMs/MACRA-MIPS-and-APMs.html

Centers for Medicare and Medicaid Services. (2017b). *Medicare claims processing manual. Chapter 12—Physicians/ nonphysician practitioners.* Retrieved from https://www.cms.gov/Regulations-and-Guidance/Guidance/Manuals/downloads/clm104c12.pdf

Gordis, L. (2013). *Epidemiology* (5th ed.). Philadelphia, PA: Saunders.

Gupta, D., Agarwal, R., Aggarwal, A. N., Singh, N., Mishra, N., Khilnani, G., . . . Jindal, S. K. (2012). Guidelines for diagnosis and management of community-and hospital-acquired pneumonia in adults: Joint ICS/NCCP (I) recommendations. *Lung India: Official Organ of Indian Chest Society*, *29*(Suppl. 2), S27. doi: 10.4103/0970-2113.99248

Institute for Healthcare Improvement. (2015). RCA2: Improving root cause analyses and actions to prevent harm. Retrieved from http://www.npsf.org/?page=RCA2

Kasper, D., Hauser, S., Jameson, J., Fauci, A., Longo, D., & Loscalzo, J. (2015). *Harrison's principles of internal medicine* (19th ed.). New York, NY: McGraw-Hill.

QSEN Institute for Nursing. (2018). Quality and safety for nurses. Retrieved from http://qsen.org/

Sherwood, G., & Barnsteiner, J. (2017). *Quality and safety in nursing: A competency approach to improving outcomes.* New York, NY: John Wiley & Sons.

Woodring, J. H., & Heiser, M. J. (1995). Detection of pneumoperitoneum on chest radiographs: Comparison of upright lateral and posteroanterior projections. *AJR: American Journal of Roentgenology*, *165*(1), 45–47. doi: 10.2214/ajr.165.1.7785629

26 Coding, Billing, and Reimbursement

NANCY MUNRO

CODING, BILLING, AND REIMBURSEMENT QUESTIONS

1. What legislation allowed NPs and CNSs to bill for their professional services for both hospital inpatients and outpatients?

   a. Rural HealthCare Protection Act of 1997
   b. Balanced Budget Act of 1997
   c. Patient Protection and Affordable Care Act of 2010
   d. Social Security Amendment of 1965

2. The AG-ACNP has been working with a hospitalist group for several years. Recently, the hospital incorporated children into the hospitalist new practice contract and the group has requested the AG-ACNP to see some children. What should the AG-ACNP do about this situation?

   a. See the children so the hospitalist group will be able to meet its contractual obligations.
   b. Meet with the hospitalists, review the consensus model with them, and consult the state NP association for further support.
   c. Ignore the situation, as the physician has approved your involvement in the expanded patient population.
   d. Immediately leave the position so that the AG-ACNP's license will be protected.

3. An AG-ACNP has just started to bill for her services. She has received a letter from the compliance department in her institution stating that her charts were audited. The compliance department has found that she was underbilling for some of her services and they are changing the CPT codes. What are appropriate actions for the AG-ANCP to pursue?

   a. Arrange an appointment with the compliance department to discuss the questioned services.
   b. Since the compliance department is more knowledgeable about CPT codes, there is no need to question its decisions.
   c. Report this incident to her supervisor immediately.
   d. Report the compliance department to CMS.

4. When an AG-ACNP is employed in an institution or group practice, he will be required to bill for his services. There is often extensive documentation requirements for proper billing. What is the first step in the process that the AG-ACNP needs to do?

   a. Most institutions or practice managers are aware of the complex process, so the AG-ACNP should not worry about this.
   b. Obtain a NPI number to start the process.
   c. Make an appointment with the billing and coding department to start the process.
   d. The compliancy departments will initiate the paperwork and notify the AG-ACNP for signatures.

5. AG-ACNPs are able to bill for services at 85% of what a physician is reimbursed; however, many practices bill under the physician's NPI number if the two are both employed by the same practice or institution. This often is a distractor in calculating the true contributions of the AG-ACNP provider to a practice. How can the AG-ACNP increase reimbursement for an institution or group practice and still practice to the full scope of his education?

   a. Make sure the AG-ACNPs bill at a higher level of care to negate the 15% loss in reimbursement.
   b. Have the AG-ACNP become trained and credentialed to perform all procedures and be reimbursed for these services.
   c. Have the AG-ACNPs see the less-complicated patients, which frees the physician time to care for more complicated patients, which results in higher reimbursement for the practice.
   d. Have the AG-ACNPs care for the patients the physicians do not want to see.

6. Appropriate documentation is the key to ensuring proper reimbursement. Complicated patient care requires more detailed documentation to include interval history, exam, and medical decision making. Components to be included for highest reimbursement are:

   a. A larger number of diagnoses
   b. Document the risks of complications, morbidity, and mortality
   c. Inclusion of all test results to demonstrate the complexity of data
   d. Number of diagnoses, complexity, risks of complications, morbidity, and mortality

7. An AG-ACNP who works in a trauma ICU will also follow patients after discharge in the trauma outpatient clinic. His physician colleagues want to follow "incident to" billing practices in order to get 100% reimbursement. The AG-ACNP must be aware of the following:

   a. A physician must be present in the clinic office when the AG-ACNP is seeing patients.
   b. A physician does not need to have participation in the care of these patients once they are seen in the clinic.
   c. A physician does not need to be present in the office but can be accessed for questions by phone.
   d. Billing can only be 100% reimbursed.

8. Inpatient CPT codes are those codes that are used when providing services for hospitalized patients. Which of the following codes are outpatient codes?

   a. 99221-99223
   b. 99231-99233
   c. 99238-99239
   d. 99495-99496

9. The majority of reimbursement for AG-ACNPs is the result of using subsequent hospital visit codes. These codes (99231-99233) can be used after an initial hospital visit code (99221-99223) note is completed. Which of these statements is correct?

    a. There is a time component for these codes.

    b. Each note must contain some level of interval history, exam, and medical decision-making components.

    c. If an AG-ACNP does the initial hospital visit note, an AG-ACNP must write all subsequent hospital visit notes.

    d. Each note must contain two of the three components of interval history, exam, and medical decision making.

10. An AG-ACNP works in the medical ICU of an institution where the AG-ACNP service provides 24/7 coverage of this unit. She has admitted a septic shock patient at 3 a.m. and initiated fluid resuscitation with vasoactive medication support and prescribed appropriate antibiotics. The patient also required a central line placed, which the AG-ACNP performed. This critical care visit note must include which of the following:

    a. Time spent performing the central line

    b. Billing language for the central line placement

    c. Clear description of the critical care assessment

    d. General description of the required interventions

11. An AG-ACNP works for a hospitalist service in a hospital and has seen one of seven patients assigned to her today. She evaluated the patient and determined that she would use the subsequent hospital visit code 99233. She was called to see the patient 6 hours later and found the patient to be acutely short of breath. She ordered chest x-ray, diagnosed pulmonary edema, and ordered diuresis; performed a bedside echocardiogram and ordered a formal study; and then transferred the patient to the ICU. What code can the AG-ACNP use for these services provided?

    a. 99231

    b. 99232

    c. 99238

    d. 99291

12. In order to bill for services provided, the AG-ACNP's salary must appear in what part of Medicare coverage?

    a. Part A

    b. Part B

    c. Part C

    d. Part D

13. RVU is a part of the reimbursement process that assists with calculating the amount of reimbursement that will be granted to a provider. It is part of a complicated equation that considers which of the following:

    a. Type of service provided

    b. Practice income

    c. Health insurance

    d. Type of provider

14. Transitional care codes 99495 and 99496 were developed in recent years to serve as another mechanism to reward coordination of care services to ensure that patients do not "bounce back" once discharged from the hospital. The patient who is being discharged and has high complexity of medical decision making must have a face-to-face visit with a physician, NP, or PA within how many days from discharge:

    a. 3 days
    b. 7 days
    c. 10 days
    d. 14 days

15. The Institute of Medicine published a consensus report titled *Dying in America* in 2014, which promoted improving the quality of and honoring individual preferences near the end of life. CMS has developed CPT code 99497 (first 30 minutes) with add-on code 99498 (each additional 30 minutes) to encourage all healthcare providers to initiate early discussion with patients about their preferences at the end of life. The CPT code 99497 can be used:

    a. 2 times
    b. 5 times
    c. 10 times
    d. No limit

■ CODING, BILLING, AND REIMBURSEMENT ANSWERS AND RATIONALES

1. **b) Balanced Budget Act of 1997**. Physician services were the original target for fee of services but there was an initiative to support NP services for patients in rural areas via the Rural HealthCare Protection Act of 1997 but this was not passed into law. The Balanced Budget Act of 1997 allowed CMS to authorize NPs and CNSs to bill for their services for both inpatients and outpatients regardless of the patients' geographic location.

2. **b) Meet with the hospitalists, review the consensus model with them, and consult the state NP association for further support**. AG-ACNPs cannot see children since they are educated to care for adults. Many states have different SOP laws, and age parameters in state laws may not always be clearly stated. However, state SOP laws do not supersede the education preparation of the AG-ACNP. The state NP association as well as SBON may be a source of support concerning the legal age of an adult. It is important for the AG-ACNP to have a discussion with the physician group because it may not understand the limits of the AG-ACNP SOP. A discussion supported with data may be the intervention needed to clarify the issue.

3. **a) Arrange an appointment with the compliance department to discuss the questioned services**. Under-billing is considered a reimbursement violation but is not recognized as frequently. Overbilling is the more common violation. Either violation is important to understand. The best way to learn about these issues is to develop a relationship with the compliance department of the institution where the AG-ACNP is employed. These professionals are expert in reimbursement topics generally and have specific knowledge about the insurance companies that are commonly associated with the institution where the AG-ACNP is employed. These departments can be an important resource regarding the best use of codes.

4. **b) Obtain a NPI number to start the process**. An NPI is a unique identification number for covered healthcare providers; it was developed to improve the efficiency and effectiveness of electronic transmission of health information. Healthcare providers and all health plans and healthcare clearinghouses must use NPIs in their administrative and financial transactions so that providers can be tracked. The process of billing for services becomes very complicated because each insurance company has separate forms that must be completed before any provider will be able to bill for their services. NPI numbers are mandatory to start the process and compliance departments are the best resource to assist with proper completion of the multiple forms of various insurance companies. Eventually, the AG-ACNP will need to sign any insurance forms the practice or institutions requires to be paid for the AG-ACNP's services.

5. **c) Have the AG-ACNPs see the less complicated patients, which frees the physician time to care for more complicated patients, which results in higher reimbursement for the practice**. The 85% reimbursement for AG-ACNPs presents a challenge to the "visibility" of the contributions of AG-ACNPs to patient outcomes. Billing should always be accurately coded and billed, not overbilled to negate the 15% difference in reimbursement percentage. Unfortunately, reimbursed at 100% for services provided takes priority in some institutions or group practices. This philosophy causes the AG-ACNP's services to be "invisible" because the AG-ACNP might provide the service, but the service will be billed under the physicians' NPI number. AG-ACNPs whose practice consists of primarily performing procedures are not working to the full extent of theAG-ACNP's education but may bring in more revenue.

6. **d) Number of diagnoses, complexity, risks of complications, morbidity, and mortality**. More complicated patients require more complex decision-making processes that must be reflected in the AG-ACNP's note. It is logical that these patients will have more diagnoses that should be addressed with a plan that has data and a discussion about risk factors, which should all reflect the thought processes of the AG-ACNP.

7. **a) A physician must be present in the clinic office when the AG-ACNP is seeing patients**. The "incident to" billing concept is a controversial concept that is closely monitored by CMS. A physician must be physically present in the office and there needs to be some evidence that

the physician has had some participation in the care plan for the patient. There is no specific frequency that the physician must participate. If these conditions are not met, the AG-ACNP can bill under his/her NPI number at 85%.

8. **d) 99495-99496**. Codes 99495 and 99496 are transitional care codes. Inpatient CPT codes are separated into three categories: Initial visit (99221-99223), subsequent hospital visits (99231-99233), and discharge (99238-99239). Initial visits involving a hospitalized patient require interval history, exam, and medical decision making. Therefore these codes will get more reimbursement for services. Once the patient is an established patient, each daily visit is then considered as a subsequent hospital visit (99231-99233). When discharging these patients, coordination of care becomes very important and reimbursement is higher than subsequent visits. Discharge codes are 99238-99239. The higher the number of the code in each category, the more involved the care delivered.

9. **d) Each note must contain two of the three components of interval history, exam, and medical decision making**. Subsequent hospital visit notes must contain detailed information in order to meet the requirement for the various levels of these codes. There is no time component that must be documented, but CMS does provide a time reference interval for approximate time spent in caring for patients using these codes. An AG-ACNP or physician can use these codes and there is no order sequence required. Each note must contain two of the three components of interval history, exam, and medical decision making and these components become more complicated as the level of the visit increases. Example: Subsequent hospital visit 99233 is the code that can receive the highest level of reimbursement, but the note must contain at least four diagnoses with associated complex data that are being addressed.

10. **c) Clear description of the critical care assessment**. The three components of a critical care note include specific descriptions of the assessment, plan, and time it took to perform these components of care. It is important to note that there are no specific criteria that must be included in the documentation of critical care services similar to subsequent hospital visit notes. The key difference is that the wording used in this type of note must reflect the life-threatening clinical situation. An example would be a 52-year-old female who presents in septic shock due to *E. coli* urinary tract infection with flank pain and dysuria for 3 days. Lactic acidosis (lactate = 6) indicated compromised tissue perfusion which was addressed using aggressive fluid resuscitation and norepinephrine at 15 mcg/min and initiating ciprofloxacin IV. The central line insertion is a separate service which can be billed but documentation must be specific and if ultrasound used, screenshot documentation may be required. Critical care time cannot include time needed to insert the central line. Documentation of time spent can be in minutes (most common method) and with the first 30 to 74 minutes, critical care code 99291 should be used and any additional 30 minutes

11. **d) 99291**. The services provided were critical care services and as long as she follows the criteria for using critical care codes, she can escalate her care when indicated. However, she cannot move from critical care codes to subsequent hospital visit codes in the same 24-hour period.

12. **b) Part B**. Medicare Part B includes physician services and outpatient care. It is important that the AG-ACNP understand that an AG-ACNP salary may appear in Part A which includes inpatient care received in a hospital or skilled nursing facility, but the salary can be switched to Part B by negotiating with hospital administration. Administration may not always understand the important contributions of the AG-ACNP role and how the role can increase reimbursement.

13. **a) Type of service provided**. The type of provider can be determined by the NPI number. The RVU calculation for reimbursement also involves the SGR formula. This formula is very complicated and was developed as a response to varying levels of cost of living depending on the area of the country. Reimbursement methodology is currently in transition. The past emphasis was the quantity of visits that would increase reimbursement, but now the emphasis is on quality of services and patient outcomes. The RVU calculation will eventually be eliminated. This is an opportunity for the AG-ACNP to demonstrate excellent patient

outcomes, which will then receive increased reimbursement. Practice expense, malpractice insurance, and complexity of service provided determines final RVUs.

14. **b) 7 days**. When the patient has a very complex care plan, the patient should be seen within 7 days of discharge to satisfy one of the criteria for CPT code 99496. Patients with moderate complexity of medical decision making should be seen within 14 days of discharge to satisfy one of the criteria for CPT code 99495. Other criteria that must be met include interactive contacts within 2 days of discharge, including phone or email mechanisms and certain nonface-to-face services.

15. **d) No limit**. These codes provide financial incentives for medical and social support services that decrease the need for ED and acute care services. This initiative will hopefully improve shared decision making and advance care planning that reduces the utilization of unnecessary medical services and those not consistent with a patient's goals for care. Flexibility with changes in patient condition was the rationale for not limiting the number of times this code can be used, but the provider must meet the documentation criteria of the add-on code 99498.

■ BIBLIOGRAPHY

American Association of Critical-Care Nurses. (2017). *AACN scope and standards for acute care nurse practitioner practice 2017* (L. Bell, Ed.). Aliso Viejo, CA: American Association of Critical Care Nurses.

American Association of Nurse Practitioners. (2013). *Fact sheet: Medicare reimbursement*. Retrieved from https://www.aanp.org/68-articles/325-medicare-reimbursement

APRN Consensus Work Group and National Council of State Boards of Nurses APRN Advisory Committee. (2008). *Consensus model for APRN regulation: Licensure, accreditation, certification and education*. Retrieved from https://www.ncsbn.org/Consensus_Model_for_APRN_Regulation_July_2008.pdf

Buppert, C. (2018). *Nurse practitioner's business practice and legal guide* (6th ed.). Boulder, CO: Jones & Bartlett.

Centers for Disease Control and Prevention. (2015). *ICD-10-CM official guidelines for coding and reporting FY 2016*. Atlanta, GA: Centers for Disease Control and Prevention.

Centers for Medicare and Medicaid Services. (2015). *Hospital value-based purchasing*. Retrieved from https://www.cms.gov/Outreach-and-Education/Medicare-Learning-Network-MLN/MLNProducts/downloads/Hospital_VBPurchasing_Fact_Sheet_ICN907664.pdf

Centers for Medicare and Medicaid Services. (2016a). *Frequently asked questions about billing the physician fee schedule for advance care planning services*. Retrieved from https://www.cms.gov/Medicare/Medicare-Fee-for-Service-Payment/PhysicianFeeSched/Downloads/FAQ-Advance-Care-Planning.pdf

Centers for Medicare and Medicaid Services. (2016b). *NPI: What you need to know*. Retrieved from https://www.cms.gov/Outreach-and-Education/Medicare-Learning-Network-MLN/MLNProducts/downloads/NPI-What-You-Need-To-KnowText-Only.pdf

Centers for Medicare and Medicaid Services. (2016c). *Transitional care management services*. Retrieved from https://www.cms.gov/Outreach-and-Education/Medicare-Learning-Network-MLN/MLNProducts/downloads/Transitional-Care-Management-Services-Fact-Sheet-ICN908628.pdf

Centers for Medicare and Medicaid Services. (2017a). *Evaluation and management services*. Retrieved from https://www.cms.gov/Outreach-and-Education/Medicare-Learning-Network-MLN/MLNProducts/Downloads/eval-mgmt-serv-guide-ICN006764.pdf

Centers for Medicare and Medicaid Services. (2017b). *MACRA: Delivery system reform, Medicare payment reform*. Retrieved from https://www.cms.gov/Medicare/Quality-Initiatives-Patient-Assessment-Instruments/Value-Based-Programs/MACRA-MIPS-and-APMs/MACRA-MIPS-and-APMs.html

Centers for Medicare and Medicaid Services. (2017c). *Medicare claims processing manual. Chapter 12—Physicians/nonphysician practitioners*. Retrieved from https://www.cms.gov/Regulations-and-Guidance/Guidance/Manuals/downloads/clm104c12.pdf

Dorman, T., Britten, F., Brown, D., & Munro, N. (2014). *Coding and billing for critical care: A practice tool*. Society of Critical Care Medicine. Mount Prospect, IL: Society of Critical Care Medicine.

Munro, N. (2013). What an acute care nurse practitioner should know about reimbursement. *AACN Advanced Critical Care, 24*(2), 110–113. doi:10.1097/NCI.0b013e31828c8890

IV

Comprehensive Practice Exam

27

Comprehensive Practice Exam: Questions

COMPREHENSIVE PRACTICE EXAM QUESTIONS

1. Close to half of those adults older than 65 years of age experience poor sleep quality and those with psychiatric problems have a more than twofold increase of insomnia. Which of the following is recommended as an intervention for good sleep hygiene?

   a. Establish a random bedtime and wake time.
   b. Take naps throughout the day when feeling tired.
   c. Maximize exposure to light during the day and minimize at night.
   d. Encourage consumption of alcohol.

2. A 28-year-old male involved in a high-speed motor vehicle crash arrived in the ED unresponsive, was intubated, and is requiring moderate ventilator settings. Injuries include grade I splenic laceration, bowel contusion. He was initially normotensive. Over the next 12 hours, his urine output diminishes to near anuria, despite 8 L of volume resuscitation. The AG-ACNP notes his abdomen is becoming distended and firm. His blood pressure drops to 90/65 and he becomes slightly agitated. PIP climbs to 30 mmHg. Based upon these findings, the AG-ACNP anticipates which priority intervention:

   a. Sedation and analgesia for ventilator management
   b. Bladder pressure monitoring with anticipation of surgical consult
   c. Fluid bolus with anticipation of vasoactive drip
   d. ECG with anticipation of cardiology consult

3. A 33-year-old woman with a 21-year history of insulin-dependent DM presents for routine follow-up. Her blood pressure has been in the 130 to 155/84 to 95 mmHg range during the past few months. A recent blood pressure taken by a nurse friend in the morning was 154/94 mmHg. She has mild proliferative retinopathy and mild sensory neuropathy. The remainder of the physical examination is unremarkable. A urinalysis reveals 2+ proteinuria. What is the most appropriate first-line treatment of her hypertension?

   a. Lisinopril (Prinivil)
   b. Atenolol (Tenormin)
   c. Doxazosin (Cardura)
   d. Diltiazem (Cardizem)

4. A 56-year-old Caucasian male with a past medical history of advanced Huntington's disease presents with several weeks of coughing, dyspnea, fever, chills, weight loss, and purulent sputum. His chest x-ray reveals infiltrates with cavitation and air-fluid levels in the bilateral lower lobes. AFB is negative, sputum culture is obtained, and a CT of the chest is pénding. The first differential diagnosis when considering treatment plans is:

   a. Lung abscess
   b. Tuberculosis
   c. Hodgkin's lymphoma
   d. Adenocarcinoma

5. A 39-year-old patient with no personal history of diabetes but a family history of noninsulin dependent DMII in multiple close relatives has a series of fasting glucose levels greater than 145 mg/dL while in the hospital for acute pyelonephritis. A HbgA1c was noted to be 8.1%. What is the next best action the AG-ACNP should initiate for the patient's plan of care?

   a. Discuss and answer questions about the test results, diagnosis, needed lifestyle changes, and medical treatments with the patient and/or family.
   b. Prescribe metformin 500 mg once daily and counsel the patient and/or family of the side effects, adverse effects, and/or complications.
   c. Advise the patient to follow up with a PCP for treatment and healthcare education upon discharge.
   d. Screen the patient for atherosclerotic cardiovascular disease risk factors and prescribe the appropriate antithrombotic and statin therapy as indicated.

6. A patient admitted with IVH develops acute hydrocephalus and an EVD is placed. Initially 20 mL bloody fluid is drained and the patient's neurologic exam improves. Over the next 3 hours, the patient becomes more lethargic, confused, has nausea, and vomits. The AG-ACNP suspects:

   a. The EVD is working fine.
   b. The EVD is clotted off.
   c. It takes time for clinical improvements to be noted.
   d. The patient developed worsening cerebral edema.

7. The treatment of choice for pericarditis chest pain occurring within 1 week post-myocardial infarction is:

   a. Aspirin
   b. Indomethacin (Indocin)
   c. Ibuprofen (Motrin/Advil)
   d. Corticosteroids

8. A 79-year-old male with advanced dementia is admitted to the medical unit with recurrent sepsis due to a UTI. The staff indicates that they are concerned the patient might be aspirating and are reluctant to feed the patient. The patient's wife indicates that she is worried that her husband is not eating and would like to have more information about a feeding tube. The AG-ACNP answer to this patient's wife is based upon which the following correct information:

   a. Percutaneous tube feedings are preferred over oral assisted feedings in patients with advanced dementia.
   b. Percutaneous tube feedings are known to prolong life in patients with advanced dementia.
   c. Percutaneous tube feedings are known to increase comfort in patient with advanced dementia
   d. Percutaneous tube feedings do not prolong life and can lead to increased use of restraints.

9. A 17-year-old male presents immediately after playing a football game, with a complaint of sudden onset of right scrotal pain associated with nausea and vomiting. It is suspected that he is experiencing testicular torsion. The next most appropriate action is:

   a. Immediately consult an urologist.
   b. Perform an ultrasound of the affected scrotum.
   c. Perform a urinary analysis.
   d. Perform radionuclide imaging.

10. A 27-year-old police officer is shot in the abdomen at close range with a .45 caliber revolver. The entrance wound is to the left flank, and the bullet is seen on x-rays to be embedded in the spleen, along with suspicion of a diaphragmatic injury. She is hemodynamically unstable with a heart rate of 145, respiration rate 22, blood pressure 80/45, and the abdomen is moderately tender to palpation. The AG-ACNP understands penetrating intra-abdominal injuries need:

   a. A CT scan of the abdomen
   b. Close clinical observation
   c. Diagnostic peritoneal lavage
   d. Exploratory laparotomy by a surgeon

11. The mechanism of action of epinephrine given for anaphylactic reaction in a patient with penicillin allergy is:

   a. Combined alpha and beta adrenergic effects
   b. Combined alpha and beta anti-adrenergic effects
   c. Beta specific adrenergic effects
   d. Alpha specific anti-adrenergic effects

12. Which term or concept is defined as the internal conflict experienced when the AG-ACNP knows what the most ethical action should be but encounters barriers discouraging him/her from carrying out the action?

   a. Care coordination
   b. Moral distress
   c. Reflective practice
   d. Shared decision making

13. A 50-year-old patient presents with an anterior myocardial infarction. He received thrombolytic therapy and is doing well. On day 3 he suddenly becomes acutely tachycardic, drops his blood pressure to 75/30, has distended neck veins with pulsus paradoxus. Rapid administration of 2 L normal saline increases the blood pressure to 95/50. The most likely diagnosis is:

   a. Cardiac tamponade due to myocardial wall rupture
   b. Cardiac tamponade due to post-myocardial pericarditis
   c. Acute papillary muscle rupture
   d. Acute pulmonary edema due to ventricular failure

14. A 53-year-old male is directly admitted to the hospital from the clinic with symptoms of fatigue, shortness of breath, and dizziness. Per the patient, these symptoms have gotten worse over the past month. On physical exam, the findings are completely normal except for pallor of the mucus membranes, tachycardia with regular rhythm, and mild dyspnea. The next step of the AG-ACNP should take is:

   a. Monitor the patient's symptoms.
   b. Check a CBC.
   c. Start a multivitamin.
   d. Order iron and total iron binding studies.

15. An older adult man presented from home with a complaint of worsening shortness of breath and white sputum production. Chest x-ray was clear and he was admitted with a COPD exacerbation and received oxygen therapy, albuterol nebulizers, and IV steroids. On hospital day 1, the AG-ACNP notes he developed a new fever, worsening leukocytosis, and increased sputum production. The AG-ACNP obtains a repeat chest x-ray that now reveals a new left lower lobe infiltrate. The AG-ACNP diagnoses the patient with:

   a. Aspiration pneumonitis
   b. Hospital acquired pneumonia
   c. Healthcare associated pneumonia
   d. CAP

16. Two types of errors occur when performing hypothesis testing and are referred to as Type I error and Type II error. A Type I error:

   a. Occurs if the null hypothesis is not rejected when it is false
   b. Is referred to as producer's risk
   c. Is due to nonsampling errors
   d. Occurs if the null hypothesis is rejected when it is true

17. Two AG-ACNPs who work in a tertiary ICU are approached by one of the ICU intensivists asking if they would be interested in working for premium pay with the telemedicine ICU service, taking calls for an out-of-state critical access hospital. Which of the following concerns would be of the LEAST importance for the practitioners in considering the offer?

   a. Licensure of their provider status across state lines
   b. Reimbursement differences across state lines
   c. Legal liability pertaining to variation in SOP
   d. Evidence of cost effectiveness in telemedicine applications

18. A 25-year-old 6-day postpartum woman presents with a temperature of 104°F, profuse diaphoresis, agitation, and hyperdefecation. The AG-ACNP suspects thyroid storm. Which agents should be AVOIDED in this patient?

   a. Acetylsalicylic acid
   b. Propanolol
   c. Acetaminophen
   d. Propythiouracil

19. A 63-year-old woman presents complaining of gradual, progressive, nonpainful enlargement of the terminal joint on fourth digit on her left hand over a 8-month period. She reports stiffness first thing in the morning that gradually improves during the day. She also reports her right knee "locks up" and is more painful after walking long distances. Examination reveals Heberden node of her fourth digit on her left hand and right knee crepitus with decreased range of motion. What is the most likely diagnosis?

   a. Osteoarthritis
   b. Gout
   c. Osteomyelitis
   d. RA

20. The AG-ACNP is working in the ED when a 19-year-old woman presents with mild shortness of breath. Her boyfriend is with her reporting she fell down the stairs injuring her ribs. Upon exam the AG-ACNP notes she has multiple ecchymosed areas in multiple stages of healing. The most important step in assessment in caring for this patient is to:

   a. Report the domestic abuse to the police.
   b. Notify child protective services.
   c. Refer her to a home for battered and abused women.
   d. Interview her separately and screen for interpersonal violence.

21. The AG-ACNP is examining a male patient with a medical history of CHF and notices bilaterally lower extremity swelling, erythema, and warmth with nondraining blisters. The patient indicates that he has been running a low-grade fever with intermittent chills. The patient also reports that this is his first episode of these symptoms and he does not have a history of recent hospitalization and lives at home. The patient's vital signs are stable except for a temperature of 100.4°F. Based on this information, the AG-ACNP prescribes which of the following medications in this patient with NKDA:

   a. IV Vancomycin
   b. IV Cefazolin
   c. IV Extended spectrum penicillin
   d. IV Fluoroquinolone

22. Which of the following is a common symptom of GAD?

   a. Anger
   b. Auditory hallucinations
   c. Difficulty falling or staying asleep
   d. Restless leg syndrome

23. The AG-ACNP has just admitted a 34-year-old male trauma patient who has sustained right-sided rib fractures after a motor vehicle crash. The patient is in no acute distress and his vital signs are stable. Upon review of the patient's chest x-ray the AG-ACNP notes a trace right-sided pneumothorax. What is the safest approach to this patient?

   a. Perform an emergent chest tube placement.
   b. Repeat the chest x-ray immediately.
   c. Follow the patient clinically, repeat a chest x-ray in 4 hours.
   d. Place a pigtail catheter.

24. An AG-ACNP working in New Jersey has practiced in the acute care setting for several years and has now moved to South Carolina. What standards will specifically govern his/her practice in the acute care setting in South Carolina?

   a. State laws regarding advanced nursing practice
   b. Institutional guidelines
   c. SOP from nursing organizations
   d. State laws regarding APRN and institutional guidelines

25. The AG-ACNP is caring for a 55-year-old male who is 2 days post-acute myocardial infarction (AMI). He is also known to be HIV-positive taking a protease inhibitor. His lipid profile is: total cholesterol: 242, triglycerides 256, LDL 142, and HDL 30. As part of secondary prevention, the AG-ACNP would initiate which of the following medication:

   a. Pravastatin (Pravachol)
   b. Atorvastatin (Lipitor)
   c. Simvastatin (Zocor)
   d. Lovastatin (Mevacor)

26. When caring for a 27-year-old female who is status post-sexual assault, a pregnancy test was positive. When giving the patient instruction regarding possible complications regarding pregnancy, the AG-ACNP correctly educates the patient when she states your baby:

   a. Is at risk of contracting gonorrhea and chlamydia as it crosses the placenta
   b. Is NOT at risk of contracting syphilis as it crosses the placenta
   c. Is at risk of contracting HIV as it crosses the placenta and can be transmitted at birth
   d. Breast feeding should also be encouraged if you are found to HIV positive

27. An 18-year-old male victim of a motor vehicle accident presents with bilateral femur fractures and a large left hemothorax. A chest tube was inserted with return of 1500 mL frank blood. He is in hemorrhagic shock with heart rate 130 and blood pressure 80/60, and declines a blood transfusion because of his religious beliefs (Jehovah's Witness). After explaining the risks and benefits, he continues to decline a transfusion. The most appropriate intervention is to:

    a. Refrain from transfusion and implement hemostasis measures.
    b. Contact his parents for consent.
    c. Perform autotransfusion of blood from the chest tube.
    d. Obtain an emergency court order to transfuse blood products.

28. Which of the following is consistent with normal age-related changes for an adult over the age of 65?

    a. Severe hearing impairment
    b. Issues with long-term memory
    c. Difficulty seeing in low-light situations
    d. Changes in personality and behavior, including intermittent agitation

29. An 18-year-old unconscious male is brought to the ED on 100% O_2 via a nonrebreather face mask, following a suicide attempt. He was found unresponsive with vomitus on his face and clothing. EMS reported a strong petroleum odor and empty furniture polish bottle next to him on the floor. Initial management should include:

    a. Endotracheal intubation
    b. Gastric lavage
    c. Activated charcoal
    d. Syrup of ipecac

30. A 74-year-old African American man presents after being found down in his home. CT scan reveals an ICH deep in the basal ganglia. The AG-ACNP suspects which of the following etiologies as the most likely cause of his ICH:

    a. Cocaine use
    b. Hypertension
    c. Arteriovenous malformation
    d. Trauma

31. A 48-year-old male with a history of SS anemia type and right humeral head osteonecrosis presents to the hematology clinic with complaints of severe painful erection for the past 6 hours. He admits to taking a friend's prescribed Viagra (sildenafil) 100 mg 8 hours ago. On examination the AG-ACNP notes the patient is in severe distress and the penis is rigid, dark blood obtained upon corporeal aspiration. There is no indication of trauma. These findings are consistent with which of the following:

    a. High-flow priapism and no immediate intervention is required
    b. High-flow priapism and treat pain
    c. Low-flow priapism and no immediate intervention is required
    d. Low-flow priapism and emergent intervention is required

32. A 68-year-old female presents to the ED with 10/10 abdominal pain. The AG-ACNP is concerned for bowel perforation given the patient underwent an outpatient routine colonoscopy earlier in the day. To assess for free air the AG-ACNP orders a chest x-ray. To obtain a quality chest x-ray, what position should the film be completed?

    a. Upright
    b. Supine
    c. Left lateral decubitus
    d. Trendelenburg position

33. A 42-year-old woman comes into the ED at 3 a.m. because she just vomited large amount of bright red blood. When the AG-ACNP approaches her to take a history, she smells of alcohol. She gives a history of all-night binge drinking with several hours of vomiting and retching that brought up clear fluid and now finally vomiting the bloody emesis. This best describes what diagnosis?

    a. Bleeding esophageal varices
    b. Mallory-Weiss tear
    c. Stress ulceration
    d. Esophageal perforation (Boerhaave syndrome)

34. A statistical power of at least _____ is considered relevant to detect a clinical difference in an outcome when a two-sided type I error rate of _____ is used.

    a. 80%, .05
    b. 70%, .05
    c. 80%, .5
    d. 85%, .10

35. Before billing for patient care, an AG-ACNP must:

    a. Establish a collaborative agreement with the physician group practice.
    b. Secure federal and state controlled-substance licenses.
    c. Obtain a national provider number and credentials with the insurance company.
    d. Obtain appropriate continuing education credits and institutional credentialing.

36. A 65-year-old male, on the palliative care service, is receiving treatment for acute exacerbation of CHF and is currently receiving milrinone (Primacor). This is the patient's third admission in 6 months. The patient's wife indicates that she has noticed a change in his mood and that he really has no interest in going out or interacting with the family. The patient continues to have a good appetite and states the he sleeps well. The patient is also conversant but makes little eye contact. The AG-ACNP caring for this patient should:

    a. Inform the wife that you will screen the patient for depression and likely start him on antidepressants.
    b. Inform the wife that this is a normal reaction and as long as he is eating well and not losing weight there is nothing to worry about.
    c. Inform the wife that the patient is likely to be at the end of his life and these symptoms are typical at this time.
    d. Inform the wife that the patient is likely experiencing a side effect from the IV medication that he is receiving for his CHF exacerbation.

37. A 23-year-old patient is admitted to the medicine service for observation after presenting to the ED with shortness of breath. He has a known history of SS anemia. The AG-ACNP is paged due to the development of acute chest pain. The patient rates his chest pain a 10/10. He is on supplemental oxygen 3 L with a SpO_2 of 94%. He is squeezing his chest and writhing in pain. Initial management includes:

    a. Order for transfusion of a unit of packed red blood cells.
    b. Call for STAT cardiology consult.
    c. Obtain an ECG and cardiac biomarkers.
    d. Obtain bedside echocardiogram.

38. A 69-year-old male is brought to the ED with severe pain in his chest that radiates to the back. Pulse is 120 beats/min and regular, blood pressure 180/100 in the right arm and 210/120 in the left arm, and respirations 36/min. The patient is diaphoretic and terrified. The remainder of the exam is notable only for decreased lower extremity pulses including femoral pulses. An anterior–posterior chest radiograph done in the ED shows displacement of intimal aortic calcification. An ECG shows ischemia in the inferior leads; initial troponin is 0.05 ng/mL. The most likely cause of this patient's symptoms is:

   a. Acute inferior wall myocardial infarction
   b. Cardiac tamponade
   c. Dissecting thoracic aortic aneurysm
   d. Cardiogenic shock

39. The ANA's Code of Ethics for Nurses states, *"The nurse promotes, advocates for, and strives to protect the health, safety, and rights of the patient."* The Public Health Code of Ethics states, *"Public health should advocate and work for the empowerment of disenfranchised community members, aiming to ensure that the basic resources and conditions necessary for health are accessible to all."* Which is the best way for the AG-ACNP to extend these two major concepts into the advocacy arenas?

   a. The AG-ACNP elects to take an assertiveness training course to improve her skills to intervene with a particularly difficult work group in her facility, which uses aggressive pain medication policies for most patients.
   b. The AG-ACNP undertakes a literature review on the scope of practice of AG-ACNPs in hospital settings as a first step to alter the credentialing privileges of AG-ACNPs in her facility to allow AG-ACNPs to direct-admit patients under their license.
   c. The AG-ACNP works as a legal consultant on scope of practice issues and quality patient care.
   d. The AG-ACNP joins his/her state and national professional AG-ACNP organization and actively participates in developing a relationship with state and national representatives to be the voice of the community.

40. An elderly woman admitted from a nursing home with septic shock related to a UTI. She had a prolonged ICU course complicated by AKI, non-STEMI and acute respiratory failure with failure to wean. She recovered from the septic shock but required prolonged mechanical ventilation for 14 days. She was about to be discharged to a long-term acute care hospital for continued ventilator weaning when she developed a new fever, tachycardia, and tachypnea. Repeat WBC was 10.5 and lactate was 2.9 mg/dL. Procalcitonin level was elevated. The AG-ACNP treats this patient with the following:

   a. Ceftriaxone (Rocephin) and azithromycin (Z-Pak)
   b. Vancomycin and piperacillin–tazobactam (Zosyn)
   c. Linezolid (Zyvox), ciprofloxacin (Cipro), and gentamycin
   d. Vancomycin, piperacillin–tazobactam (Zosyn), and levofloxacin (Levaquin)

41. A new AG-ACNP will quickly understand that appropriate documentation is the key to ensuring proper reimbursement. ICD codes are an important component of the documentation process. The new revision of these codes (ICD 10) has:

   a. Little impact for documentation in critical care areas
   b. Led to longer and more complex codes for more specific disease identification
   c. Decreased the number of codes
   d. Impacted outpatient codes primarily

42. While caring for an intubated 54-year-old male trauma patient on hospital day 6 who is on high levels of positive pressure ventilation, the AG-ACNP notices the patient's fever curve and leukocytosis are increasing. Additionally she identifies increased bilateral diffuse opacifications on a morning chest x-ray, increased peak/plateau inspiratory pressures, and increasing oxygenation requirements. What is the most likely diagnosis and associated management strategy?

    a. Spontaneous pneumothorax; needle decompression to second intercostal space midclavicular line and placement of a thoracotomy tube

    b. Acute CHF exacerbation; administration of IV diuretic with consult to cardiology and transthoracic echocardiogram

    c. ARDS; adjust mechanical ventilator to low tidal volume protocol and lung protective ventilation measures with a VAP protocol

    d. Bilateral post-obstructive atelectasis; consult to pulmonology for immediate bronchoscopy

43. The AG-ACNP's misunderstandings about a patient's cultural beliefs can cause confusion, misperception of illness, and disrupt the AG-ACNP-patient therapeutic relationship. Which action demonstrates an AG-ACNP's cultural competence?

    a. Ask the patient closed-ended questions and actively listen to the responses.

    b. Individualize care to the patient's cultural influences as much as possible.

    c. Impose one's own beliefs onto the patient while remaining nonjudgmental.

    d. Avoid inquiring about the patient's religious beliefs and practices.

44. A 51-year-old male is brought to the hospital status post-motor vehicle accident. It is suspected that the patient's chest hit the steering wheel. The patient is noted to have an anterior chest wall hematoma and the following blood pressure changes: blood pressure at the end of expiration 135/90 mmHg and at the end of inspiration 110/92 mmHg. Which of the following conditions is most likely?

    a. Aortic insufficiency

    b. Cardiogenic shock

    c. LV failure

    d. Cardiac tamponade

45. The AG-ACNP is discharging 74-year-old with a new diagnosis of hypothyroid and treatment with levothyroxine (Synthroid). As part of the patient teaching, the AG-ACNP instructs the patient to call the AG-ACNP if:

    a. Her heart rate is above 100.

    b. Her heart rate is below 70.

    c. Her blood pressure is less than 100/70.

    d. She experiences cold intolerance.

46. A 27-year-old man presents with complaint left shoulder pain. He was playing football 3 days ago and was tackled, landing on his left shoulder. Physical examination reveals a positive "empty can" and Neer sign test. The AG-ACNP diagnoses him with:

    a. Rotator cuff tear

    b. Acute bursitis

    c. Adhesive capsulitis

    d. Dislocation

47. Which of the following acts provides federal privilege and confidentiality protections for patient safety information, called the patient safety work product, to encourage reporting and analysis of medical errors?

    a. HIPPA

    b. PSQIA

    c. COBRA

    d. Patient Self-Determination Act

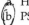

48. In patients with severe COPD, a chest x-ray will often demonstrate which of the following changes?

    a. An increase in vascular markings
    b. Flattening of the diaphragm
    c. Hypoinflation
    d. Hypolucency

49. A 54-year old male diabetic patient is admitted to the medical unit secondary to left lower extremity cellulitis with an infected ulcer. The patient was working in his garage and sustained a small scratch to his left leg. The scratch quickly increased in size with noted redness and swelling to the left lower extremity. The wound was cleansed in the ED, the patient was started on IV clindamycin and ceftriaxone and admitted to the medical unit. On day 2 of admission the AG-ACNP notes the patient to be febrile, with an increasing WBC count. The patient verbalizes worsening pain with a tingling sensation to the lower extremity without relief from oral Vicodin. Upon exam, the left lower extremity increased from prior demarcation with persistent erythema and palpable crepitus to the lateral aspect of the leg. Based on this information the most important intervention at this time would be to:

    a. Increase pain medication to intravenous Dilaudid.
    b. Change to penicillin G 4 million units IV Q 4H and clindamycin 900 mg IV Q 8H.
    c. Add IV vancomycin 20 mg/kg IV BID to antibiotic regimen STAT, goal trough 15 to 20.
    d. Order a STAT x-ray of the patient's left leg.

50. Not all states have autonomous practice yet for AG-ACNPs, thus SBON or state boards of medicine have criteria specifying the level of collaboration between the AG-ACNP and a supervising physician. With this in mind, which of the following should the AG-ACNP seek when selecting an employment setting?

    a. Standard hourly rate as provider staff
    b. Specifics of the agency's AG-ACNP practice guidelines
    c. Expectation for net revenue generation
    d. Standard benefit package offered to staff

51. In caring for patients with chronic illnesses it is important for the AG-ACNP to integrate palliative care into the overall management of patients as appropriate in order to:

    a. Assist patients toward understanding their illness trajectory.
    b. Provide seamless care coordination into hospice.
    c. Prepare the family for the dying process and death.
    d. Aid patients and families to comprehend the illness trajectory and dying process.

52. Which of the following factors is associated with increased risk of hospital associated delirium?

    a. Polypharmacy
    b. Short hospital stay
    c. Young age
    d. Normal albumin level

53. Which AG-ACNP professional competency and term is defined as the purposeful and collaborative interpersonal process aimed to support and facilitate the patient and family through health-related experiences to facilitate achieving health-related mutually determined goals?

    a. Quality
    b. Leadership
    c. Policy
    d. Coaching

54. The AG-ACNP is asked to evaluate a 51-year-old female who is scheduled for an elective knee replacement. Her past medical history is significant for hypertension, DM, and a myocardial infarction 4 months ago. The next appropriate step would be to:

    a. Schedule an ECG and echocardiogram.
    b. Order a cardiology consult.
    c. Postpone surgery for 2 months.
    d. Proceed with the evaluation.

55. A 68-year-old Spanish-speaking Hispanic male with a history of hypertension is brought to the ED by his family for evaluation of difficulty speaking and left arm weakness that has persisted for several hours. The AG-ACNP concerned that the patient may be experiencing an ischemic stroke. The AG-ACNP has difficulty obtaining accurate and detailed history and timing of the development of symptoms. Which factor most likely contributed to the delay in care?

    a. High health literacy
    b. Not having an interpreter available
    c. Hispanics tend to have a lower awareness of strokes than the general population
    d. Hispanics are more likely to use EMS

56. A female patient is admitted to the hospital after falling ill after travel from a foreign country. She is diagnosed with a highly contagious infection that can be fatal. The decision to place her in strict isolation and limit the number of healthcare providers who encounter her would most closely demonstrate which ethical principle?

    a. Nonmaleficence
    b. Beneficence
    c. Utilitarianism
    d. Autonomy

57. A 76-year-old female with a past medical history of Lewy body dementia is being treated on a medical unit for sepsis due to a UTI. The patient's baseline is confusion with hallucinations. The nurse caring for the patient informs the AG-ACNP that the patient is agitated and thrashing about in bed. The sitter is concerned the patient may harm herself. On exam the AG-ACNP notes a well-developed, well-nourished female who is thrashing about in bed and calling out to persons that are not present. The patient's vital signs are stable, and a resting tremor is noted. Which of the following interventions would be the most appropriate for this patient?

    a. Prescribe lorazepam (Ativan)
    b. Prescribe quetiapine (Seroquel)
    c. Apply loose restraints to prevent self-harm
    d. Verbal comfort with frequent reorientation

58. Formulating a clinical research question is the first step associated with EBP. Clinical research questions are asked in PICOT format. Which element represents the usual standard of care:

    a. Population (P)
    b. Intervention (I)
    c. Comparison (C)
    d. Outcome (O)

59. A 24-year-old female presents with complaints of shortness of breath, chest tightness, wheezing, and nonproductive cough 3 to 4 times a week for the past month. This resolves within 30 minutes with the use of her albuterol inhaler and rest. She has a past medical history of asthma that has been well controlled with an albuterol metered dose inhaler. She states that she thought that it would improve, but has failed to do so. She denies fever, chills, chest pain, dizziness, syncope, or hemoptysis. A chest x-ray is negative for any acute processes. What would be the next step in management?

    a. Add an ICS
    b. Add an ICS and a LABA
    c. Add a LABA and a systemic corticosteroid
    d. Add an ICS and a systemic corticosteroid

60. Immunizations are examples of which type of prevention?

    a. Primary prevention
    b. Secondary prevention
    c. Tertiary prevention
    d. Rehabilitation prevention

61. An AG-ACNP is seeing a new patient with a new diagnosis of MS. The patient reports she had had three episodes each lasting a few days over the past 2 months, but has fully recovered in between. Her episodes consist of fatigue accompanied by diplopia, visual blurring, leg weakness with intermittent spasm, and ataxia. AG-ACNP recognized this description of MS is:

    a. Primary progressive
    b. Progressive relapsing
    c. Relapsing/remitting
    d. Secondary progressive

62. Outpatient CPT codes are used by AG-ACNPs who see patients in an office or clinic setting. Which of these codes are codes for inpatient use only?

    a. 99201-99205
    b. 99211-99215
    c. 99241-99245
    d. 99291-99292

63. A 22-year-old college student presents to the ED's fast track to be seen and evaluated for complaints of painful urination and right testicular pain. The social history reveals he has unprotected MSM and has been sexually active since age 15. During examination the AG-ACNP notes a watery to mucus penile discharge. The first-catch urinary specimen indicates a positive NAAT. He has NKDA. Which of the following would be the most appropriate treatment regimen?

    a. Doxycycline 100 milligrams (mgs) by mouth every 12 hours for 14 days AND high-risk sexual counseling
    b. Azithromycin 1 gram (g) oral single dose AND high-risk sexual counseling
    c. Levofloxacin 500 milligram (mg) by mouth daily for 14 days
    d. Augmentin 500 mg by mouth every 8 hours for 14 days

64. A 40-year-old female with previous medical history of morbid obesity, DMII, and hyperlipidemia (HLD) presents with a 4-day history of right upper quadrant, dull, colicky pain that is worse after eating that radiates to the shoulder with associated nausea, emesis, fever, anorexia, and fatigue. Her labs are notable for a leukocytosis and a mild aspartate aminotranferase (AST)/alanine transaminase (ALT) elevation. Upon exam, she has a positive Murphy's sign with point tenderness to her right upper quadrant, which is also present on ultrasound imaging of the gallbladder. Based on this clinical picture, the AG-ACNP is concerned that she has:

    a. Acute appendicitis
    b. Acute cholecystitis
    c. Gallstone pancreatitis
    d. Diverticulitis

65. An AG-ACNP is caring for an admitted patient. To prevent complications during hospitalization, the AG-ACNP prescribes stress ulcer prophylaxis for which of the following indications:

    a. Hypercoagulable state
    b. Mechanical ventilation less than 48 hours
    c. High-dose steroid use
    d. Admission to ICU

66. What is the current recommendation for a healthy 68-year-old female who has not received the pneumococcal vaccine?

    a. PPSV23 only
    b. PCV13 only
    c. PPSV23 first and 8 weeks later PCV13
    d. PCV13 first then 1 year later PPSV23

67. A 55-year-old female was admitted to the medicine service for numbness of the extremities and difficulty maintaining balance. Her past medical history is significant for vitamin B_{12} deficiency. Upon further discussion with the patient, the AG-ACNP discovers the patient has not been on any of her medications for the past month. Laboratory studies are obtained and the patient's vitamin B_{12} level was found to be 150 pg/mL. The management plan of this patient would include:

    a. Vitamin B_{12} 1 mg subcutaneous for the first week, then monthly maintenance therapy
    b. Vitamin B_{12} 10,000 nanograms orally daily
    c. Taking a multivitamin daily
    d. Education to the patient regarding the importance of dietary intake of B_{12}

68. A 19-year-old male presents with a complaint of sudden hearing loss. After taking a thorough history with no specific abnormalities, the AG-ACNP evaluates his inner ear canal, which yields no specific findings. The next step in evaluating this patient involves the use of a tuning fork. When questioned by the patient to the intent of the tuning fork, the AG-ACNPs response should be: The tuning fork allows for:

    a. Evaluation of any fractures in your skull; if you sense pain then you likely have a fracture that could be the source of your pain
    b. Evaluation of vibration and hearing loss; it allows for evaluation of sensorineural or conductive hearing loss
    c. Evaluation of pitch discrimination and vocal variability; if you can hear the tuning fork then there is loss of pitch discrimination
    d. Evaluation of CSF leakage, if there is otorrhea or rhinorrhea after the placement of the tuning fork then the fluid loss could be attributing to conduction loss

69. When the AG-ACNP is being credentialed by the hospital, what governs the flexibility of the AG-ACNP practice?

    a. Laws created by statutes from federal legislative action bills
    b. Regulations written by the board of nursing for the state of employment
    c. Specific hospital job description and privileges requested
    d. National certification and educational preparation of the AG-ACNP

70. A 62-year-old male patient is admitted following an anterior wall STEMI and subsequent placement of a drug-eluting stent. Several hours after his coronary intervention, the nurse reports
bradycardia with a heart rate of 30 beats/ min. The patient is alert but diaphoretic, blood
pressure is 82/48 with complaints of dizziness and nausea. Which intervention should the
AG-ACNP do first?

    a. Start a dopamine drip at 5 mcg/kg/min
    b. Crash cart to bedside to begin transcutaneous pacing
    c. Alert the catheterization team of his need to return for in-stent restenosis
    d. Order glucagon for reversal of severe beta blockade

71. A 30-year-old woman presents with a carbuncle on her back. She reports it happened a day
after being at the gym, when she was lifting weights on the bench. She saw her PCP who treated
it with 7 days of (cephalexin) Keflex, but did not note any improvement. On exam, it is a 2 inch
area of firm, erythematous carbuncle that is warm to touch and is fluctuant. The AG-ACNP
next step is:

    a. Incision and drainage
    b. Perform a biopsy
    c. Decolonize the skin
    d. Obtain qSOFA score

72. The AG-ACNP is interviewing for a position with a pulmonology group and will be making
rounds in the hospital on all new inpatient consults. It is the physician's plan to bill for the AG-
ACNP's services as "incident to" so that services provided by the AG-ACNP are reimbursed at
100% of the physician's rate. The AG-ACNP's best response is:

    a. The physician must be physically present in the hospital when the AG-ANCP renders the
service to bill "incident to."
    b. "Incident to" billing cannot be used to bill for inpatient services under any circumstances.
    c. "Incident to" billing cannot be used for new consults, only for care of existing hospitalized
patients.
    d. The physician must be immediately available by electronic means when the AG-ACNP
renders the service to bill "incident to."

73. A patient takes his blood sugar at 3 a.m. and it is noted to be 50 mg/dL despite his am blood
sugars having been high over the past week. The treatment for this would be:

    a. Reduce the bedtime insulin
    b. Increase the bedtime insulin
    c. Add a long-acting agent at night
    d. Decrease the carbohydrates at night

74. A 23-year-old male presents to the ED appearing fearful, is disoriented to self and place, and
with rapid, incoherent verbose speech. He is accompanied by a college friend who reports the
patient has not slept for the past 2 days and is being unusually afraid of people and places. The
friend reported the patient also began acting erratically toward him regarding the use of his
textbook and notes from a shared class. For instance, the patient accused the friend of stealing
notes from his binder and conspiring with the teacher to make sure he failed. The patient has
not shown aggression. These behaviors began about 4 days ago and have increasingly gotten
worse. The patient has no recent history of substance abuse or personal history of psychiatric
illness. What crisis management technique is most appropriate for the AG-ACNP to initiate
next for this patient?

    a. Advise the patient for the need to seek psychiatric evaluation.
    b. Explain everything that will be done with calm but firm direction.
    c. Order quetiapine (Seroquel) 50 mg by mouth once now.
    d. Order STAT lab collection of a toxicology screen, chemistry, and hematology panel.

75. The AG-ACNP is rounding on an 84-year-old woman admitted to the hospital for dehydration. The AG-ACNP finds the patient sitting in a chair near the bed, alert and oriented to person, place, and time. Which of the following instruments would provide the AG-ACNP with the most information about her fall risk in the hospital?

    a. St. Thomas risk assessment tool (STRATIFY)
    b. The Timed Up and Go Test (TUG) of 15 seconds
    c. A score of 4 on the SPICES instrument
    d. A score of 6 on KATZ Index of Independence in ADL

76. A 72-year-old female patient with dementia presents following a fall and is unable to verbalize if she hurts anywhere. On assessment she has a right shortened externally rotated leg. The AG-ACNP suspects the patient has a/an:

    a. Hip fracture
    b. Pelvis fracture
    c. Patella dislocation
    d. Ankle sprain

77. A 58-year-old obese female is admitted to the medical unit with acute exacerbation of CHF. Upon completing the assessment the AG-ACNP notes bilateral lower extremity edema with scaling and pruritus especially concentrated over the medial aspect of the ankles. The lower extremities are also noted to be erythematous with increased pigmentation and no warmth. The patient is afebrile and vital signs are stable. Based upon this assessment, the best treatment recommendation is:

    a. Anti-embolism hose
    b. IV vancomycin
    c. Compression stockings with a gradient of 30 to 40 mmHg
    d. Oral glucocorticoids

78. To most important step in EBP is for the AG-ACNP to:

    a. Search the best databases and collect the best evidence.
    b. Critically appraise the evidence.
    c. Formulate a clinical research question.
    d. Integrate the best evidence with one's clinical expertise and patient preferences.

79. A 70-year-old female is brought in to the ED after being found wandering out into traffic. She has no shoes on but appears unharmed. She states her name but cannot tell you what happened. Her daughter states that her mother has been increasingly forgetful over the past year and recently requires help to pay her bills. Her mother usually walks to the senior center by herself three times per week which is four doors down the street from her home. Her wandering behavior is new. She is able to continue to play the piano at the senior center. What is the most likely diagnosis for this patient?

    a. Normal age-related changes
    b. Vascular dementia
    c. Alzheimer's dementia
    d. Delirium

80. A 27-year-old female presents to the ED with dysuria, green vaginal discharge, and pain during sexual intercourse. This is the patient's third ED visit in the past year for similar complaints and she was not able to make follow-up women's health appointments. The patient is diagnosed with pelvic inflammatory disease and simple cystitis secondary to suspected gonorrheal and chlamydial sexually transmitted infection. What is the AG-ACNP's next best action?

    a. Assess the patient's level of health literacy and barriers for self-care.
    b. Provide the patient with written educational material about her diseases appropriate to her reading level.
    c. Order a pregnancy test and pelvic ultrasound, and prescribe empiric antimicrobial therapy.
    d. Consult case management to make a follow-up women's health appointment for the patient.

81. A 92-year-old patient is being cared for on the medical unit for aspiration pneumonia. In addition to the patient's multiple comorbidities and age, the AG-ACNP understands which of the following risk factors contribute to adverse drug occurrences in older adults:

    a. Six or more doses of medications per day
    b. BMI 22
    c. Creatinine clearance 45 mL/min
    d. Male gender

82. A 70-year-old Cambodian female is brought in by her family for evaluation of fever, cough, and chest discomfort due to frequent coughing over the past 4 days. When the AG-ACNP auscultates to her chest, he/she notices red inflamed circles in a symmetrical pattern across her upper back. Which is the most appropriate question for the AG-ACNP to ask:

    a. Have you been burned by someone in your family?
    b. Tell me about these reddened areas on your back?
    c. How long have you had this rash on your back?
    d. When did you fall down and injure yourself?

83. When assessing for obstructive sleep apnea-hypopnea syndrome using the Mallampati Airway Classification, one would visualize the following in a patient with a class III:

    a. Hard palate
    b. Hard palate, soft palate, base of uvula
    c. Hard palate, soft palate, uvula, tonsillar pillars
    d. Hard palate, soft palate, uvula

84. A 78-year-old female patient with a past medical history of COPD presents with shortness of breath. Her chest x-ray reveals a small pneumothorax. This generally can be treated with inpatient observation without a chest tube unless the patient:

    a. Coughs
    b. Requires intubation
    c. Develops pneumonia
    d. Has a positive tuberculosis history

85. A 64-year-old male with a history of chronic heart failure with reduced ejection fraction presents to clinic for a reassessment after having been in clinic 1 week prior with increasing diuretic requirements. Despite careful fluid and sodium restriction and escalating doses of furosemide (Lasix) and metolazone (Zaroxolyn), the patient is found to have marked JVD, diffuse bilateral crackles, andpink, frothy sputum; he remains dyspneic. The AG-ACNP's initial action is to

   a. Increase the furosemide dose to 200 mg orally twice per day
   b. Obtain sputum specimen and order culture and sensitivity testing
   c. Arrange for inpatient admission
   d. Order chest CT scan to rule out pulmonary thromboembolus

86. A 55-year-old woman presents with headaches. Review of systems was positive for fever, fatigue, and muscle aches that started with stiffness, pain in her neck, and through her shoulders, low back, and hips. Workup reveals an elevated ESR and CRP. The most likely diagnosis is:

   a. Meningitis
   b. Temporal arteritis
   c. Migraine
   d. Brain tumor

87. A 61-year-old female with a history of CAD with complaints of epigastric discomfort is suspected to have an abdominal aortic aneurysm. Her blood pressure is stable at 128/76. Which diagnostic study should the AG-ACNP order for initial screening for abdominal aortic aneurysm?

   a. Abdominal ultrasound
   b. Abdominal (kidneys-ureter-bladder) x-ray
   c. Contrasted abdominal CT
   d. Endovascular ultrasound

88. A patient underwent a CT angiogram for evaluation of a possible pulmonary embolus. The patient is being evaluated for contrast-induced AKI. Contrast-induced AKI is considered if which of the following occurs:

   a. The serum creatinine rises by 1.5 fold or greater from the baseline value.
   b. The urine output is less than 600 milliliters over a 12-hour period.
   c. The BUN level remains unchanged.
   d. The serum creatinine rises by greater than or equal to 5 millimoles per L within 48 hours

89. The AG-ACNP has been asked by a drug company to make a presentation about its new drug. The company agrees to pay an honorarium but tells the AG-ACNP he/she can only speak about their drug's research study showing greatly improved response rates over other products. What ethical principle is in conflict this situation?

   a. Fidelity
   b. Veracity
   c. Autonomy
   d. Justice

90. An AG-ACNP is working for a cardiology consult service in a community hospital. He/she usually covers the service with one cardiologist who will see patients as well as perform interventional procedures in the cardiac catheterization lab. The group has decided that the AG-ACNP patient visits will be "shared" so that there can be 100% reimbursement. Which of the following components is correct to meet the criteria of a shared visit?

a. The physician and AG-ACNP do not have to be part of the same service
b. AG-ACNP practices within his/her SOP
c. Face-to-face MD encounter is optional
d. Proper MD note separate from the AG-ACNP note

91. A 57-year-old female is seen in urgent care for respiratory distress. She has a history of RA and GERD, is a moderate social drinker, and she also has a 20-pack-year smoking history. She is post-menopausal and has a surgical history of total hip replacement 4 years ago. Her review of systems is negative except for generalized joint stiffness, right knee pain, and heartburn and belching. She is on Ultram for management of her RA, and omeprazole for her GERD. Her exam is positive for substernal chest pain and wheezing, but no clinical exam findings for pneumonia. An aerosol bronchodilator treatment relieves the bronchospasms and her chest x-ray is normal. The AG-ACNP feels a GI medicine referral is appropriate. Which of the following should the AG-ACNP order to help make an accurate diagnosis of complications of GERD?

a. CT scan chest and abdomen
b. 24-hour pH esophageal and pharyngeal pH monitoring
c. EGD and colonoscopy
d. Nissen fundoplication

92. A 45-year-old male is admitted to the medicine service for fatigue, fever, chills, and weight loss. He has a known history of AIDS. He has been off all of his medications for the past 6 months. His CD4+ count is less than 50/cells/μL. The AG-ACNP should:

a. Immediately start previous regimen of ART.
b. Treat current infection and delay ART until improved.
c. Start a new regimen of ART.
d. Start broad-spectrum antibiotics and begin ART when afebrile.

93. A young adult male involved in a motorcycle crash presents with flail chest. Chest x-ray demonstrates dense opacity in the right lung field with loss of the hemidiaphragm. Breath sounds are significantly diminished. CT demonstrates presence of a hemothorax. A thoracostomy tube is inserted. The AG-ACNP should prepare the patient for surgical intervention when the chest tube output reaches:

a. .5 L (500 mL)
b. 1.0 L (1000 mL)
c. 1.5 L (1500mL)
d. 2.0 L (2000 mL)

94. A 70-year-old male patient presents with occasional cramping pain in his right calf with exercise. After undergoing ABI testing, the patient has recently been confirmed to have peripheral arterial disease. Which intervention is the most appropriate in the initial management of this patient?

a. CT angiogram for endovascular stent
b. Smoking cessation
c. Referral for consideration of bypass surgery
d. Institute warfarin therapy for anticoagulation

95. The AG-ACNP is evaluating a 46-year-old female who presents to the ED with fever, chills, malaise, shortness of breath and increased sputum production for 2 days prior to presentation. What test is the most cost effective diagnostic test to confirm a diagnosis?

a. Chest radiograph
b. Chest CT scan without IV contrast
c. Flu swab and RVP
d. Chest CT with intravenous contrast

96. The AG-ACNP is seeing a patient with a history of HIV who is admitted for treatment of pneumonia. His CD4 count upon admission is less than 50 cells/µL. He sees a story on the news about a measles outbreak in the state. He inquired about receiving the MMR vaccine to protect himself. The AG-ACNP's best response is:

   a. "The MMR is a live vaccine and with your low CD4 count, you may become infected."
   b. "Yes, we can give you the MMR at the time of discharge."
   c. "We can consider the MMR once your pneumonia is resolved."
   d. "The MMR is contraindicated for you because your CD4 count is so high."

97. A 40-year-old patient presents to the ED reporting an unintentional pregnancy and need for confirmatory tests before she has an abortion. Without informing the patient, the AG-ACNP has emotionally charged personal beliefs that abortion goes against his/her religious practices and values. What approach can the AG-ACNP take to maintain a therapeutic relationship with the patient?

   a. Identify if the patient is married and notify her spouse of the issue.
   b. Explore the patient's social support system to help with decision making.
   c. Elicit behavior coaching techniques to assess the patient's readiness to change her mind.
   d. Acknowledge personal distress and determine if another provider should assume care.

98. The AG-ACNP may bill "incident to" in a cardiology practice, in which of the following situations?

   a. Rounding on newly admitted patients in the coronary care unit on the same day as the physician
   b. In the cardiac care unit as long as the AG-ACNP is directly supervised by the physician
   c. The physician must perform the initial plan of care, subsequent follow-up frequency that reflects his/her active participation in the clinic
   d. When writing the follow-up management plan when rounding with the physician in the hospital setting

99. Using the Parkland formula, what is the first 24-hour fluid resuscitation amount for a 45% TBSA burn in a 70-kg patient?

   a. 12,600
   b. 13,500
   c. 14,380
   d. 17,800

100. An elderly client presents to the ED with 1-week history of dyspnea. Assessment reveals cool, clammy skin; weak peripheral pulses; and increased work of breathing. The client is hypotensive with blood pressure 88/60 and disoriented. The client is urgently transported to the ICU and a pulmonary artery catheter is placed. Hemodynamics reveals PCWP of 28 mmHg and CI 1.6 L/min/m². Which of the following diagnoses is most likely for this client?

   a. Septic shock
   b. Cardiogenic shock
   c. Hypovolemic shock
   d. Neurogenic shock

101. A 20-year-old college student presents with a chief complaint of a fever and sore throat. The patient reports these symptoms began yesterday. She reports her intake has been reduced due to painful swallowing. She denies cough, rash, shortness of breath. Vital signs: temperature 102°F, heart rate 100, respiration rate 20, blood pressure 116/68. The AG-ANCP's exam reveals cervical lymphadenopathy and erythematous pharynx with white exudate. The AG-ACNPs next step is to:

    a. Obtain rapid antigen detection test

    b. Prescribe amoxicillin 500 mg PO daily

    c. Obtain throat culture

    d. Prescribe metronidazole (Flagyl) 500 mg TID

102. When practicing evidence-based nursing, which of the following strategies is expected of AG-ACNPs?

    a. Replicating previous research studies

    b. Reading and understanding published research reports

    c. Preparing an integrative literature review

    d. Devoting a specific amount of time working with a researcher

103. An 82-year-old woman is admitted after a fall. The AG-ACNPs workup reveals she had a syncopal episode, secondary to anemia. Her admitting chest x-ray shows a large left upper lobe lung mass. She tells the AG-ACNP that she knows she has lung cancer and has declined treatment. She also does not want her family to know of this diagnosis. The AG-ACNP maintains her confidence while supporting the family. This is an example of:

    a. Informed consent

    b. Fidelity

    c. Beneficence

    d. Nonmaleficence

104. An 18-year-old patient is admitted to the ICU with a TBI and Glasgow Coma Score of 5T ("T" for intubated). What can the AG-ACNP do to facilitate communication and a therapeutic relationship with the patient?

    a. Order continuous sedation and analgesic infusions to ensure comfort and facilitate rest.

    b. Ask visiting family members to speak on the patient's behalf and communicate to the patient on the AG-ACNP's behalf.

    c. Pay attention to nonverbal expressions of the patient and communicate explanations of care and reassurance to the patient.

    d. Allow 24-hour visitation by at least one family member to provide the patient with social support.

105. A 41-year-old male client has a 5-year history of hypertension. He is admitted to the hospital with complaints of exertional dyspnea, requiring three pillows for sleep, and episodes of breathlessness that nightly wakes him. His blood pressure on admission was 180/106, pulse rate 104, respiration rate 30. He has JVD to the angle of his jaw, and 1+ lower extremity edema bilaterally. A transthoracic echocardiogram was performed and reveals normal systolic function, but the transmitral Doppler flow pattern demonstrates grade 2 diastolic dysfunction with increased septal and posterior wall dimensions. Which diagnosis is the most likely etiology for the client's condition?

    a. Coronary atherosclerosis

    b. Renal artery stenosis

    c. Aortic dissection

    d. Hypertensive cardiovascular disease

106. A patient has a history of "incidental" discovered thyroid nodules, with no symptom. The patient asks how often an ultrasound needs to be performed.

    a. 3 to 6 months

    b. Yearly

    c. Every 5 years

    d. Every 10 years

107. A 25-year-old basketball player presents with complaint of "ankle sprain." The right ankle is swollen, tender, and unable to bear weight. The X-ray of the ankle is negative for fracture. The AG-ACNP suspects high ankle (syndesmotic) sprain. What test should be performed to confirm the diagnosis?

   a. Squeeze test
   b. Talar tilt test
   c. Anterior drawer test
   d. Hawkin's test

108. A 20-year-old college student presents with complaints of pelvic pain after unprotected sex over the weekend. The AG-ACNP takes a full sexual history, including inquiries about number and gender of sexual partners, along with the following:

   a. Practices, past history of sexually transmitted diseasesTDs, protection for STDs, pregnancy plans
   b. Practices, past history of STDs, penile discharge of partners
   c. Pregnancy plans, protection for STDS, history of placenta previa
   d. Past history of STDs, history of placental abruption

109. A restrained driver who was T-boned on the driver's side presents with severe abdominal pain. The AG-ACNP should expect which of the following injuries:

   a. Large intestines
   b. Liver
   c. Spleen
   d. Small intestines

110. The AG-ACNP is seeing an ischemic stroke patient in clinic post discharge from the hospital. His wife is concerned about his behavior change. She explains his behavior is inappropriate because he burst into tears often, even at happy times. Sometimes he laughs when she is trying to discuss serious financial and family matters. He is cognitively intact and denies anhedonia or blue mood when questioned. He is physically unable to participate in the things he enjoyed before the stroke and unable to go back to work due to left-sided hemiparalysis. What is the most appropriate teaching to give to the patient and his family?

   a. The confusing outbursts are common in patients after they have a stroke, and it is known as PBA.
   b. Many times patients have posttraumatic stress disorder after a major event like a stroke, and this will be a new reality for them to deal with.
   c. Emotional outbursts are part of the post-stroke depression and can be treated with psychotherapy.
   d. Anxiety is common after a stroke and this behavior should resolve in 8 to 12 weeks

111. A 52-year-old female patient was involved in a motor vehicle collision and sustained blunt trauma to her chest. She was unresponsive and intubated at the scene. Upon presentation in the ED, the patient is coughing, and pink frothy secretions are noted in the endotracheal tube. Her blood pressure is 60/30, heart rate 134. She has markedly elevated JVD. An echocardiogram revealed a flail mitral valve and torrential regurgitation, consistent with mitral valve rupture. Which intervention is most important in this client's plan of care?

   a. Urgent left heart catheterization
   b. Immediate cardiac surgery for repair
   c. STAT intravenous diuretic dose
   d. Initiation of intravenous inotrope therapy

112. The AG-ACNP is seeing a 71-year-old-male in medical ICU with an acute exacerbation of chronic bronchitis. The AG-ACNP knows that the pulmonary function assessment of chronic bronchitis is the same as that of emphysema. Which one of the following clinical findings is associated with chronic bronchitis, but not emphysema:

a. Hypochloremia
b. Increased AP diameter
c. Polycythemia
d. Respiratory acidosis

113. A patient presents with new onset ST segment elevation and T wave inversion in leads II, III, and aVF. The most appropriate diagnosis is

a. Anterior myocardial infarction
b. Inferior myocardial infarction
c. Lateral myocardial infarction
d. Septal myocardial infarction

114. A 70-year-old African American male with history of diabetes and hypertension is admitted for CAP. On hospital day 2, the bedside nurse calls the AG-ACNP stating that the patient has a right facial droop and aphasia. His blood pressure is 165/85 and he is awake, alert, and oriented to person, place, and time. He is able to ambulate. What is the AG-ACNP's next step?

a. Call a rapid-response code.
b. Order STAT noncontrast head CT, ECG, tPA.
c. Evaluate the patient; identify when the patient was last seen normal.
d. Order a STAT basic metabolic panel.

115. The AG-ACNP has successfully extubated a 55-year-old male who had been on mechanical ventilation due to respiratory failure. The patient is now experiencing postextubation stridor due to upper airway edema. Which of the following treatments should the AG-ACNP order?

a. Oxygen at 100%
b. Aerosolized racemic epinephrine
c. Reintubation
d. Tracheostomy

116. A 58-year-old patient is considering peritoneal dialysis for the management of his end-stage renal disease. Which of the following places the patient at an increased risk for peritonitis?

a. Depression
b. Chronic back pain
c. Diverticulitis
d. CHF

117. Value-based purchasing is a CMS initiative that emphasizes "quality versus quantity" in patient care. The MACRA of 2015 is the legislation that is directing the value-based purchasing initiative. Which of the following is included the MACRA:

a. HIPAA
b. RBRVS
c. Fee-for-service payment program
d. Quality Payment Program

118. The AG-ACNP's SOP is:

   a. Governed by the ANA
   b. Governed by the nurse practice act
   c. The same from state to state
   d. Rarely based on state and national standards

119. A 56-year-old male patient is post op day 2 from a CABG × 3. The AG-ACNP is called with the following data: temperature 39.2°C (102.5°F), WBC15,000, respiration 25, blood pressure 97/54, decline in mental status. The AG-ACNP initially treats with normal saline 30 cc/kg. After initial fluid resuscitation measures, MAP remains less than 60 mmHg and blood pressure remains84/54. The patient currently meets the criteria for:

   a. Cardiogenic shock
   b. SIRS
   c. Sepsis
   d. Septic shock

120. An 85-year-old patient returns from the cath lab following a TAVR procedure and is currently in atrial fibrillation with a ventricular rate of 110 and blood pressure 130/78. The patient has right-sided hemiplegia and global aphasia. Of the following, which differential diagnosis is likely:

   a. Hemorrhagic stroke involving the basal ganglia
   b. Subarachnoid hemorrhage
   c. Embolic event to the right middle cerebral artery
   d. Embolic event to the left middle cerebral artery

121. AA is the most common abdominal emergency. Diagnosing AA is often hampered by diagnostic uncertainty and the need for risk stratification. Which of the following diagnostic studies is the most helpful in diagnosing AA?

   a. Low-grade fever, nausea, and vomiting
   b. Abdominal ultrasound
   c. CT imaging of the abdomen
   d. KUB x-ray

122. A 54-year-old male patient, currently receiving chemotherapy for squamous cell carcinoma of the lung, is being treated for post obstructive pneumonia. During rounds, the patient indicates to the AG-ACNP that he is quite constipated and has not had a bowel movement in 5 days. Additionally, the patient also reports a poor appetite. In addition to the pain medication that the patient is receiving, the AG-ACNP suspects which of the following factors contribute to constipation:

   a. Hyperuricemia
   b. Hyperkalemia
   c. Hypercalcemia
   d. Hypermagnesemia

123. Mobitz type I or Wenckebach is characterized by:

   a. A prolongation of PR interval (PRI) from beat to beat until a P wave is not conducted
   b. Random dropped beat with no change in the QT interval
   c. Prolongation of the QT interval
   d. PRI less than 0.12 seconds followed by a dropped beat

124. The AG-ACNP is evaluating a 58-year-old male who presents to the ED with complaints of right lower quadrant pain that initially started in the periumbilical region. The AG-ACNP suspects acute appendicitis but needs an additional evidence-based test to order to confirm the suspicion. What is the best test to order?

    a. Radiograph of the abdomen (KUB)
    b. Focused assessment with sonography for trauma
    c. Abdominal ultrasound with vascular duplex
    d. CT scan of the abdomen with IV contrast

125. A young adult presents to the ED with a 2-day history of sore throat, now complaining of shortness of breath. The AG-ACNP observes he is sitting on the stretcher, leaning forward, is drooling and appreciates audible stridor. The highest priority is:

    a. Obtain a lateral x-ray of the neck
    b. Perform direct visualization of the larynx
    c. Secure the airway with expert consultation
    d. Obtain CBC with differential and blood cultures

126. The AG-ACNP's patient is seen for follow-up evaluation. Four months ago, laboratory studies showed a TSH concentration of 8.0 mU/L; free T_4 was within the normal reference range. Current laboratory evaluation shows TSH concentration remains elevated; free T_4 is within the reference ranges. The presence of which of the following in this patient is most likely to warrant treatment for subclinical hypothyroidism:

    a. Age older than 65 years
    b. TSH concentration of 11 mU/L
    c. Undetectable TPO antibodies
    d. Weight loss of 10 lbs

127. An 83-year-old female is found unresponsive in her home, which had minimal heat. She is known to have heart failure with preserved ejection fraction (EF) of 40%, chronic kidney disease, stage 3, and mild dementia. She is intubated and transported to the hospital. On arrival, she is unresponsive, with a rectal temperature of 30°C (86°F), blood pressure 88/50, respiration rate 12 via bag valve mask (no spontaneous respirations), SpO_2 94% on FiO_2 of 60%. Laboratory work is pending. Which of the following rewarming techniques are most appropriate?

    a. Forced air warming blanket and warm IV fluids
    b. Warm blankets, gastric lavage with warm fluids
    c. Heated humidified oxygen and cardiopulmonary bypass
    d. Forced air rewarming and hemodialysis

128. The AG-ACNP would be found guilty of malpractice in a lawsuit over which situation:

    a. She let it slip that a patient has gonorrhea, damaging his reputation.
    b. He acts hastily in treating an aneurysm, resulting in otherwise avoidable partial paralysis.
    c. He notices symptom of syphilis, but does not work to diagnose or treat the underlying condition, resulting in central nervous system damage.
    d. She aims to subdue an unruly patient by striking her in the face with her hand.

129. An African American patient presents with a history of hypertension. The patient is currently receiving monotherapy with hydrochlorothiazide, and has a blood pressure of 160/94. The most appropriate treatment for this patient is

    a. Start the patient on amlodipine (Norvasc).
    b. Double the dosage of the hydrochlorothiazide (Microzide) and add furosemide (Lasix).
    c. Start lisinopril (Zestril).
    d. Start metoprolol (Lopessor).

130. A 55-year-old woman is complaining of pain and tingling that radiates up her left arm. The pain began 2 weeks ago in her left wrist. Pain is reproduced with Tinel and Phalen's sign. The best initial intervention to reduce her pain is:

    a. Cortisone injection
    b. Use of night splint of wrist and forearm
    c. Refer for orthopedic consult
    d. Short arm cast

131. A patient's sociodemographic background and history can create significant amounts of _____, which can further affect her health status outcome.

    a. Stress
    b. Racial discrimination
    c. Depression
    d. Anxiety

132. A 62-year-old male is admitted with a COPD exacerbation. He is on home oxygen and has had three other episodes of COPD exacerbation requiring hospitalization this year alone. He continues to smoke two packs of cigarettes per day. What technique may be helpful for this patient?

    a. Cognitive behavioral therapy
    b. Motivational interviewing
    c. Electroconvulsive therapy
    d. Psychotherapy

133. The AG-ACNP is leading a quality improvement project aimed to increase home blood pressure monitoring patient education provided by nursing staff upon discharge when the hypertension medication regimen is changed or has been initiated during the admission. During unit rounds, the AG-ACNP overhears statements made during patient education sessions. Which statement is correct teaching to patients about blood pressure monitoring at home?

    a. Sit in a recliner chair with feet elevated and legs uncrossed before measuring your blood pressure.
    b. Rest at least 20 minutes before taking your blood pressure at home to avoid a falsely elevated measurement.
    c. Measure the blood pressure daily in both arms at least 1 minute apart and record the lower blood pressure reading.
    d. Avoid smoking, caffeinated beverages, or exercise within 30 minutes before taking your blood pressure.

134. A 60-year-old man presents to the ED after 3 hours of chest pain. His history is notable for hypertension, diabetes, and benign prostatic hypertrophy. In the ED, his blood pressure is 145/90 mmHg and heart rate is 92 beats/min. His lungs are clear. An ECG shows 2-mm ST-segment elevations in the anterior leads. Which of the following interventions should be initiated?

    a. Tissue plasminogen activator (TPA)
    b. Aspirin, heparin, and beta-blockers without TPA
    c. Aspirin, heparin, and beta-blockers only
    d. Immediate cardiac catheterization

135. A new AG-ACNP joins a new team of interprofessional providers. The AG-ACNP recognizes professional collaboration in healthcare as:

    a. An imbalance of power relations among leaders and subordinates
    b. Communication among individuals that fails to recognize alternative views
    c. True partnership that values expertise, power, and respect on all sides
    d. Strategic planning that excludes perspectives from all employees

136. An AG-ACNP working in the ICU observes a bedside nurse instill 5 mL normal saline via endotracheal tube and then ambu bag the patient followed by suctioning the endotracheal tube. The AG-ACNP's best intervention is to:

    a. Write an incident report.
    b. Talk with the nurse.
    c. Email the manager.
    d. Inform the charge nurse.

137. Legal authority for advanced practice nursing rests with:

    a. Federal statues
    b. Certifying bodies
    c. State laws and regulations
    d. Insurance company credentialing processes

138. The AG-ACNP is evaluating a patient for possible extubation. Which of the following tests would be the best indicator for successful extubation?

    a. Daily interruption of sedation and spontaneous breathing trials
    b. Decreasing fraction of inspired oxygen
    c. NIF and cuff leak test
    d. Removing pressure support

139. The AG-ACNP is managing a 54-year-old-female with ARDS. Her ABG is: pH 7.45, $PaCO_2$ 35, PaO_2 60, HCO_3 25, O_2 Saturation 90%, Base Excess 0. The best evidence for the AG-ACNP to implement is which of the following type of ventilatory assistance:

    a. 100% nonrebreather mask
    b. BiPAP
    c. Volume control with low tidal volumes
    d. Volume control ventilation with increased tidal volumes

140. A 54-year-old female involved in a motor vehicle crash presented with complaints of diffuse abdominal pain and back pain. Vital signs upon arrival were blood pressure 80/60, heart rate 110, with a noted deteriorating mental status (Glasgow Coma Score 13). Upon evaluation of the patient, the AG-ACNP visualizes Grey Turner's sign and notes a tense, firm abdomen upon light palpation which causes the patient to moan/cry out in pain. Which is the most appropriate initial diagnostic imaging selection for the AG-ACNP to select?

    a. CT chest/abdomen/pelvis without contrast
    b. KUB x-ray
    c. Diagnostic peritoneal lavage with warmed .9% normal saline solution
    d. Bedside focused assessment with sonography for trauma examination

141. The AG-ACNP is caring for a 79-year-old man who has been successfully resuscitated. He had a sudden, witnessed collapse in a shopping mall where he was found to be in pulseless VT. He has a prior history of CAD with a single coronary stent placed 2 years ago. He now has stable vital signs but remains comatose. His 12-lead ECG shows ST segment depressions in the

anterior leads. Which statement regarding the role of cardiac catheterization in his care is true? Cardiac catheterization is:

a. Contraindicated secondary to his neurologic status
b. Advisable in the setting of ST-segment myocardial ischemia
c. Indicated based on his presentation
d. Advisable after the patient is stabilized

142. A 60-year-old male (70 kg) brought to ED by EMS for a generalized tonic clonic seizure. He was given a second dose of lorazepam 4 mg IV approximately 5 minutes ago with no effect. The attending physician verbally orders phenytoin (Dilantin) 1400 mg (20 mg/kg) to be given over 5 minutes. The AG-ACNP's response is to:

a. Agree with the attending's decision to pursue a second-line antiepileptic.
b. Discuss the need to adjust the infusion rate to be given over 30 minutes.
c. Suggest trying another dose of lorazepam before going to a second-line antiepileptic.
d. Change the dose to 100 mg Q 8 hours.

143. An AG-ACNP is caring for a patient who is recovering from sepsis due to pneumonia. The patient's course has been complicated by AKI, requiring hemodialysis. The AG-ACNP anticipates which of the following complication during hemodialysis:

a. Nausea and vomiting
b. Headache
c. Hypotension
d. Muscle cramps

144. Ulcerative colitis and Crohn's disease are similar in most of the conventional treatment, except one of the following is used in the management of Crohn's disease, but is NOT needed for ulcerative colitis:

a. Corticosteroids
b. Adalimumab (Humera)
c. Nutritional therapy
d. Immunomodulators

145. A 72-year-old male presents to the ED with acute exacerbation of COPD. Review of systems is benign other than symptoms related only to the COPD exacerbation. The patient states that he has had some weight loss secondary to early satiety and night sweats over the past several weeks. Physical exam findings include barrel chest, diminished breath sounds, tachypneic with speaking, and painless, mobile, cervical lymphadenopathy. A CBC revealed: WBC 26,000, hemoglobin 10.2, hematocrit (Hct) 30.6, platelets 88,000, neutrophils 28%, lymphocytes 70%. Vital signs were recorded as the following: heart rate 92 and regular, blood pressure 140/86, respiration rate 22, temperature 98.6°F. The AG-ACNP caring for this patient is most suspicious this is:

a. CAP
b. Myelodysplastic syndrome
c. CLL
d. CML

146. During damage control resuscitative surgery and splenectomy for a splenic laceration, a patient required 6 units of packed red blood cells and 2 units of FFP. Post-operative lab values show stable hemoglobin/hematocrit values, but the patient continues to require increased levels of oxygen, is hypertensive to 170/60, and increased crackles are heard on auscultation of the lungs. Post-operative chest radiograph demonstrated cardiomegaly with diffuse pulmonary edema,

which is changed from before. What is most likely the cause of the patient's hypertension and increased oxygen demands?

a. TACO
b. Dependent atelectasis secondary to a prolonged intraoperative case
c. TRALI
d. Acute myocardial infarction (type II NSTEMI-supply/demand mismatch)

147. A 60-year-old woman presents with complaints of right upper quadrant pain and fever for 24 hours. The patient reports nausea, but no vomiting. She denies weight loss, diarrhea, constipation, change in stool, travel out of the country, and change in diet. Vital signs are: temperature 102.5°F (39.2°C), heart rate 118, respiration rate 24, blood pressure 90/50, O_2 saturation 95%. Upon examination, the AG-ACNP notes scleral icterus, right upper quadrant tender to palpation. WBC 16,200 with 18% bands, lactate 3.4. The most likely diagnosis is:

a. Acute cholecystitis
b. Hepatitis
c. Ascending cholangitis
d. Gastric outlet obstruction

148. A 53-year-old man with long-standing ischemic cardiomyopathy is admitted to the ICU with hypotension following a 24-hour episode of viral gastroenteritis. He is given intravenous fluids. The following day he develops chest pain, shortness of breath, and mental status changes. On physical examination, temperature is 38.2°C (100.8°F), heart rate is 100/min, blood pressure is 75/45 mmHg, respiration rate is 12/min, and he is mildly lethargic. Jugular venous pressure is difficult to assess. He has bilateral crackles heard on auscultation. Cardiac examination reveals regular rhythm, a normal S_1 and S_2, and the presence of an S_3. There is peripheral edema bilaterally to the thighs, and his extremities are cool. A pulmonary artery catheter is placed and provides the following data:

|1|1| heightCVP
12 mmHg (normal, 0–5 mmHg)
PAOP
19 mmHg (normal, 6–12 mmHg)
CI
2.0 L/min/m^2 (normal, 4–8 L/min)

Which of the following is the most likely diagnosis?

a. Cardiogenic shock
b. Hypovolemic shock
c. Septic shock
d. Toxic shock

149. A deeply unconscious man presents via ambulance to the ED. Family reports he has had a 30-pound weight loss over the past 2 months. Medical history is significant for obesity and metabolic syndrome. On exam, his skin and mucus membranes are quite dry. Vital signs are: temperature 37.5°C, heart rate 120, blood pressure 98/60, unlabored respirations 30/min. Laboratory values include: WBC 21,300; hemoglobin and hematocrit (H/H) = 16.2/51; ABG: pH 7.39/PaCO$_2$ 42/PaO$_2$ 68/Bicarb25/Sat 92%/Base excess-0; basic metabolic profile (BMP) reveals sodium 153; potassium 4.0; chloride 102; carbon dioxide 25; BUN 68, creatinine 2.3; glucose 1020. The most likely diagnosis is:

a. HHS
b. DKA
c. Myxedema coma
d. Alcoholic ketoacidosis

150. The AG-ACNP is managing the care of an obese 45-year-old male with ventilator dependency who was underwent a tracheostomy 14 days ago. The patient has a size eight tracheostomy tube with a cuff. Today the patient was successfully weaned from the ventilator and is now on a trach collar. The AG-ACNP plans to change out the cuffed tracheostomy tube to a size six cuffless tracheostomy tube. What complication should the AG-ACNP be concerned about in this patient?

    a. Tracheal collapse
    b. Tracheal malacia
    c. Tracheal stenosis
    d. Tracheoinnominate artery fistula

151. The AG-ACNP is seeing a 47-year-old female with complaints of dyspnea, nonspecific chest pain and syncope. On examination the AG-ACNP detects crackles in the bases and an increase in the pulmonary component of the second heart sound P2. The P2 is split and intensified and is stronger than the aortic component A2. The gold standard to diagnose pulmonary hypertension is:

    a. Chest x-ray
    b. ECG
    c. Cardiac catheterization
    d. Transthoracic echocardiogram

152. The AG-ACNP is caring for a 50-year-old female who has persistently elevated total cholesterol and LDL despite lifestyle modifications over several months. The patient is prescribed an HMG-CoA reductase inhibitor to reduce the risk of coronary events. The treatment goal is:

    a. LDL less than 100
    b. LDL less than 70
    c. Get the patient to a maximum HMG-CoA reductase inhibitor dose
    d. Reduce LDL while preventing hepatotoxicity

153. A 21-year-old male is brought into the ED from a large, loud dance party and is experiencing a focal seizure of the right hand. Which recent use of a drug of abuse would the AG-ACNP consider to be the most likely cause of his condition?

    a. Marijuana
    b. Heroin
    c. Nicotine
    d. Cocaine

154. A 71-year-old man presents having been instructed to come to the ED by his PCP, due to recent lab results. The AG-ACNP reviewed his labs and noted a creatinine of 3.4 and blood urea nitrogen of 32. Which of the following of his medications most likely caused these laboratory findings?

    a. Amlodipine (Norvasc)
    b. Diclofenac (Zorvolex)
    c. Hydralzine (Apresoline)
    d. Multivitamin with iron

155. A 36-year-old male trauma patient status post motor vehicle crash was taken to the operating room for an exploratory laparotomy for multiple abdomen injuries, after aggressive resuscitation in the emergency room. Postoperatively, the patient is in the ICU on mechanical ventilation and adequately sedated. Six hours postoperatively, the patient develops increased peak airway pressures, distended abdomen, decreased urine output, with blood pressure 80/62 mmHg. What is the most appropriate first step for the AG-ACNP?

    a. Adjust vent settings to decrease PEEP.
    b. Administer fluid bolus of 500 mL saline.
    c. Assess for intra-abdominal hypertension.
    d. Start vasopressin to support low blood pressure.

156. In a burn patient with inhalation injury, an endotracheal tube was placed by anesthesia and placement confirmed via chest x-ray. The patient is successfully sedated with low dose dexmedetomidine hydrocholoride (Precedex) with a RASS goal of 0 to –1. Twenty minutes later, the nurse reports his SPO₂ is 90% on 50% FIO₂ and five PEEP and his heart rate and blood pressure begin to downtrend although his RASS score is +1. When reviewing the patient's medical history he is found to be on no medications and without a significant medical history. Should the AG-ACNP be alarmed at the blood pressure and heart rate trend?

a. No, he is young and likely a marathon runner, so his heart is just returning to baseline.
b. Yes, he is likely experiencing hypoxemia and needs and immediate bronchoscopy.
c. No, this is an anticipated side effect of dexmedetomidine hydrochloride (Precedex).
d. Yes, he may be exhibiting neurogenic shock secondary to his upper airway burns.

157. An 80-year-old man with a history CHF due to ischemic cardiovascular disease is comfortable at rest. However, when walking to his car, he develops dyspnea, fatigue, and sometimes palpitations. He must rest for several minutes before these symptoms resolve. His New York Heart Association classification is which of the following?

a. Class I
b. Class II
c. Class III
d. Class IV

158. A 56-year-old patient with known HIV, and a documented CD4 count of 180, asks the AG-ACNP about vaccinations. Vaccination recommendations for this patient include all of the following EXCEPT:

a. Zostavax
b. Pneumococcal
c. Tdap (tetanus, diptheria, and whooping cough)
d. Influenza

159. The AG-ACNP is managing the care of a patient with a pulmonary embolism. What findings would the AG-ACNP likely see on an ECG of a patient with a pulmonary embolism?

a. Bradycardia
b. Right bundle branch block
c. Left bundle branch block
d. Precordial T wave elevations

160. A 37-year-old woman brought to ED by the police for "vomiting." Per report the patient was arrested for erratic driving, resisting arrest, and refusing a breathalyzer. Once the patient was in the holding cell, she continued to vomit and was complaining of the "worst headache of her life." The patient reports she has been having headaches for the past month or so but that this headache was the worst pain ever, 10/10 and this is a first to have nausea and vomiting. Vital signs are: heart rate 98, blood pressure 184/104, respiration rate 16, temperature 98°F, O₂ saturation 90% on RA. Noncontrast head CT reveals a frontotemporal SAH. The AG-ACNP's first action is to:

a. Stat neurosurgical consult.
b. Start labetalol drip.
c. Give Keppra 500 mg IV drip over 10 minutes.
d. Give oxygen and order basic labs.

161. A 64-year-old female with a past medical history of breast cancer and recent 18-hour air travel from vacation presents to the hospital with complaints of chest pain, syncope, and acute onset of shortness of breath. She underwent a CTA and was noted to have a large filling defect in the posterior-basal segment of the right lower lobe artery. She was admitted to the hospital and started on weight-based Lovenox (enoxaparin sodium) subcutaneous injections every 12 hours.

The following is the result of laboratory tests 36 hours after admission: Sodium 138, Chloride 102, Potassium 3.8, Bicarbonate 22, BUN 55, Creatinine 3.0, Glucose 72. The AG-ACNP reviews previous lab values from 3 months ago, which show the following: Sodium 137, Chloride 100, Potassium 4.2, Bicarbonate 25, BUN 22, Creatinine 1.0, Glucose 70. The most likely cause of the changes in the laboratory results is:

a. Lovenox (Enoxaparin)
b. Extended travel
c. Contrast nephropathy
d. Protein C deficiency

162. A 48-year-old obese Hispanic diabetic female presents to the ED with a gradual onset of right upper quadrant pain with fever, anorexia, nausea, and vomiting for 2 days. She states the pain is worse with inspiration and is radiating to her right shoulder. She denies any history of the same. Physical exam reveals right upper quadrant tenderness to palpation, and a positive Murphy's sign. The AG-ACNP suspects this is acute:

a. Cholecystitis
b. Pancreatitis
c. Pyelonephritis
d. Appendicitis

163. A 77-year-old male with a history of atrial fibrillation develops an acute abdomen. When finally seen and examined 4 days after onset of the abdominal pain, he has no bowel sounds with diffuse tenderness and mild rebound. There is a trace of blood on the rectal exam. He is acidotic and developing signs of sepsis. The most likely diagnosis is:

a. Acute pancreatitis
b. Mesenteric ischemia
c. Primary bacterial peritonitis
d. Cholecystitis

164. The AG-ACNP is managing the care of a 64-year-old female with a massive pulmonary embolism who is hemodynamically unstable in the ICU. The AG-ACNP knows that the treatment of choice in this patient is:

a. Alteplase (tPA)
b. Enoxaparin (Lovenox)
c. Heparin
d. Warfarin (Coumadin)

165. A 57-year-old woman is brought to the ED by her son. He states that she has been acting strangely for the last day or so. According to her records, her usual antihypertensive regimen consists of lisinopril/hydrochlorothiazide 20/25 mg daily (Prinizide), extended-release nifedipine (Procardia XL) 90 mg daily, and sustained-release metoprolol 50 mg every day. Her son indicates that she ran out of her medication about 1 week ago. On examination, the patient is confused, somnolent, and complaining of headache. Her blood pressure is 230/114 mmHg bilaterally. Funduscopic examination shows arteriolar narrowing and no distinct optic disk margins. The lung examination reveals no crackles; the cardiac examination is significant for an S_4 gallop and a grade 2 midsystolic ejection murmur at the right upper sternal border. The abdomen is soft, not tender, and without bruits. No peripheral edema is present. Appropriate management would be to:

a. Observe in the emergency room and administer clonidine (Catapres) 0.3 mg by mouth every 6 hours.
b. Admit to the telemetry unit and treat with intravenous hydralazine (Apresoline).
c. Admit to the ICU and treat with intravenous labetalol (Trandate).
d. Admit to the telemetry unit and resume outpatient oral antihypertensive regimen.

166. Which population is most affected by health disparities in the United States:

    a. Asian
    b. Caucasian, non-Hispanic
    c. Pacific Islander
    d. Hispanic

167. The AG-ACNP is writing orders for assist control (AC) mechanical ventilation for a 57-year-old male who is has just been intubated for hypoxic and hypercapneic respiratory failure. The AG-ACNP knows that AC is different than synchronous intermittent ventilation (SIMV) in that the patient will receive:

    a. Peak expiratory pressure at the beginning of exhalation
    b. Pressure support during inspiration
    c. Tidal volume with only set breaths
    d. Tidal volume with set breaths and triggered breaths

168. An older adult male patient is admitted after a fall. Physical therapy is assessing the patient to determine rehabilitation needs. The AG-ACNP observes the patient is ambulating slowly, has a stiff gait with minimal arm swing, and his face appears "mask-like." The occupational therapist note informs the AG-ACNP of hand tremors when at rest, micrographia, and microphonia. Both therapists recommend inpatient rehabilitation for strength training and help with activities of daily living. The AG-ACNP is concerned he has:

    a. Parkinson's disease
    b. Alzheimer's disease
    c. Huntington's disease
    d. MG

169. The AG-ACNP is seeing a patient in the ED with complaints of loss of appetite, fatigue, swelling of the lower extremities and abdomen, and frothy urine. The patient reports a history of lupus and hypertension. Laboratory tests indicate severe albuminuria, hypoalbuminemia, and hyperlipidemia. The most likely cause of the patient's symptoms and laboratory findings is:

    a. Nephrotic syndrome
    b. Pyelonephritis
    c. Nephrolithiasis
    d. Cystitis

170. A 65-year-old-male presents with fever, anorexia, productive cough, night sweats, and weight loss. The AG-ACNP suspects the patient has tuberculosis. Which test will confirm the diagnosis of tuberculosis?

    a. Chest x-ray
    b. CT scan of the thorax
    c. Positive intradermal PPD
    d. Positive sputum for mycobacterium tuberculosis

171. A 65-year-old man is admitted for elective hip replacement. On hospital day 3, the nurse calls to report the patient is agitated, tremulous, and diaphoretic. Vital signs are: temperature 98.6°F, heart rate 110, respiration rate 20, blood pressure 160/80. Upon review of his lab data the AG-ACNP notes normal chemistries except for a low magnesium level of 1.2 mEq/L, WBC 7.5, hemoglobin 8.1, hematocrit 26, platelet count 150,000. Red blood cell indices show low mean corpuscular volume. The AG-ACNP is most concerned he:

    a. Is septic
    b. Is experiencing alcohol withdrawal
    c. Has malnutrition
    d. Has an anxiety disorder

172. A patient has been diagnosed with latent tuberculosis. The AG-ACNP prescribes which of following drug therapy:

    a. Isoniazid + vitamin B_6 × 6 months
    b. Isoniazid, rifampicin, ethambutol, and pyrazinamide × 3 months
    c. Rifampicin, pyrazinamide, and ethambutol × 6 months
    d. No treatment necessary; it is latent

173. A 63-year-old woman with a history of cirrhosis was brought to the ED with acute hematemesis and altered mental status. She is hypotensive, tachycardic, and vomiting blood. After intubation and fluid resuscitation, she is taken to endoscopy where multiple large varicosities seen. The gastroenterologist infuses octreotide and vasopressin, attempts band ligation, sclerotherapy and a Minnesota tube, all of which are slow to stop the bleeding. Her laboratory studies reveal the following: hemoglobin 5.8 g/dL, platelets 90,000/mm^3, international normalized ratio (INR) 2.8. After blood product resuscitation, she remains borderline hypotensive at 90/55 mmHg and continues to bleed. What would be the next best intervention?

    a. Another Sengtaken-Blakemore tube
    b. TIPS
    c. Hepatic transplantation
    d. Continue fluid resuscitation and transfusion

174. A 33-year-old-male is brought to the ED following a car crash into a tree. Upon examination, he has a Glasgow Coma Score of 13, right chest wall deformity associated with diminished left breath sounds, and abdominal tenderness. His pulse rate is 120, blood pressure is 110/60 mmHg, respiratory rate is 30. Which of the following is the most appropriate next step?

    a. Endotracheal intubation
    b. CT scan of the brain
    c. Chest tube placement
    d. Focused assessment with sonography for trauma (FAST)

175. A 20-year-old man stumbles into the ED complaining of shortness of breath and chest pain after he fell onto a pile of sharp rocks striking his right anterior chest wall. Upon presentation he is observed to be gasping for air, clutching his right chest, complaining of extreme shortness of breath that is worsening with each breath he takes. The AG-ACNP notices that his trachea is moving to the left side. The primary diagnosis is_____and immediate action is to _____.

    a. Right tension pneumothorax, insert a needle into his right second intercostal space, midclavicular line
    b. Acute coronary syndrome, give an aspirin 325 mg by mouth STAT
    c. Left tension pneumothorax, insert a needle into his left second intercostal space midclavicular line
    d. Pericardial tamponade, perform pericardiocentesis

28

Comprehensive Practice Exam: Answers and Rationales

COMPREHENSIVE PRACTICE EXAM ANSWERS AND RATIONALES

1. **c) Maximize exposure to light during the day and minimize at night.** Proper light exposure establishes regular rhythms to improve sleep. Establishing a regular sleep schedule increases sleep quality at night. Avoiding naps will improve sleep quality, taking naps decreases sleep quality. Avoiding alcohol, caffeine, and nicotine improve sleep quality. If these interventions do not work and underlying causes have been ruled out, refer to a sleep laboratory for assessment.

2. **b) Bladder pressure monitoring with anticipation of surgical consult.** This patient has developed abdominal compartment syndrome, likely due to third spacing into the bowels, due to the associated injury. With increasing intra-abdominal pressure, the patient is exhibiting signs of slowed perfusion distally shunting blood flow for essential body processes. Normal abdominal compartment pressure is 0 mmHg; however, as pressure climbs above 20 mmHg, blood flow is impeded. In addition, volume presses upward on the diaphragm causing an increase in PIP.

3. **a) Lisinopril (Prinivil).** Patient is a type 1 diabetic with complications including diabetic nephropathy. Due to the fact that ACEIs delay the progression to end-stage renal disease, they are the agents of choice in persons with type 1 diabetes and evidence of renal dysfunction. Thus lisinopril, an ACEI, is the correct choice. The other medications can be added on if her blood pressure remains uncontrolled; however, they are not first-line medications as none of them prevent progression of end-stage renal disease.

4. **a) Lung abscess.** Aspiration of oral flora typically results in lung abscesses that present similar to tuberculosis. The negative AFB is the determining factor. There are other infections that may produce a false negative, but none produce a false positive. Hodgkin's lymphoma presents without cough and with painless lymphadenopathy in cervical or supraclavicular areas. Adenocarcinoma does not usually present with fever, chills, or purulent sputum, which are indicative of infection process.

5. **a) Discuss and answer questions about the test results, diagnosis, needed lifestyle changes, and medical treatments with the patient and/or family.** Summarizing findings, providing feedback, and promoting the social support of family members being involved in the patient's care facilitates behavior coaching for long-term change and aims to reduce the burdens of chronic illness. The AG-ACNP should engage this style of communication before initiating treatments to facilitate patient and family-centered care thereby allowing

the patient and family to participate in the medical treatment decisions collaboratively with the AG-ACNP. Initiating behavioral coaching before beginning new therapies without the patient/families input also reinforces the therapeutic patient-AG-ACNP relationship. All other responses may be appropriate after coaching/counseling of the results, and so on, is performed by the AG-ACNP.

6. **b) The EVD is clotted off.** The patient initially demonstrated clinical improvement, indicating the EVD had been working, but an acute change occurred. The return of bloody fluid is concerning and a known risk for clotting off or obstructing the outflow from the EVD. Cerebral edema is a possible cause and manifests as described here, but is less likely in this scenario.

7. **a) Aspirin.** In patients without pain, often no treatment is required. However, aspirin (650 mg every 4–6 hours) will usually relieve the pain. NSAIDs such as indomethacin and ibuprofen, along with corticosteroids, can cause impaired infarct healing and predispose to myocardial rupture, and therefore should be avoided in the early post-myocardial infarction period.

8. **d) Percutaneous tube feedings do not prolong life and can lead to increased use of restraints.** In the ABIM "Choosing Wisely" initiative, the first recommendation from the AGS, the AAHPM, and the Society for Post-Acute and Long-Term Care Medicine (AMDA) includes a statement that addresses the use of percutaneous feeding tubes in patients with advanced dementia. This collaborative group supports the use of oral assisted feedings over percutaneous tube feedings in patients with advanced dementia. Studies suggest that percutaneous feeding tubes are not known to prolong life and often times lead to increased agitation because of restraints used to prevent the patient from pulling out the feeding tube.

9. **a) Immediately consult a urologist.** Testicular torsion, which primarily affects males ages 10 to 20, is considered a urologic emergency which can cause severe testicular ischemia. Immediate surgical exploration is the first line of management. The ultrasound has high sensitivity and specificity for testicular torsion, but the delay in obtaining imaging studies can contribute to extended time of testicular ischemia.

10. **d) Exploratory laparotomy by a surgeon.** Gunshot wounds to the abdomen require exploratory laparotomy for repair of intra-abdominal injuries (not necessarily to "remove the bullet"). Any entrance or exit wound below the level of the nipple line is considered to involve the abdomen. In very select cases of abdominal trauma due to a small-caliber gunshot wounds involving the right upper quadrant, conservative management may be used if the patient is properly monitored with close follow-up of clinical signs and serial abdominal CT scans. However, in a hemodynamically unstable patient with suspected diaphragmatic injury and possible hollow viscus perforation, exploratory laparotomy is indicated.

11. **a) Combined alpha and beta adrenergic effects.** Patients suffering from an anaphylactic response have mast cell degradation, which causes a histamine-mediated response that includes vasodilation and bronchospasm. Epinephrine is a nonspecific alpha/beta adrenergic medication helping reduce vasodilatation (alpha-1) and bronchospasm (beta-2).

12. **b) Moral distress.** Moral distress is increasingly recognized among AG-ACNPs who frequently experience patient refusal of appropriate treatments. The conflict often arises for AG-ACNPs when attempting to promote shared decision making and patient autonomy and maintaining the ethical principle of beneficence. Care coordination involves the AG-ACNP navigating healthcare delivery systems to facilitate optimal patient care. Reflective practice involves the AG-ACNP reflecting upon understanding prior experiences better to identify new insight intended to be used in the next relevant case. Shared decision making is a patient-centered communication strategy used to facilitate patient autonomy and reinforce a trusting AG-ACNP-patient relationship.

13. **a) Cardiac tamponade due to myocardial wall rupture.** This patient does not have any chest discomfort, pain on inspiration, or a pericardial rub to suggest pericarditis. There is no mention of a systolic murmur or rales that would suggest either papillary muscle rupture or acute pulmonary edema. Ventricular septal rupture is associated with a harsh holosystolic murmur with a thrill and pericardial discomfort. Tamponade secondary to rupture of the

ventricular free wall (myocardial wall rupture) is frequently associated with JVD and pulsus paradox.

14. **b) Check a CBC**. A patient presenting with pallor of the mucous membranes, tachycardia, and no other clinical symptoms should have routine blood work checked prior to obtaining specialized studies. A CBC will reveal the patient's hemoglobin to confirm or rule out anemia. Iron studies would not be warranted without knowing what is causing the symptoms (hemoglobin, hematocrit, MCV). The patient is having clinical symptoms and requires monitoring but also intervention. One would not start a pharmacologic intervention until a diagnosis is made.

15. **d) CAP**. CAP is defined as pneumonia that incubates within 48 hours of admission. The concept of healthcare-associated pneumonia was removed in the 2016 HAP and VAP guidelines. Hospital-acquired pneumonia is defined as pneumonia that is not incubating at the time of hospital admission and occurs 48 hours or more after admission. VAP is defined as a pneumonia occurring greater than 48 hours after endotracheal intubation. There is no indication in the stem indicating this patient aspirated, furthermore, aspiration typically is seen in the right lower lobe because the left mainstem bronchus is more angulated due to the location of the heart.

16. **d) Occurs if the null hypothesis is rejected when it is true**. If the null hypothesis is rejected when it is true, then a type I error has occurred. For example, a type I error has occurred if we claim that drug A reduces mortality when in fact there is no difference between drug A and the placebo in the reduction of mortality. The probability of committing a type I error is known as the level of significance.

17. **d) Evidence of cost effectiveness in telemedicine applications**. It is not the issue that tele-ICU programs have shown to lower patient mortality and increase quality and decrease cost (Lilly et al., 2014). It is the liability issue of APRNs' variation in SOP, licensure, and legal liability that cannot be delegated by protocols or on-the-job training that should be of concern.

18. **a) Acetylsalicylic acid**. In thyroid storm, regardless of the patient population, it's best to avoid ASA or other nonsteroidal anti-inflammatory agents as they interfere with the binding of T4 and thyroid binding globulin, make the "storm" worse. Propanolol and propylthiouracil are the mainstay of treatment. Acetaminophen is helpful for the fever and patient comfort, but does little for the treatment of this syndrome.

19. **a) Osteoarthritis**. This patient has OA. It is the most common joint disease in adults. It affects more women than men, particularly after the age of 50. OA is slow process that may eventually lead to disability, recurrent falls, inability to live independently, and significant mortality. Stiffness of OA lasts 15 to 30 minutes in the morning. This is in contrast to patients with RA, whose stiffness last 1 to 2 hours and often requires warming or soaking to improve. Gout and osteomyelitis involve inflammation, pain, and swelling of the joint.

20. **d) Interview her separately and screen for interpersonal violence**. The AG-ACNP should screen for interpersonal violence. Abuse has not been diagnosed, so reporting to police is premature. In addition, reporting domestic violence varies among states. There is no need to notify child protective services, as she would be considered a competent adult. Providing information for safe shelter may be one tool/resource to provide, but not the best first step in managing the situation. The most important initial step is assessment of the situation; that takes the highest priority.

21. **b) IV cefazolin**. The patient likely has cellulitis, which is a superficial inflammation of the skin and underlying tissues and is characterized by erythema, warmth, and tenderness of the involved area. The most common organisms associated with this presentation are streptococci or methicillin-sensitive staphylococcal aureus. According to the IDSA, cefazolin is the recommended drug of choice among others that do not include broad spectrum penicillin or fluoroquinolones. There is no need for extended spectrum in a patient with a first episode; in addition, one must also consider common organisms that are likely causing the

cellulitis. Vancomycin is recommended for MRSA skin and soft tissue infections, and the patient does not have risk factors of concern for MRSA.

22. c) **Difficulty falling or staying asleep.** Restlessness, irritability, and difficulty falling asleep or staying asleep are common features of GAD. The diagnostic criteria of GAD include excessive worry and anxiety associated with at least three of the following symptoms: sleep disturbance, irritability, being easily fatigued, restlessness or feeling keyed up or on edge, difficulty concentrating or mind going blank, and muscle tension. The worry is difficult to control and there is decline in ability to function related to the symptoms. Auditory hallucinations, anger, and restless leg syndrome are not associated with GAD.

23. c) **Follow the patient clinically, repeat a chest x-ray in 4 hours.** The best answer is to follow the patient clinically and repeat a chest x-ray with any concerns of worsening. The patient is not in distress and vitals are stable. An emergent chest tube placement is not indicated and not preferred given the patient is stable. Repeating the x-ray immediately is not appropriate as findings will not change. A pigtail catheter may not be indicated.

24. d) **State laws regarding APRN and institutional guidelines.** Standards of practice for the ACNP are developed by the American Association of Critical-Care Nurses, the American Association of Colleges of Nursing, and the NONPF. These standards serve as general guidelines for practice for the AG-ACNP. It is the state laws that provide specific parameters that will guide AG-ACNP practice in each state. Those state laws will then guide each institution's practice guidelines so that providers in each institution are compliant with state laws.

25. a) **Pravastatin (Pravachol).** Since this patient is post-AMI, he requires a statin (HMG-COA reductase inhibitor) medication for secondary prevention. Part of his HIV treatment is a PI. All of the PIs are extensively metabolized by CYP34A. This class of drugs is known to interact with statins that use the cytochrome P450 system. The 34A-dependent statins (atorvastatin, simvastatin, and lovastatin) tend to accumulate in plasma in the presence of drugs that inhibit or compete for the 3A4 cytochrome. As such, the area under the curve would be increased for the statin and the patient is at risk for myopathy. Of all the statins listed, pravastatin is the only drug that is not catabolized through CYP34A and is safe to use in this situation.

26. c) **Is at risk of contracting HIV as it crosses the placenta and can be transmitted at birth.** Syphilis and HIV can cross the placenta and can be contracted during the birthing process. Gonorrhea and chlamydia do not cross the placenta, but can be contracted at birth. Erythromycin ointment is typically prescribed at birth to reduce risk of neonatal blindness associated with chlamydia. HIV can be passed in breast milk.

27. a) **Refrain from transfusion and implement hemostasis measures.** The patient has the right to refuse a medical intervention, including blood transfusion. The AG-ANCP must honor this wish. There is no need to contact his parents as he is of legal age. Autotransfusion may be an option that could be considered; there are varying views within the religion, but is not accepted by all. A court order is not indicated.

28. c) **Difficulty seeing in low-light situations.** Difficulty seeing in low-light situations are among normal changes seen with aging. Personality traits are typically stable over time. Mild to moderate hearing loss is associated with normal aging; severe hearing loss is pathological. Having issues with short-term memory loss is associated with normal aging, but not long-term memory.

29. a) **Endotracheal intubation.** The patient is unresponsive and has been vomiting. Endotracheal intubation is necessary first to protect the lungs from initial and/or repeated aspiration. Ipecac and gastric lavage are contraindicated because of the high risk of aspiration. Activated charcoal poorly absorbs hydrocarbons.

30. b) **Hypertension.** Hypertension accounts for 60% to 70% of all primary ICH. Coagulopathy, sympathomimetic drugs, and cerebral amyloid angiopathy cause the remaining portion of

ICHs. Incidence is particularly high in African Americans and Asians. Advanced age and heavy alcohol consumption are contributing factors.

31. **d) Low-flow priapism and emergent intervention is required**. Priapism is pathological condition characterized by persistent penile erection that continues for greater than 4 hours, or is unrelated to sexual stimulation. Priapism is characterized as ischemic, nonischemic, or stuttering priapism. Ischemic is a persistent, painful erection with little to no cavernous blood flow, and nonischemic is a persistent, nonpainful erection with high arterial blood blow. Stuttering or intermittent priapism is a recurrent ischemic priapism characterized by nonsexual painful erections and periods of detumescence. Patients with SS disease are at increased risk of priapism due to hemolysis, low flow state, and abnormal regulation of the nitric oxide pathway. Ischemic priapism is considered a urological emergency to restore blood flow to prevent cavernosal fibrosis and permanent erectile dysfunction.

32. **a) Upright**. The best position to obtain a quality image and answer the clinical picture is the upright position, as air rises and will be best visualized on chest x-ray under the diaphragm. Supine, left lateral decubitus, and Trendelenburg positions do not provide the optimal evaluation of free air below the diaphragm on chest x-ray as the air is less likely to rise under the diaphragm.

33. **b) Mallory-Weiss tear**. A Mallory-Weiss tear occurs after prolonged, forceful vomiting and, eventually, bright red blood comes up. Endoscopy establishes diagnosis and allows photocoagulation.

34. **a) 80%, .05**. In general, the current standard is to have at least 80% statistical power to detect a clinically relevant difference in an outcome using a two-sided type I error rate of .05. Negative results in small, underpowered studies do not provide compelling evidence of no effect.

35. **c) Obtain a national provider number and credentials with the insurance company**. An AG-ACNP must first apply for a national provider identifier online through the NPPES and then credential with each individual insurer. The NPI is a unique identifier while credentialing is a process that generally collects educational, license, malpractice, employment, and certification data on individual providers.

36. **a) Inform the wife that you will screen the patient for depression and likely start him on antidepressants**. Depression is often underrecognized, as many health providers place it in the context of a normal consequence of a terminal illness. Patients with poor prognoses will often demonstrate mood changes or loss of interest instead of the specific depression symptoms of insomnia, anorexia, and weight change. The patient should be screened for depression and started on antidepressant therapy even though it may take 2 to 6 weeks for symptoms to improve. Psychostimulants are also recommended, as they are considered safe and effective in the short term. Improving the patient's mental status will improve his overall quality of life. Milrinone does not have a side effect profile that supports mood changes.

37. **c) Obtain an ECG and cardiac biomarkers**. The patient is presenting with chest pain of unknown etiology but has a history of SS anemia, thus ACS is high in the differential diagnosis. The priority should be to rule out a cardiac component to his shortness of breath, thus an ECG and cardiac biomarkers. Although a two-dimensional echocardiogram would demonstrate wall motion abnormalities, this would not be the initial management. Consulting cardiology is premature as a diagnosis has not been made yet. Ordering analgesia for pain control is appropriate in this patient's situation and history of SS anemia. Transfusing a unit of red blood cells is inappropriate now as the hemoglobin is not known,;additionally, with a known past medical history of SS anemia, ACS/chest pain need to be ruled out urgently.

38. **c) Dissecting thoracic aortic aneurysm**. This patient presents with typical signs and symptoms of acute aortic dissection—excruciating, severe at onset, pain of a sharp and tearing nature, blood pressure differential of 20 to 30 mmHg between two extremities along with an abnormal chest x-ray. Although there is mention of ischemia on the ECG, cardiac enzymes do not indicate an infarction. There are no symptoms in the stem that would indicate either cardiac tamponade or cardiogenic shock such as hypotension.

39. d) The AG-ACNP joins his or her state and national professional NP organization and actively participates in developing a relationship with state and national representatives to be the voice of the community in which he or she works. Patient advocacy is larger than just at the bedside, and although assertiveness training may supplement the lack of skills when individuals are barriers to best practice, this is insufficient to move along the public health code of ethics The education arena uses literature reviews frequently to assess for best practice, but the issue of disenfranchised community members is bigger than institutions limited credentialing scope. Knowing the public health code in the state in which you are practicing and the statute definition of your standard operating procedure might be the better first step. We need quality individuals to be the legal advocates for AG-ACNPs and the public and although this can be done in the litigation arena, it is usually a case-by-case basis and not very efficient. The best way to advocate on a larger scale is through the policy arena, which requires you actively engage with the players who are your representatives in the state and national level.

40. d) Vancomycin, piperacillin-tazobactam (Zosyn) and levofloxacin (Levaquin). This patient has VAP. Treatment needs to include coverage for MRSA and double coverage for pseudomonas and Gram-negative organisms. Thus, vancomycin or linezolid would be appropriate coverage for MRSA. And piperacillin-tazobactam (Zosyn) and levofloxacin (Levaquin) would provide double coverage one from beta-lactam-based antibiotic and one without beta-lactam-based agents. Cipro and gentamycin are both nonbeta-lactam-based agents. Ceftriaxone and azithromycin are common treatments for CAP.

41. b) Led to longer and more complex codes for more specific disease identification. The ICD-10 codes are much more complex to improve the categorization of symptoms and diseases. They have also increased in number, especially in areas such as orthopedics, to help determine the specific location of the problem. The compliance and medical record departments are the best resources for this type of information.

42. c) ARDS; adjust mechanical ventilator to low tidal volume protocol and lung protective ventilation measures with a VAP protocol. The patient has developed ARDS and needs low tidal volume ventilation. Patients may develop a spontaneous pneumothorax due to ARDS or high levels of positive pressure ventilation, but pnuemothoracies cause increased PIP, not increased plateau pressures. Acute CHF additionally can present gradually, and may cause increased bilateral infiltrates on radiograph. CHF, however, usually does not cause an increase in PIP/plateau pressures along with an uptrending leukocytosis/fever curve. Bilateral postobstructive atelectasis can also cause increased PIP and bilateral obscuration on chest radiograph; however, it does not present with upward trending leukocytosis/fever curve.

43. b) Individualize care to the patient's cultural influences as much as possible. The AG-ACNP should avoid making assumptions about a patient's cultural beliefs that are based upon the patient's physical/ethnic differences, appearance, or dress. A patient may have apparent cultural indications externally but many are less obvious. Therefore, the AG-ACNP should ask open-ended questions related to the patient's cultural beliefs and practices in an effort to demonstrate cultural sensitivity, acknowledgement, and respect for the patient's preferences, and avoid imposing one's own beliefs onto the patient while remaining nonjudgmental. Demonstrating cultural competence strengthens the AG-ACNP-patient therapeutic relationship.

44. d) Cardiac tamponade. This patient has sustained a steering wheel injury and blunt cardiac trauma. There is no mention of any new onset murmurs, thus ruling out aortic insufficiency, nor is there mention of any symptoms of LV failure. The patient has a paradoxical blood pressure typical for cardiac tamponade. A blood pressure of 135/90 is atypical of cardiogenic shock.

45. **a) Her heart rate is above 100**. The geriatric patient may have developed hyperthyroidism secondary to the treatment of hypothyroidism. The patient needs to be instructed to call if any symptoms occur. A heart rate of below 70 is too vague; low blood pressure and cold intolerance are symptoms that are not specific to the medication side effects.

46. **a) Rotator cuff tear**. Both a positive empty can and Neer's sign is consistent with the diagnosis of torn rotator cuff. Acute bursitis is a result of trauma to the burse that may happen but would have a negative empty can and Neer's sign. Adhesive capsulitis occurs slowly over 4 to 6 months. Dislocations happen immediately related to trauma with patient unable to lift the affected arm.

47. **b) PSQIA**. HIPPA is the protection of health information which protects personal information sharing. PSQIA provided for the establishment of PSOs to receive reports of patient safety events or concerns from healthcare providers and to provide analyses of these events to the reporting providers. COBRA is related to an individual's or family's ability to obtain insurance for up to 18 months after loss of a job. The Patient Self-Determination Act requires that all patients entering the hospital be given information on their right to execute advance directives.

48. **b) Flattening of the diaphragm**. In severe COPD there is a hyperinflation of the lungs causing them to push downward, flattening the diaphragm. Increased vascular markings are seen in CHF and pulmonary edema. Hypoinflation is seen in atelectasis and shallow respirations due to abdominal or rib pain and depressed mental status.

49. **b) Change to penicillin G 4 million units IV Q 4H and clindamycin 900 mg IV Q 8H**. Diabetic patients are at increased risk for necrotizing fasciitis. Necrotizing fasciitis is a progressive and rapidly spreading inflammatory reaction that involves the tissue between the skin and the muscle (superficial fascia). The initial skin lesion is often small and trivial but rapidly spreads. Patients report increased pain out of proportion to what one might expect for this type of injury. The signs and symptoms are readily apparent (do not need radiology to confirm; CT would be diagnostic test of choice) in this situation and time is of essence. Immediate change to high-dose penicillin and clindamycin is imperative to treat streptococcus. Surgical intervention is a major therapeutic modality for necrotizing fasciitis and should also be obtained. Vancomycin is narrow spectrum and would not cover possible anaerobic or Gram-negative bacilli organisms.

50. **b) Specifics of the agency's NP practice guidelines**. Some states have no legal requirement for physician involvement in NP practice. However, in the majority of states, there is some legal requirement for physician involvement at some level. Some states define the scope specifically and others vaguely, thus agencies develop more definitive guidelines.

51. **d) Aid patients and families to comprehend the illness trajectory and dying process**. Palliative care provides a structured foundation for delivery of healthcare in order to meet several outcomes. These outcomes include assisting BOTH the patient and families to obtain information related to the current health condition that includes the illness trajectory. The information should be provided in a manner in which the patient is able to comprehend the treatment plan and possible outcome. Palliative care is delivered by an interdisciplinary team that assists with seamless care coordination, not just to transition into hospice. Ultimately, palliative care provides the opportunity for BOTH the patient and family to prepare for death in a manner that allows for personal reflection and growth, hospice, and bereavement.

52. **a) Polypharmacy**. The following are risk factors for hospital acquired delirium: old age, male sex, dementia, severe illness (determined by acute physiologic assessment and chronic health evaluation [APACHE] score), visual impairments, urinary catheterization, polypharmacy, low albumin, and length of hospital stay.

53. **d) Coaching**. Coaching is a competency involving the interpersonal, clinical, and technical skills aimed to assist the patient and family achieve goals to attain higher levels of wellness,

risk reduction, and improved quality of life. Policy is a competency involving the advocacy and understanding of how policy impacts ethical, legal, and social factors influencing healthcare, or vice-versa. Quality is a competency involving the evaluation, synthesis, and translation of evidence-based resources/research into clinical practice aimed to improve and deliver the highest quality of care. Leadership is a competency involving the assumption of leadership roles in advanced practice and performance of leadership skills.

54. **c) Postpone surgery for 2 months**. There is no urgency noted in the aforementioned question. As such the recommendation is that 60 days should elapse after a myocardial infarction before noncardiac surgery. A recent MI, defined as having occurred within 6 months of noncardiac surgery, was also found to be an independent risk factor for perioperative stroke, which was associated with an eight-fold increase in the perioperative mortality rate.

55. **c) Hispanics tend to have a lower awareness of strokes than the general population**. Evidence supports a lower health literacy regarding strokes exists in Hispanic, as well as African American patients when compared with the general population. Cultural competence must be practiced in order to increase stroke awareness. Disparities in stroke outcomes are affected by healthcare access and cultural practices. Because of this, underrepresented minorities may delay seeking care for signs and symptoms of stroke. In addition, males, African Americans, and Hispanics are less likely to use the EMS, which contributes to delay in seeking care.

56. **c) Utilitarianism**. This is an example of utilitarianism, which is the belief that the right act for the greatest good for the greatest number of people. Nonmaleficence is the duty to do no harm. Autonomy deals with the respect for individual's rights and beneficence is the duty to prevent harm and promote good.

57. **d) Verbal comfort with frequent reorientation should be attempted first**. Antipsychotics are indicated in the treatment of severe agitation and are noted to be superior to benzodiazepines; however, atypical antipsychotics have a black-box warning for treatment of Lewy body dementia and Parkinson's disease. Lorazepam is considered to be a second-line agent and is used to treat alcohol withdrawal and neuroleptic malignant syndrome. Studies support the use of haloperidol for the treatment of agitation; however, the patient has a history of Lewy body Parkinson's dementia that would place the patient at risk for increased extrapyramidal symptoms.

58. **c) Comparison** The intervention is the issue of interest that is being compared to the standard of care. Population delineates the patient group of interest and the outcome is the effect of the interventions.

59. **a) Add an ICS**. Daytime symptoms greater than 2 days per week require one step up. This patient was on step 1 with as-necessary SABA use only, but now requires step 2, which is the addition of an ICS.

60. **a) Primary prevention**. Categories of prevention include primary, secondary, and tertiary prevention. Primary prevention aims to remove or reduce risk factors for disease (e.g., immunizations); secondary-prevention strategies promote early detection of disease (e.g., Pap smear screening to detect carcinoma or dysplasia of the cervix); and tertiary-prevention measures are aimed at limiting the impact of an established disease (e.g., mastectomy for breast cancer).

61. **c) Relapsing/remitting**. There are four clinical types of MS: RRMS, SPMS, PPMS, and PRMS. RRMS accounts for 85% of MS cases at onset. PPMS do not experience attacks; rather, they have a steady functional decline. SPMS begins as RRMS, but the patient experiences a steady deterioration unassociated with acute attacks. PRMS experience a steady deterioration, but unlike SPMS, have occasional attacks superimposed on the progressive course.

62. **d) 99291-99292**. The codes 99291 and 99292 are critical care codes and can be used only with an inpatient or hospitalized patient. The outpatient codes are separated into two categories: new patient (99201-99205) and established patient (99211-99215). New patients require more time, data collection, and medical decision making. Therefore these codes will get more

reimbursement for services. Once the patient is an established patient in a practice, codes 99211-99215 will be used. Consultation services in observation status are reported with the outpatient consultation codes 99241–99245. The range of codes in both categories signifies the level of care been provided from Level 1 to Level 5. There are specific documentation criteria for each level that demonstrate more complicated patient care.

63. **b) Azithromycin 1 gram (g) oral single dose AND high-risk sexual counseling**. Chlamydia is a common sexually transmitted disease among those 15 to 24 years of age, who account for two-thirds of new cases. Chlamydia is common among MSM and those who engage in high-risk unprotected sexual behavior. Chlamydia can be transmitted during unprotected sex in the absence of ejaculation, or during oral or anal sex. Symptoms of *Chlamydia trachomatis* in men include a watery to mucus penile discharge, burning sensation during urination, and pain and swelling in one or both testicles. Diagnoses of chlamydia in men can be made by either obtaining a urethral swab, or first catch urine specimen using NAAT. This method is recommended due to the ease of testing as well as sensitivity and specificity. High-risk sexual education is recommended to reduce the risk for reinfection and minimize disease transmission, and sexual partners should be referred for evaluation, testing, and presumptive treatment if there has been a sexual encounter during the 60 days prior to the patient's onset of symptoms. Anyone diagnosed with chlamydia should be tested for HIV, gonorrhea, and syphilis. Recommended treatment includes the following: azithromycin 1 g orally single dose (recommended therapy onsite, which facilitates directly observed single-dose therapy) OR doxycycline 100 mg orally every 12 hours for 7 days. Alternative regimens are erythromycin base 500 mg orally every 6 hours for 7 days OR erythromycin ethylsuccinate 800 mg orally every 6 hours for 7 days OR levofloxacin 500 mg once daily for 7 days OR ofloxacin 300 mg by mouth every 12 hours for 7 days.

64. **b) Acute cholecystitis**. The diagnosis is made on a characteristic history and physical examination including the classic triad of onset of sudden, sharp pain to the right upper quadrant, fever, and leukocytosis. Ultrasound is the best choice of imaging for diagnosis, which will demonstrate calculi in many cases and is useful for detection of signs of gallbladder inflammation including thickening of the wall, pericholecystic fluid, and dilatation of the bile duct. In those with calculous cholecystitis, the classic presentation is the Charcot's triad of fever, right upper quadrant pain, and jaundice. The pain may radiate to the scapula or shoulder areas, especially on the right side. Other symptoms that may occur are anorexia, nausea, and emesis. Acute pancreatitis is characterized by severe, persistent, epigastric abdominal pain that may radiate to the flank and worsens while lying supine and improves with knees sitting up and flexed. AA pain may start as a mild periumbilical cramping that becomes more severe and radiates to right lower quadrant with associated nausea, emesis, abdominal swelling, and fever with a positive McBurney's point.

65. **c) High-dose steroid use**. Stress ulcer prophylaxis is indicated for mechanical ventilation greater than 48 hours, coagulopathy, high-dose steroid use. ICU admission, hypercoagulable states and mechanical ventilation less than 48 hours are not clear indications for PPI.

66. **d) PCV13 first, then 1 year later PPSV23**. According to the CDC guidelines, the recommendation for a healthy person is to receive the PCV 13, then 1 year later, PPSV23.

67. **a) Vitamin B_{12} 1mg subcutaneous for the first week, then monthly maintenance therapy**. Either subcutaneous or oral vitamin B_{12} therapy are appropriate options for this patient. However, the oral dose is 1000 ng orally daily, not 10,000 ngrams. The ongoing management plan will need to be discussed. Education is a very important factor as the patient had not been taking her medications and has developed symptoms of vitamin B_{12} deficiency. This patient needs proper education about taking daily medications for a chronic condition, but not on dietary intake of B_{12}, thus this is not the best answer. A multivitamin could be considered but is not part of the initial treatment plan.

68. **b) Evaluation of vibration and hearing loss; it allows for evaluation of sensorineural or conductive hearing loss**. The AG-ACNP will perform the Weber (sensorineural) and Rhinne (conductive) tests to see if there are any structural or conductive deficits. The use of a tuning

fork will allow for pitch discrimination but multiple forks will be needed. Tuning forks are not used to check for CSF leakage or focal pain in a skull fracture.

69. **c) Specific hospital job description and privileges requested.** Laws created by statutes from legislative bills are broader and more general, whereas regulations are more specific with details on how the legislation is enforced, but do not dictate to facilities what privileges they allow. Therefore, regulations may be more restrictive or lenient depending on the regulatory atmosphere of the state. It is the specific credentialing rules of the hospital and their interpretation, usually based on physician credentialing, that control the specific job description and privileges. Depending on the employer interpretations, more than certification and educational preparation control credentialing.

70. **b) Crash cart to bedside to begin transcutaneous pacing.** In a patient with bradycardic arrhythmia in the setting of ACS, the concern should be for high-degree AV block (either second-degree Mobitz II block or complete heart block). High-degree AV block is an absolute indication for transvenous pacing. In the urgent situation, the immediate answer would be to resort to ACLS measures, which indicates transcutaneous pacing. Dopamine might be indicated for unstable bradycardic arrhythmias, but vasoconstriction and increasing SVR is high-risk for this postmyocardial infarction patient. This complication is not an indication of in-stent restenosis. There is no indication that this complication was related to beta-blocker administration.

71. **a) Incision and drainage.** Incision and drainage is the recommended treatment for inflamed epidermoid cysts, carbuncles, abscesses, and large furuncles. This scenario is concerning for community-acquired MRSA due to treatment failure.

72. **b) "Incident to" billing cannot be used to bill for inpatient services under any circumstances.** Medicare rules are very specific for "incident to" billing. "Incident to" billing cannot be used for new patients, must be limited to the defined office-suite, and cannot be used in the inpatient setting.

73. **d) Decrease the carbohydrates at night.** Nocturnal hypoglycemia is a result of a surge of counterregulatory hormones resulting in a.m. hyperglycemia, thought to be the intake of excessive carbohydrate intake that results in the rebound hyperglycemia. The appropriate treatment is to reduce bedtime carbohydrates. Reducing the insulin will worsen the a.m. hyperglycemia. Adding a long-acting agent at night would not be helpful. Diet is the most efficacious method to deal with this issue.

74. **b) Explain everything that will be done with calm but firm direction.** The patient in the scenario is demonstrating acute psychosis of unclear etiology. The patient had not demonstrated aggressive or agitated behaviors and did not warrant a tranquilizer being ordered first. Advising the patient to seek psychiatric evaluation before making a complete assessment is premature management and does not address the acute psychosis. Ordering STAT lab tests will aid in excluding medical etiologies for the acute psychosis but should be done after an explanation of what to expect is done in an effort to show the patient respect and establish a trusting the relationship.

75. **a) St. Thomas risk assessment tool (STRATIFY).** In the hospital setting STRATIFY has been shown to have intermediate-to-high accuracy in discriminating fallers from nonfallers. This screening tool consists of five clinical factors related to falling with a simple scoring system. A positive score on ≥2 of the 5 items indicates an increased risk of falls. Another tool to use to assess fall risk in the hospital setting is Hendrick II Fall Risk model, which may have higher accuracy, but has not been widely adopted yet. A score of 5 or greater indicates high risk for fall. The TUG test is used in the community setting and a of score less than 20 seconds is normal and low risk for falls. The SPICES instrument is designed to prevent health alterations in several categories and is an alert system. The KATZ index provides information about activities of daily living and independent function.

76. **a) Hip fracture.** An external rotation of the leg is highly suspicious for a hip fracture or femur fracture. A leg may be shortened with a pelvic fracture but not usually rotated. Patella dislocation or ankle sprain does not shorten the leg.

77. **c) Compression stockings with a gradient of 30 to 40 mmHg.** Patient has stasis dermatitis as evidence by edema, erythema, scaling, and increased pigmentation. Findings associated with stasis dermatitis are typically seen over the medial aspect of the ankles. Patients with stasis dermatitis benefit from compression stockings with a compression gradient of 30 to 40 mmHg. Antiembolism hose will not provide that type of support. Antibiotics are not indicated in the case of stasis dermatitis unless there is concern for underlying infection. In this case the legs are not warm and the patient is afebrile. Topical glucocorticoids may be used to decrease pruritus but systemic glucocorticoids are not indicated as treatment.

78. **c) Formulate a clinical research question.** The most important step in the EBP to identify the best and most relevant evidence is to formulate a specific PICOT question.

79. **c) Alzheimer's dementia.** The patient has a classic presentation of Alzheimer's dementia. There is a slow insidious onset with short-term memory loss and problems completing more complex activities of daily living, such as bill paying. Normal age-related changes do not include the described scenario. Vascular dementia is differentiated by a history of stroke temporally related to the symptoms. Delirium is an acute process without a history of the gradual and insidious decline in cognitive function. The ability to get to the senior center to volunteer and play the piano do not rule out Alzheimer's, as procedural memory may stay intact for extended length of time.

80. **a) Assess the patient's level of health literacy and barriers for self-care.** The assessment of a patient's health literacy with evidence-based and validated tools has proven to improve the quality and usefulness of patient education materials. This is the best choice because this is the third visit in a relatively short period of time in a young and otherwise healthy female for the same medical problem. Addressing the patient's health literacy can help to effectively reduce health disparities and improve the patient's quality and safety of care. The other choices provided may be appropriate after the patient's health literacy is assessed and validated.

81. **c) Creatinine clearance 45 mlL/min.** Twelve or more medication doses per day are typically associated with adverse drug reactions. Patients with a low body mass index (<18.5 BMI) would also be a risk factor especially in older adults. A person with a BMI of 22 has adequate body weight. A creatinine clearance of less than 50 mL/min places an individual at risk for an adverse drug reaction because elimination of medication is decreased. This decrease is related to smaller renal size, decreased blood flow, and functioning nephrons. Gender has no impact on adverse drug reactions.

82. **b) Tell me about these reddened areas on your back?** Involving the patient in the treatment plan helps build trust between the AG-ACNP and patient and increases the patient's adherence to the course of treatment. The most effective models for providing patient-centered approach to care start with a nonjudgmental or assumption-based question that offers the patient the opportunity to explain her situation/experience and give the AG-ACNP the opportunity to listen. The other answers are based on assumptions. Two prominent models are LEARN: Listen, Explain, Acknowledge, Recommend, Negotiate, and ETHNIC: Explanation, Treatment, Healers, Negotiate, Intervention, Collaboration.

83. **b) Hard palate, soft palate, base of uvula.** The higher the Mallampati score, the more obstructed the view is in the posterior oropharynx, thus, the more severe the OSA.

84. **b) Requires intubation.** If a patient requires intubation, a chest tube needs to be placed because positive pressure ventilation can turn a small pneumothorax into a life-threatening tension pneumothorax. The other conditions do not warrant a chest tube to be placed.

85. **c) Arrange for inpatient admission.** The assessment findings of JVD, bilateral crackles, and pink-frothy sputum should lead the AG-ACNP toward a likely diagnosis of fluid volume overload, which is evidence of acute decompensation of his chronic heart failure. Patients

with excess fluid volume refractory to outpatient therapies should be considered for inpatient admission to facilitate further evaluation and fluid volume management. Further escalation of oral furosemide doses is unnecessary at this point, and will likely not be of benefit, as absorption of oral medications is lessened in the setting of severe fluid volume overload. There is no indication in this scenario for immediate suspicion of infectious or embolic processes.

86. **b) Temporal arteritis**. Giant cell arteritis is more common in women who are older than 50 years and patients of Scandinavian descent; rarely in African American populations. Classic signs are similar to polymyalgia rheumatic pain and stiffness of the neck, shoulders, low back, hips, and thighs. Signs of inflammation include elevated sedimentation rate and CRP. While meningitis has a fever, there is no change in mental status. In addition, the neck pain in meningitis is nuchal rigidity with Kernig or Brudzinski's sign that indicate meningeal irritation. Migraines do not typically have fevers, increased ESR, or CRP. Brain tumors may cause headaches, but they do not typically present with fevers and muscle aches. They usually have focal neurological symptoms that occur dependent on the location of the tumor location.

87. **a) Abdominal ultrasound**. Abdominal ultrasonography is the diagnostic study of choice for initial screening for the presence of an abdominal aortic aneurysm. Calcifications within the aneurysmal sac can sometimes be noted on plain-film x-rays, but this is not indicated as the initial diagnostic tool. A contrasted CT scan will provide more detailed information about aneurysm diameter, and should be done when the aneurysm nears 5.5 cm. Endovascular ultrasound is not indicated for the diagnosis of abdominal aortic aneurysm.

88. **a) The serum creatinine rises by 1.5 fold or greater from the baseline value**. The definition of contrast-induced AKI, according to the Renal Association, British Cardiovascular Intervention Society, and the Royal College of Radiologists, is when one of the following criteria is met: (1) serum creatinine rises by greater than or equal to 26 millimoles within 48 hours, (2) serum creatinine rises greater than or equal to 1.5-fold from the baseline value which known or presumed to have occurred within 1 week, or (3) urine output is less than .5 milliliters per kilogram per hour for greater than six consecutive hours.

89. **b) Veracity**. Veracity is the duty to be truthful. In this situation you would be expected to present all studies related to the approval of the medication by the FDA. Justice is the duty to be fair and fidelity is the duty to be faithful. Autonomy is the duty to respect an individual's thoughts and actions.

90. **b) AG-ACNPs practice within their SOP**. Shared visits are a concept used in reimbursement practice but it is not a code. The physician and NP or physician assistant (PA) can "share" the development and implementation of a plan of care for a patient, but strict criteria need to be met. The providers need to be in the same practice, the AG-ACNP must be practicing within his/her SOP, and it must be a same-day encounter. The AG-ACNP can see patients, develop a plan, and document that plan in a note. The physician must link his/her assessment with the AG-ACNP note and one of the following three components must be documented: history, exam, or medical decision making. The critical criterion that is often overlooked is that the physician must have a face-to-face encounter with the patient IF 100% reimbursement is desired. If any of these criteria are not satisfied, the AG-ACNP can bill at 85% under his/her NPI. CMS is closely monitoring this reimbursement practice to assure compliance.

91. **b) 24-hour pH esophageal and pharyngeal pH monitoring**. The classic hallmark symptoms of GERD are substernal burning or warmth that is aggravated by the supine position and ingestion of large meals. Most diagnosis and treatment can be started with acid reduction and lifestyle alterations. This patient can still use counseling for the latter. However, some patients with known GERD require more involved diagnostic tests, which included a barium swallow, pH monitoring, and, often, a flexible endoscopy, all which the GI medicine referral will help her with. The Nissen fundoplication is a surgical treatment for GERD, not

a diagnostic test. CT scan is not indicated. While an EGD is appropriate, a colonoscopy is not indicated.

92. **b) Treat current infection and delay ART until improved.** No treatment should be started when the patient is sick if the patient has been off a medication regimen, due to fear of reconstitution syndrome. In HIV infections, an exaggerated inflammatory response to a disease-causing microorganism can occur when the immune system starts to recover following treatment with ART. IRIS occurs in two forms: "unmasking" IRIS refers to the flare-up of an underlying, previously undiagnosed infection soon after ART is started; "paradoxical" IRIS refers to the worsening of a previously treated infection after ART is started. IRIS can be mild or life-threatening.

93. **c) 1.5 L (1500 mL).** When chest tube drainage exceeds 1.5 L it is considered massive and surgical intervention needs to be considered.

94. **b) Smoking cessation.** Initial attempts to manage PAD are conservative, focusing on risk-factor modification such as smoking cessation, blood pressure management, weight loss, and exercise. Revascularization attempts with stents or bypass surgery are reserved for patients with significant disability and failure of conservative therapies. There is no indication for warfarin therapy solely related to PAD.

95. **a) Chest radiograph.** While CAP can be diagnosed in the absence of chest radiograph, it is recommended to obtain one. CT scans will provide additional information and can be useful in diagnosing lung pathology it is not required in suspected CAP, nor are they cost effective. Flu swab and RVP may be appropriate based on history; it will not confirm a diagnosis of pneumonia.

96. **a) "The MMR is a live vaccine and with your low CD4 count, you may become infected."** The MMR is a live vaccine and is contraindicated in patients with CD4 count less than 200 cells/μL. It is also contraindicated in patients who are receiving chemotherapy.

97. **d) Acknowledge one's own distress and determine if another provider should assume care.** Reflective practice of one's own beliefs and affective responses to patient's healthcare decisions can cause moral distress and provoke strong emotions within the AG-ACNP. The provider must be self-aware and reflective enough to identify when the therapeutic AG-ACNP-patient relationship is threatened by opposing views. Informing the patient's spouse of the patient's plan would be unethical and a breach of the patient's privacy and confidentiality. Inquiring of the patient about her support system's availability to assist with her decision making may lend the patient to perceive the AG-ACNP's motive is judgmental and is inferring she is not capable of making the decision on her own. Behavior coaching techniques are aimed to facilitating long-term lifestyle changes related to high-risk behaviors leading to chronic illness. This technique would not be indicated for this scenario.

98. **c) The physician must perform the initial plan of care, subsequent follow-up frequency that reflects his/her active participation in the clinic.** The key to answering this question is when "incident to" evaluation and management (E/M) billing is allowed. It is never allowed in a hospital setting. Either the AG-ACNP bills under his/her NPI, at 85% of the allowable medical billing, or in most settings the E/M is billed after physicians' attestation under the physician's NPI number. Care provided in the physician's office on established patients can be under the "incident to" billing rules as long as the physician is immediately available, and the physician must perform the initial service or plan of care and establish frequency of follow-up reflecting his/her active participation in care of the patient. The patient usually sees the physician once a year.

99. **a) 12,600.** The Parkland formula is 4 mL/kg/TBSA percentage burn.

100. **b) Cardiogenic shock.** Cardiogenic shock is defined by both clinical signs of a low-flow state and associated hemodynamic measurements. This client's left ventricular filling pressure is very elevated, and CI is very low. There is no evidence of hypovolemia. The client's hypotension is most likely mediated by poor cardiac performance. Sepsis may present with hypotension as well, but the key findings here are the hemodynamic disturbances.

101. **a) Obtain rapid antigen detection test,** to assess for streptococcus group B, which has a specificity >90%. Treatment can be considered with amoxicillin; however, dosing is 500 mg by mouth daily. When rapid antigen detection tests are negative, the CDC does not recommend obtaining backup cultures in adults. Metronidazole is commonly used to treat anaerobic organisms found in the mouth; however, it will not treat streptococcus.

102. **b) Reading and understanding published research reports**. A foundational skill for nurses and AG-ACNPs is to be able to read and understand clinical trials, systematic reviews, and clinical practice guidelines. Performing research or integrative reviews requires more advanced skills and education in research methodology. Working with a researcher may not be part of the position description.

103. **b) Fidelity**. Fidelity is the commitment of faithfulness and our obligation to others. If the patient is competent, the patient has the right to determine who has access to personal information about the patient's health, regardless of the outcome.

104. **c) Pay attention to nonverbal expressions of the patient and communicate explanations of care and reassurance to the patient**. Research findings indicate comatose patients have reported being able to hear and understand statements spoken to them while unconscious. The AG-ACNP should continue communicating with the unconscious patient to not only provide the patient with information but also provide the patient with emotional support, thereby reinforcing the patient-AG-ACNP therapeutic relationship. Sedation and analgesia will provide comfort but will not facilitate the AG-ACNP–patient relationship. The family can certainly communicate to the AG-ACNP information that the AG-ACNP may not know; however, it is important for the AG-ACNP to communicate to the patient on his/her own behalf.

105. **d) Hypertensive cardiovascular disease**. This client is displaying signs of volume overload and heart failure, likely secondary to long-standing arterial hypertension. There is no indication of coronary atherosclerosis, though his heart failure exacerbation and hypertension certainly may produce demand ischemia. Renal artery stenosis is a potential etiology for his hypertension, but not directly responsible for his current condition. Aortic dissection is another potential complication of hypertension, but his current symptoms do not seem to suggest this diagnosis. Diastolic dysfunction and LV hypertrophy are associated with hypertensive cardiac disease.

106. **a) 3 to 6 months**. Thyroid nodules are frequently found incidentally, depending on the imaging modality. If discovered and the patient is asymptomatic and the nodule is of borderline concern, follow up with ultrasound is recommended every 3 to 6 months. Yearly or every 5 and 10 years are too long a time period for follow-up.

107. **a) Squeeze test**. The squeeze test is a confirmatory provocative test for syndesmotic ankle sprain. The examiner supports the lateral fibula and tibia with one hand and gently forces external rotation with the other. Pain at the distal syndesmosis (at lateral malleolus) confirms distal syndesmotic ligamentous injury. The Talar tilt test is done to determine joint instability. Anterior drawer test of the ankle detects excessive anterior displacement of the talus on the tibia. Hawkins test is used to determine rotator cuff impingement.

108. **a) Practices, past history of sexually transmitted diseasesTDs, protection for STDs, pregnancy plans**. The CDC recommends the "five Ps" for taking a sexual history: assessment of numbers of *partners* and their gender, *practices* (referring to social habits), *past* history of STDs, *protection* from STDs, and *pregnancy* plans.

109. **c) Spleen**. Understanding mechanism of injury is key to anticipating injuries. The spleen is the most commonly injured organ in blunt trauma. Liver trauma can be blunt or penetrating; large and small intestines are more commonly injured in penetrating trauma.

110. **a) The confusing outbursts are common in patients after a stroke, and it is known as PBA.** PBA is very common in poststroke patients and should not be confused with depression, posttraumatic stress disorder, or anxiety.

111. **b) Immediate cardiac surgery for repair.** Immediate surgical repair of the ruptured valve is essential for the client's survival. There is no indication for left heart catheterization. Efforts to manage heart failure will not be effective without mitral valve repair, and may complicate her condition further.

112. **c) Polycythemia.** Chronic bronchitis is a condition of excess mucus production causing hypoxemia causing compensatory increase in red blood cell production resulting in polycythemia. Both chronic bronchitis and emphysema are conditions resulting in carbon dioxide retention causing respiratory acidosis and metabolic retention of bicarb. As a result, chloride is excreted producing, hypochloremia. Emphysema is a condition of alveolar distention, loss of elastic recoil, and air trapping that causes increase in AP diameter. Both chronic bronchitis and emphysema are conditions resulting in carbon dioxide retention causing respiratory acidosis.

113. **b) Inferior myocardial infarction.** ST segment elevation in Leads II, III, and aVF represents an inferior myocardial infarction. An anterior myocardial infarction would be leads V3 and V4, a septal myocardial infarction would be leads V1 and V2, and a lateral myocardial infarction would be V4 and V5 as well as including Leads aVL and I.

114. **c) Evaluate the patient; identify when the patient was last seen normal.** Bedside physical assessment of the patient with NIH stroke score by the AG-ACNP is critical and an accurate history must be obtained to determine if the patient is experiencing a CVA prior to ordering diagnostic tests and lab work.

115. **b) Aerosolized racemic epinephrine.** Stridor that is due to upper airway edema can be treated with cool mist, aerosolized racemic epinephrine, parenteral steroids, and heilox. Place the amount of oxygen at the level the patient was receiving unless there is desaturation. The patient does not have vocal cord paralysis. Edema due to vocal cord paralysis would require reintubation. Tracheostomy would be performed for mechanical ventilation dependency.

116. **c) Diverticulitis.** Bowel source infections such as diverticulitis can contribute to enteric peritonitis and should be considered if two or more enteric organisms are noted in the culture. If the culture indicates an anaerobe or a fungus, it suggests an intra-abdominal cause of the peritonitis.

117. **d) Quality Payment Program.** Resource-based relative value scale is part of the system that allows the calculation of RVUs. MACRA will eventually eliminate the RVU calculation. The implementation of this legislation will occur over several years. Outpatient services are the initial focus of these changes but inpatient services will also be eventually affected. The AG-ACNP needs to become familiar with the QPP reporting systems that will be used by insurance companies and become more efficient in reporting patient outcomes. MIPS, Advanced Alternative Payment Models, and the QPP are all part of MACRA.

118. **b) Governed by the nurse practice act.** SOP is governed by state laws, which vary widely from state to state. ANA sets the standard for all nursing professionals but does not govern practice. There are many states with FPA and many without; unfortunately, this is not based on standards but on legislative statutes, which is frequently controlled by influence of various entities, some which may not be supportive of APRNs.

119. **d) Septic shock.** The patient is exhibiting septic shock with fever, tachypnea, mental status changes, and hemodynamic instability. If the patient was in early stages, such as infection, SIRS, or sepsis, the response to the fluid resuscitation would have normalized the patient's vital signs.

120. **d) Embolic event to the left middle cerebral artery**. Atrial fibrillation places the patient at high risk for embolic stroke and may be associated with cardiac surgery. With occlusion of the left middle cerebral artery, the signs and symptoms present contralaterally with right-sided hemiplegia. A hemorrhagic stroke is most commonly associated with hypertension and a subarachnoid hemorrhage typically presents as the "worst headache of a patient's life."

121. **c) CT imaging of the abdomen**. CT is the most accurate mode of imaging in suspected appendicitis; however, radiation is a concern. Ultrasound is beneficial while decreasing the need for CT in some situations, but is operator dependent. Laboratory markers and clinical signs have very limited diagnostic utility on their own but show promise when used in combination, such as the Alvarda score. Plain films are rarely helpful and not routinely obtained. Low-grade fever, nausea, and vomiting are too generalized to be diagnostic for appendicitis alone.

122. **c) Hypercalcemia**. Hypercalcemia is a paraneoplastic syndrome associated with squamous cell carcinoma of the lung. Symptoms of hypercalcemia are constipation, nausea, and poor appetite. Patients with hypercalcemia will typically have hypomagnesemia. Hyperkalemia will cause muscle weakness and nausea; it does not typically cause constipation. Hyperuricemia will cause joint pain and does not cause constipation.

123. **a) A prolongation of PR interval from beat to beat until a P wave is not conducted**. Wenckebach is characterized by prolongation of the PR interval from beat to beat until a P wave is not followed by a QRS, but no change in QT interval. A randomly dropped beat is more typical of a Mobitz II. A PR interval less than normal (<0.12 seconds) is a first-degree heart block, but there is no dropped beat.

124. **d) CT scan of the abdomen with IV contrast**. The reported positive-predictive values of CT is 95% to 97% and the overall accuracy is 90% to 98%. Neither (FAST) focused assessment with sonography for trauma or abdominal ultrasound with vascular duplex will aide in the diagnosis of acute appendicitis.An x-ray of the abdomen is rarely of value except when an opaque fecalith (5% of cases) is observed in the right lower quadrant.

125. **c) Secure the airway with expert consultation**. This patient likely has epiglottitis. Securing the airway is the highest priority by experts in airway management. Direct visualization of the larynx in the ED with tongue depressor and laryngoscopy can cause laryngospasm and complete airway obstruction. Intubation with fiberoptic laryngoscopy should be performed in a controlled environment (i.e., operating room). Obtaining plain films or labs would delay the management of the airway. X-ray may demonstrate a "thumbprint" sign, whereas labs would demonstrate leukocytosis with bandemia and commonly positive blood cultures for *H. influenza*.

126. **b) TSH concentration of 11 mU/L**. TSH concentration of 11 mU/L as a TSH greater than 10 mU/L warrants treatment for subclinical hypothyroidism, as does the presence of symptoms, TPO antibodies, or risk factors in younger patients with a TSH concentration of 4 to 10 mU/L.

127. **a) Forced air warming blanket and warm IV fluids**. The choice of rewarming is influenced by several factors, including clinical condition, heart rhythm, and availability of resources. This patient is in the ED, and rewarming with forced air blankets and warm fluids is appropriate. Bypass and hemodialysis take additional resources that may not be readily available.

128. **b) Acts hastily in treating an aneurysm, resulting in otherwise avoidable partial paralysis**. Malpractice is failing to render services/care with the same diligence and precaution that another AG-ACNP would render under similar situation, thus permanent damage occurred by acting hastily in care of the patient. Failure to act in a reasonable fashion, resulting in an injury, is negligence. Releasing information about a patient's medical condition damaging his reputation is slander. Hitting someone is battery.

129. **a) Start the patient on amlodipine (Norvasc).** Calcium channel blockers are preferred over ACE inhibitors and beta-blockers in the African American population. In addition, lisinopril is less effective in African Americans, and while hydrochlorothiazide may be effective in controlling blood pressure by decreasing circulating blood volume, adding furosemide places the patient at risk for hypokalemia. The current recommendation is to have the patient on a diuretic and a calcium channel blocker.

130. **b) Use of night splint of wrist and forearm.** Carpal tunnel is caused by compression of the median nerve. Splinting the wrist in a neutral position provided the best relief and is the first line of treatment. If splinting is not effective, then cortisone injection is beneficial.

131. **a) Stress.** Scientific knowledge has found causal pathways and physiologic mechanisms that can explain the links between socioeconomic factors and health. One of the biggest factors is the physiologic damage to multiple vital organ systems caused by chronic stress, through neuroendocrine and immune pathways. While anxiety and depression can adversely affect ones report of overall health, it does not cause the same level of physical responses.

132. **b) Motivational interviewing.** The patient has ongoing risk-taking behavior (i.e., smoking) that is negatively impacting his health. Motivational interviewing has been found to be helpful in these types of risk-taking behaviors.

133. **d) Avoid smoking, caffeinated beverages, or exercise within 30 minutes before taking your blood pressure.** The patient should be instructed to sit in a straight-backed chair with feet flat on the floor. Rest at least 5 minutes before taking the blood pressure is needed, not 20 minutes. Home blood pressure measurements should identify if there is a significant difference of blood pressure readings between the patient's arms. However, AG-ACNPs should instruct the patient to use the arm with the highest blood pressure for consistency.

134. **d) Immediate cardiac catheterization.** The patient is having an acute anterior STEMI and needs immediate reperfusion therapy. Given that he is presenting late, at 3 hours, the first choice, if possible, is primary angioplasty. If this procedure cannot be performed quickly, he has no absolute contraindications to thrombolytic therapy and should receive it as soon as possible. He should be immediately considered for cardiac catheterization. Immediate cardiac catheterization is preferable, especially in someone who is presenting more than 3 hours after the onset of symptoms.

135. **c) True partnership that values expertise, power, and respect on all sides.** It is a balance of power among leaders and subordinates. Communication among the team recognizes and appreciates alternative viewpoints and includes perspectives from all levels of employment.

136. **b) Talk with the nurse.** This is no longer an acceptable SOP for clearing airways. The nurse needs immediate coaching to correct the behavior. Addressing this one on one with the nurse is the best avenue to maintain safe patient care and a professional relationship with the nurse.

137. **c) State laws and regulations.** Some states regulate the SOP bylaws, while others give that authority to the individual SBON.

138. **a) Daily interruption of sedation and spontaneous breathing trials.** Daily interruption of sedation and SBT are the best predictor of liberation from mechanical ventilation. Patients should be able to follow you with eyes, grasp tongue, and lift head off of the bed. While decreasing the level of oxygen near the level of atmospheric oxygen is recommended, the level of inspiratory capacity should be at least 15 mL/kg. The leak test and NIFs are not good indicators of assessing extubation; a patient may still have a normal leak test and fail extubation. Air leak tests assess for the presence of airway edema and inflammation. The leak test is the amount of expired air with cuff inflated over the next six breaths. Take the mean of the lowest three expired tidal volumes minus the expired tidal volume with the cuff deflated. This is the cuff leak volume. A cuff leak volume ≥ 110 milliliters is predictive of postextubation stridor. Pressure support of 5 to 10 cm H_2O is used during weaning trials.

139. **c) Volume control with low tidal volumes**. Volume control with low tidal volumes 4 to 6 mL/kg is a protective lung strategy to prevent volutrauma. Addition of PEEP is also needed to maintain mean airway levels. The goal FiO_2 is less than or equal to 50%. 100% nonrebreather will cause additional atelectasis and not improve gas exchange. The patient does not need to augment inspiration with higher inspiratory pressure. Volume control ventilation with increased tidal volumes will put the patient at risk for volutrauma.

140. **d) Bedside-focused assessment with sonography for trauma examination**. This is the fastest/most specific way to evaluate for acute abdominal bleeding. CT chest, although good at detecting abdominal bleeding, will take time to complete and the patient is presently unstable. Radiography will take too long and is not specific enough to evaluate for abdominal bleeding. Peritoneal lavage used to be the standard of practice but is not as specific as thought and can actually cause more trauma if not done by a skilled clinician.

141. **c) Indicated based on his presentation**. Because of the evidence linking early PCI to improved survival outcome, the 2015 American Heart Association guidelines recommend that all patients successfully resuscitated from cardiac arrest of suspected cardiac etiology should be considered for emergent coronary angiography. The patient in this scenario has known CAD. This recommendation applies regardless of neurologic status or presenting arrest rhythm.

142. **b) Discuss the need to adjust the infusion rate to be given over 30 minutes**. Dilantin infusion cannot exceed 50 mg/min due to cardiac depression, hypotension, and bradycardia. The faster it is administered the more likely these will occur. The dose of 70 kg*20 mg = (1400 mg)/(50 mg/min) = 28 minutes. The patient has already received two doses of lorazepam, thus pursuing a second-line agent is correct; however, there is a problem with his order as is that needs to be corrected. Lorazepam has already been given twice and a total dose should not exceed 0.1 mg per kg. Loading dose for new onset seizures is 20 mg/kg, whereas 100 mg Q 8 hours can be the maintenance dose to maintain therapeutic levels.

143. **c) Hypotension**. Hypotension is the most common complication of hemodialysis due to fluid and shifts. Decreasing flow rates or reducing the amount of volume being removed can reduce the hypotension. Albumin is commonly used to treat hypotension. Muscle cramps can occur due to electrolyte fluctuations, but it is not the most common complication seen in hemodialysis.

144. **c) Nutritional therapy**. CD and ulcerative colitis are both chronic, relapsing inflammatory disorders of the GI tract. In both CD and ulcerative colitis, there is leukocyte infiltration of the GI mucosa which causes epithelial damage. Conventional therapy aims at managing the immune system response. Ulcerative colitis is localized to the colon, whereas any part of the GI track can be affected by CD. Nutritional therapy is often essential in CD due to the development of short bowel syndrome, strictures, and enteric fistulae being the underlying pathology. Nutrition therapy is also used to augment malnutrition before surgical interventions to decrease surgical risks. CD is the second common indication for HPN. With development of intestinal failure, nutritional management including HPN is required as a rescue therapy.

145. **c) CLL**. CLL is a malignancy of mature B cells characterized by progressive lymphocytosis, lymphadenopathy, splenomegaly, and cytopenias. The patient is experiencing "B" related symptoms that are specific to night sweats and lymphadenopathy. The WBC is elevated related to lymphocytosis. In a patient with CAP, leukocytosis would be expected; however, neutrophilia would be the cause. CML is characterized by an increase in the granulocytic cell line (leukocytosis) and platelet hyperplasia, thus thrombocytosis. Myelodysplastic syndrome supports cell dysplasia; therefore, a decrease in WBC, red blood cells, and platelets would be expected.

146. **a) TACO**. Although dependent atelectasis can arise from a prolonged operation (e.g., CABG/MVR/AVR) procedures, TACO is the most likely source here given the transfusion of 6 units packed red blood cells and 2 units FFP. TRALI is also related to blood product

transfusion; however, there is usually hypotension and leukocytosis in this immune medi-ated response. Acute myocardial infarction (AMI) may occur but likely will not cause car-diomegaly with associated pulmonary edema.

147. **c) Ascending cholangitis.** The most likely diagnosis is ascending cholangitis caused by obstruction of the common bile duct. Seventy percent of patients present with Charcot's triad of jaundice, fever, and abdominal pain. Additional sign of shock and confusion is Reynold's pentad, which is associated with high mortality rates. While this patient may also have acute cholecystitis, it does not typically present with jaundice. Hepatitis can cause jaundice but not typically the sepsis-like picture. Gastric outlet obstruction does not cause this clinical picture.

148. **a) Cardiogenic shock.** Clinical signs of cardiogenic shock include evidence of poor car-diac output with tissue hypoperfusion (hypotension, mental status changes, cool mottled skin) and evidence of volume overload (dyspnea, rales, JVD). Hemodynamic criteria for cardiogenic shock include (1) sustained hypotension (systolic blood pressure <90 mmHg), (2) reduced CI (<2.2 L/min/m^2), and (3) an elevated (>18 mmHg) PAOP.

149. **a) HHS.** HHS typically presents in patients with DMII. Patients may be with a change in mental status ranging from lethargy to coma and have a several-week history of polyuria, polydipsia, and weight loss. Because there is no development of acidosis, there is usu-ally not nausea, vomiting, abdominal pain, or Kussmaul respirations. Hallmark findings in HHS are severely elevated glucose levels, elevated osmolality, and prerenal azotemia due to severe volume loss. It's not uncommon for patients to present in hypovolemic shock. DKA and alcoholic ketoacidosis would demonstrate acidosis, ketosis, and ketonuria. Myxedema coma may present with depressed mental status or even coma, but not with the same elec-trolyte and glucose abnormalities.

150. **a) Tracheal collapse.** Changing out a tracheostomy tube can cause the trachea to collapse in an obese patient. The trachea can also collapse in patients who have a neck mass. Tra-cheal malacia is softening of the tracheal rings. A patient with tracheal malacia would have issues with returning volumes on mechanical ventilation. Tracheal stenosis can occur due to mucosal necrosis and scarring from weeks to months after decannulation. Chest x-ray may show a narrowing airway. Treatment is humidified oxygen and nebulized racemic epinephrine and steroids. Surgical procedure is rigid bronchoscopy with laser excision, stenting and even tracheal reconstruction. Tracheoinnominate artery fistula is caused from pressure from the tracheal tube or cuff on the innominate artery. This usually presents in the first 3 weeks of a tracheostomy. It also can occur in tracheostomies that are placed lower in the trachea, which is closer to the innominate artery. Management includes hyperinflating the tracheostomy cuff to control the bleeding while preparing for surgery.

151. **c) Cardiac catheterization.** Diagnostics to confirm the diagnosis of pulmonary hypertension are transthoracic echocardiogram, and other diagnostics to identify other pulmonary causes as pulmonary function studies and CT of the chest. However, the gold standard is a cardiac catheterization. A chest x-ray would identify lung pathology, not pulmonary hypertension. ECG is with 55% sensitivity and specificity of 70%. The ECG will show right axis deviation, right axis deviation with a right bundle branch block, and an R/S ratio $\geq$1 in lead V, an S wave greater than 7 mm deep in V5 or V6, incomplete right bundle branch block. MRI is an important diagnostic in assessing diseases of the heart, mediastinum, pleura, and chest wall, but is not sufficient to diagnose pulmonary hypertension.

152. **c) Get the patient to a maximum HMG-CoA reductase inhibitor dose.** The 2013 American College of Cardiology/American Heart Association guideline for the treatment of blood cholesterol does not recommend treating to specific LDL targets. Instead, appropriate statin therapy should be selected based on risk category. The goal is to get the patient to a max-imal dose of statin and not a specific LDL. The FDA no longer recommends periodic liver enzyme testing while on a statin. Statin-related hepatotoxicity is an idiosyncratic reaction that is extremely rare and completely unpredictable, so there is no point in routinely check-ing transaminases.

153. **d) Cocaine**. Cocaine can cause seizure due to alteration of neuronal excitability and can therefore lower the seizure threshold in a patient. Marijuana would be concerning for the potential to be laced with another drug of abuse, but itself is not a cause of seizures. Heroin withdrawal could cause seizures, but use of heroin itself does not cause seizures. Nicotine usage has numerous long-term effects on the body, but recent usage is not a trigger for seizure activity.

154. **b) Diclofenac (Zorvolex)**. Older adults are at increased risk for AKI. Polypharmacy and drug toxicity pose an increased susceptibility to AKI and chronic kidney disease. Drugs commonly associated with AKI among older adults are NSAIDs, diuretics, ACE inhibitors, ARBs, antibiotics, and contract agents. Older patients who are started on an NSAID face double the risk for AKI at 65 years of age or older, and have an increased risk of being hospitalized within the first 45 initiating NSAID therapy.

155. **c) Assess for intra-abdominal hypertension**. Patients undergoing emergent surgery requiring aggressive resuscitation are at risk for third spacing, as well as intestinal edema. This may occur minutes to hours after surgery, especially when continued resuscitation is ongoing. The closed and recently operated-on abdomen has decreased compliance and as a result intra-abdominal hypertension can develop. If unchecked, intra-abdominal hypertension progresses to abdominal compartment syndrome, which is shown with numerous clinical signs and symptoms. These include increased peak airway pressure, decreased tidal volume, hypoxia, decreased urine output, and hypotension, to name a few. If symptoms are identified early, medical management may avert the need for surgical decompression. Intra-abdominal pressures can be quickly measured via a bladder pressure, hence the first step in assessing this patient.

156. **c) No, this is an anticipated side effect of dexmedetomidine hydrochloride (Precedex)**. It is very likely he is exhibiting signs of dexmedetomidine use, which includes hypotension and bradycardia. Although his RASS is +2 without hypertension and tachycardia, this can be muted by sedation. Although he has no medical history, it is unknown if he is a marathon runner so it is not safe to assume this. Hypotension and bradycardia are signs of neurogenic shock, but the mechanism of injury does not necessarily support this diagnosis, making it more likely to be a side effect of dexmedetomidine. Bradycardia is a side effect of hypoxemia; however, his SPO_2 of 90% at 50% FIO_2 is a P:F of 180 which is a moderate lung injury; as with neurogenic shock, dexmedetomidine is most likely the cause of his bradycardia and hypotension. The AG-ACNP should anticipate the use of a synergistic analgesic medication and/or change to a different sedative agent.

157. **c) Class III**. The New York Heart Association classification is a tool to define criteria that describe the functional ability and clinical manifestations of patients with heart failure. These criteria have been shown to have prognostic value with worsening survival as the class increases. They are also useful to clinicians when reading studies to understand the entry and exclusion criteria for clinical trials. Class I is used for patients with no limiting symptoms; Class II for patients with slight or mild limitations; Class III implies no symptoms at rest but dyspnea or angina or palpitations with little exertion, patients are moderately limited; Class IV is for severely limited, so that even minimal activity causes symptoms. This patient has symptoms with mild exertion that is comfortable at rest; therefore, he is New York Heart Association Class III.

158. **a) Zostavax**. Live vaccines should be avoided in persons with CD4 counts lower than 200. Zostavax (shingles vaccine) is a live vaccine. Patients who are immunocompromised and receive a live vaccine are at increased risk for developing the actual disease. Pneumococcal, Tdap, and influenza are examples of inactivated vaccines.

159. **b) Right bundle branch block**. Right bundle branch block is seen in patients who are having a pulmonary embolism. Sinus tachycardia is commonly seen in patients with pulmonary embolism. A right bundle branch is seen on ECG and not a left bundle branch block. A patient with a pulmonary embolism will show precordial T wave inversions.

160. **b) Start labetalol drip**. This patient likely has an aneurysmal SAH. Classic signs include "worse headache of life," nausea, vomiting, photophobia, and nuchal rigidity as well as seizures. The patient's blood pressure is too high and needs to be addressed first to prevent rebleeding. Thus, labetalol is fast acting and can easily be titrated. A commonly used alternative is a nicardipine (Cardene) infusion. The aneurysm needs to be secured, but can be done intravascularly rather than open craniotomy, as the aneurysms are usually deep in the brain. Seizure prophylaxis is important, especially given the location of the SAH. This patient could likely seize and will need to be given an anticonvulsant, but this is not the highest priority. This patient could benefit from oxygen therapy, as hypoxia should not be tolerated in this patient and basic lab work will be crucial, but again, not the FIRST thing to do.

161. **c) Contrast nephropathy**. Contrast-induced nephropathy is defined as renal failure which occurs within 48 hours of undergoing diagnostic testing in which intravascular radiographic contrast was utilized. No other identifiable cause can be associated with the changes in serum creatinine. Contrast-induced nephropathy can be defined as a 0.5 to 1.0 mg/dL increase in serum creatinine from baseline. Renal dosing is recommended in patients who have severe renal impairment and are at increased risks for hyperkalemia and bleeding. Protein C deficiency is a hematological disorder which increases the risk for the development of deep vein thrombosis or other thrombolic events.

162. **a) Cholecystitis**. Patients with biliary disease may present with symptoms ranging from mild to severe, intermittent or constant, and physical exam reveals right upper quadrant tenderness to palpation of the epigastrum, and Murphy's sign (increased pain or inspiratory arrest during deep subcostal palpation of the right upper quadrant during inspiration). Acute pancreatitis occurs more often in alcoholics, and is characterized by mid-epigastric, constant pain that radiates to the back. Physical exam findings may be mid-epigastric, right upper quadrant, or left upper quadrant pain but without a positive Murphy's test. Acute pyelonephritis presents with fever, chills, and flank pain. Physical exam findings of fist percussion of the back over the CVA's with fever and chills may support pyelonephritis. AA may present with diffuse abdominal pain which may begin in the periumbilical or epigastric region which progresses over time to the right lower quadrant with maximal point of tenderness at the McBurney's point (the intersection of a line between the umbilicus and the right anterior superior iliac spine in the right lower quadrant).

163. **b) Mesenteric ischemia**. Mesenteric ischemia is seen predominately in the elderly, but another key is the development of an acute abdomen in the presence of a patient with atrial fibrillation or a recent myocardial infarction (MI) (the source of the clot that breaks off and lodges in the superior mesenteric artery.) The elderly do no mount impressive acute abdomens, often the diagnosis is made late, when there is blood in the bowel lumen (the only condition that mixes acute pain with GI bleeding) and acidosis and sepsis have developed. In very early cases, arteriogram and embolectomy may be an option.

164. **a) Alteplase (tPA)**. Patients who are unstable with massive pulmonary embolism should receive thrombolysis; alteplase is a commonly used thrombolytic drug. Enoxaparin (Lovenox) is a low molecular weight heparin that is an anticoagulation therapy that is used in patients with venous thromboembolism. Although heparin is an anticoagulation therapy that is used in patients with venous thromboembolism, alteplase is needed to reverse the shock state. Warfarin (Coumadin) is an anticoagulation therapy that is used in patients with venous thromboembolism and would not stabilize the hemodynamics.

165. **c) Admit to the ICU and treat with intravenous labetalol (Trandate)**. This patient presents with signs and symptoms of hypertensive encephalopathy—a hypertensive emergency. In patients with the clinical syndrome of malignant hypertension, encephalopathy is related to failure of autoregulation of cerebral blood flow at the upper pressure limit, resulting in vasodilation and hyperperfusion. Malignant hypertension is a syndrome associated with an abrupt increase of blood pressure in a patient with underlying hypertension or related to the sudden onset of hypertension in a previously normotensive individual.

Signs and symptoms of hypertensive encephalopathy may include severe headache, nausea, and vomiting focal neurologic signs, and alterations in mental status. Untreated, hypertensive encephalopathy may progress to stupor, coma, seizures, and death within hours. It is important to distinguish hypertensive encephalopathy from other neurologic syndromes that may be associated with hypertension, such as cerebral ischemia, hemorrhagic or thrombotic stroke, seizure disorder, mass lesions, delirium tremens, and so on.

Appropriate initial management includes admission to the ICU, and administration of intravenous agents to lower blood pressure. The initial goal of therapy is to reduce mean arterial blood pressure by no more than 25% within minutes to 2 hours or to a blood pressure in the range of 160/100–110 mmHg. This may be accomplished with IV nitroprusside, a short-acting vasodilator with a rapid onset of action that allows for minute-to-minute control of blood pressure. Parenteral labetalol and nicardipine are also effective agents for the treatment of hypertensive encephalopathy. Administration of oral agents may result in unpredictable rates of blood pressure lowering and is not recommended.

166. **d) Hispanic**. Over the past few decades, a large and growing body of evidence has significant racial and ethnic disparities in health in the U.S. Racial or ethnic disparities are more evident than socioeconomic disparities, because routine public health data in the United States generally have been reported by racial or ethnic group but less often by socioeconomic influences such as income and education. African Americans, and then closely followed by Hispanics, are the most disproportionately represented among the more socioeconomically disadvantaged groups, followed by American Indians, as well as some Pacific Islander and Asian-American groups.

167. **d) Tidal volume with set breaths and triggered breaths**. In assist control mechanical ventilation, the patient receives preset tidal volume with a set respiratory rate and patient triggered breaths deliver full tidal volumes. Peak expiratory pressures at the beginning of exhalation are used to provide better gas mixing in the alveoli, which provides an increase in oxygenation.Pressure support is applied in synchronous intermittent mechanical ventilation and continuous positive pressure ventilation to augment the patient's own tidal volume. Controlled mechanical ventilation provides tidal volume with only set breaths.

168. **a) Parkinson's disease**. Classic signs of Parkinson's disease are resting tremor, rigidity, and bradykinesia. Other common features are hypomimia or mask-like face, sleep disorders, micrographia, and microphonia. MG typically affects women in their early 20s to 30s and men in their 50s to 60s. Hallmark features include weakness later in the day or with repeated usage.

169. **a) Nephrotic syndrome**. Symptoms of nephrotic syndrome are loss of appetite, fatigue, ascites, and lower extremity edema. Diagnostic tests reveal proteinuria (albuminuria), low blood albumin level, and hyperlipidemia. Common causes of secondary nephrotic syndrome are lupus and diabetes.

170. **d) Positive sputum for mycobacterium tuberculosis**. Send three sputum specimens for AFB smears and cultures. Tuberculosis confirmation is made with a positive AFB smear along with a positive nucleic acid amplification (NAA) test for mycobacterium complex which is confirmed on culture. Chest x-rays on older adults may show parenchymal infiltrates, whereas younger adults may show upper lobe infiltrates. Cavitary lesion may be seen, but are not diagnostic. CT scans are used to detect occult diseases, as in a differential diagnosis of parenchymal lesions. Positive intradermal PPD indicates exposure to tuberculosis, not confirmatory for the infection.

171. **b) Is experiencing alcohol withdrawal**. Alcohol withdrawal peaks two to three days after cessation of alcohol intake. Classic signs are anxiety/agitation, tachycardia, hypertension, diaphoresis, and tremors. Laboratory findings consistent with alcohol withdrawal include low MVC and electrolyte abnormalities, including hypokalemia and hypomagnesemia. He is not likely to be septic with this presentation, including normal WBC and temperature. Bandemia is not reported. While he may have malnutrition, it is not the most likely diagnosis. Anxiety is a sign of alcohol withdrawal, but is not the best answer.

172. **a) Isoniazid + Vitamin B$_6$ × 6 months**. Latent tuberculosis infection (LTBI) can be treated with single-drug therapy using isoniazid. Peripheral neuropathy, an adverse reaction of isoniazid, occurs in 2% of cases and as a result, concomitant treatment with pyridoxine (vitamin B$_6$) can be implemented.

173. **b) TIPS**. TIPS is the best option for this patient classified as a Child-Pugh class C cirrhotic. The Blakemore tube would only be a temporary measure. The fluid administration and transfusion is likely to lead to a consumptive coagulopathy and progressing into disseminated intravascular coagulation (DIC). She is not a good transplant candidate in an acute state.

174. **c) Chest tube placement**. Chest tube placement is the most important initial intervention in this patient with chest wall deformity and diminished breath sounds after blunt trauma with possible hemo/pneumothorax.

175. **a) Right tension pneumothorax and insert a needle into his right second intercostal space, mid-clavicular line**. This patient has a tension pneumothorax on the right side. Proper emergency intervention is to insert a 14- or 16-gauge angio-catheter into the second intercostal space midclavicular line.

■ REFERENCE

Lilly, C. M., Zubrow, M. T., Kempner, K. M., Reynolds, H. N., Subramanian, S., Eriksson, E. A., ... Cowboy, E. R. (2014). Critical care telemedicine: Evolution and state of the art. *Critical Care Medicine*, *42*(11), 2429–2436.

V

After the Certification Exam

29

When You Pass the Certification Exam

DAWN CARPENTER, ALEXANDER MENARD,
AND NIKHIL RASWANT

There are only two possible outcomes upon completion of the certification exam. You will find out right away whether you have passed or failed. This chapter outlines the next steps needed to transition into clinical practice as an adult-gerontology acute care nurse practitioner (AG-ACNP).

Chapter 30 offers suggestions on what to do should you fail the examination. While we do not like to think negatively, it is unfortunately a harsh reality that some graduates do fail the exam. They will need information on how to regroup and move on after the disappointing news along with how to optimize preparation for the next attempt.

■ CELEBRATE

Congratulations when you pass! Be sure to take time to celebrate this important accomplishment! A lot of hard work went into achieving this important milestone in your career. Whether you choose to celebrate over a dinner at your favorite restaurant, at a big party, or with a vacation away, it's extremely important to recognize this achievement, both for yourself and for those who are closest to you.

■ RECOGNIZE YOUR SUPPORTERS

While you bask in the glory of your achievement, acknowledge the people who have helped and supported you in this endeavor. Family, friends, coworkers, preceptors, and faculty have been on this journey with you. Spouses, children, parents, siblings, and friends have taken a backseat to allow you time and space to complete your program. They may have picked up extra household duties or child care responsibilities to make time for you to focus on school. Recognize their sacrifices and thank them for supporting your dream. Acknowledge your coworkers and managers who may have picked up shifts or swapped schedules to allow you time off to study, write papers, or do clinical time.

■ NEXT STEPS

Passing the certification exam is the first step toward the rest of your career as an APRN. There are multiple additional steps between passing the exam and starting your first day of employment as an AG-ACNP. These steps can take time to complete, thus, it is suggested to continue working in your current nursing position until you are fully credentialed in the new role. The onboarding process is a fairly prescriptive sequence of steps that can take 3 to 4 months or more to complete to be fully credentialed and ready to start practice as a nurse practitioner (NP) in an acute care setting.

These steps vary from state to state, but the general components and sequencing are discussed in this chapter. Upon passing the national certification exam, the next steps are:

- Step 1: Apply for state licensure
- Step 2: Obtain a national provider identifier (NPI) number
- Step 3: Identify supervising/collaborating physician, if applicable
- Step 4: Sign a contract/practice agreement
- Step 5: Apply for a federal Drug Enforcement Agency (DEA) registration number
- Step 6: Obtain a state controlled-substance license, if applicable
- Step 7: Subscribe to the state prescription drug-monitoring program
- Step 8: Institutional credentialing
- Step 9: Begin employment

Some steps are contingent upon a previous step being completed. New graduates frequently experience delays during at least one step in this process. For this reason, we again encourage you *not* to resign from your nursing position too soon or you could find yourself without an income or insurance while the onboarding process is completed.

■ INTERVIEWING FOR POSITIONS

Exploring employment opportunities and interviews can arise during your educational program, many times even before you finish coursework or clinical rotations. Alternatively, you may choose to wait until after graduation to pursue employment. For this reason, materials and content regarding job search, resume and curriculum vitae preparation, interviewing, and negotiating for positions are discussed separately in Section V, Chapter 31 of this book.

Step 1: Apply for State Licensure

After passing the certification exam, the very first step toward employment as an AG-ACNP is to obtain state licensure in the state where you plan to work. Please visit your respective state board of nursing (SBON) website for information and processes on obtaining state licensure. Do not delay your application for state licensure. Depending on your state, this process can take up to 4 to 6 weeks.

You must obtain state licensure first, and then you must have actually accepted a job offer from an institution or group practice before proceeding.

Step 2: Obtain an NPI Number

After obtaining state licensure, you'll need to obtain an NPI number at nppes.cms.hhs.gov/#/. NPI is a unique, 10-digit number given to each healthcare provider and healthcare organization by the Centers for Medicare and Medicaid Services (CMS). The NPI was established in 1996 as a part of HIPAA. All healthcare providers or organizations covered by HIPAA must obtain an NPI number (CMS, 2015). This number will follow you from practice site to practice site.

You need to be hired in order to complete this step. Some institutions will do this for you as part of the onboarding process; others require you to apply on your own. The online process is outlined here:

- Enter personal identifiers and whether or not you are a "sole proprietor."

  - A sole proprietor is an individual and only owner of a business that is not incorporated. An unincorporated business is called a sole proprietorship. This will be important only if you are opening your own healthcare business or practice (Buppert, 2018).

  - Enter business information, including hiring organization and practice site address.

  - You can enter additional practice sites and organizations if you are affiliated with multiple organizations.

- Enter Medicaid identifiers.

- Identify the type of practice site, called a taxonomy code, which describes the type, classification, and area of specialization. Healthcare provider taxonomy code sets can be found at www.wpc-edi.com/reference/codelists/healthcare/health-care-provider-taxonomy-code-set/.

- Enter provider type, including your license number and state of licensure.

- Enter personal contact information, in case someone needs to contact you with questions or clarifications.

Step 3: Identify Supervising/Collaborating Physician (if Applicable)

Several states are still pursuing independent practice. As of this writing there are 23 states that have independent practice, 16 states with reduced practice, and 12 states that have restricted practice (American Association of Nurse Practitioners [AANP], 2018). There are varying levels of NP independence and physician collaboration requirements, ranging from no supervision to direct supervision, including a gradating approach based on amount of experience.

The federal definition of "collaboration" states that collaboration is a "process by which an NP works with a physician to provide healthcare within the providers' scope of practice and expertise, whereby the physician provides medical direction and supervision as provided by jointly developed guidelines that are in congruence with the state laws where the services are provided" (42 U.S.C.S. § 1395x(aa)(6) in Buppert, 2018). This definition does not imply that direct or onsite supervision is required. Rather, state boards of registration in nursing define the level of supervision required. Check with your specific state website to obtain the most up to date information.

If you are applying for positions in a state that does not have independent practice, clearly identify who will be your supervising or collaborating physician. You need this information to complete the next few steps.

Step 4: Sign a Collaborative Practice Agreement (if Applicable)

The requirements vary by state as to if, when, and how long NPs must have a collaborating physician. State-specific regulations and requirements are defined in collaborative practice agreements and may include some or all of the following:

a. The parties who are involved in the agreement and cite the state laws governing the NP practice

b. The scope of practice (SOP), including:

   i. The patient population and age groups

   ii. The range of health/illness conditions to be diagnosed and managed, including actual or potential health problems, health counseling, teaching, and supportive care

   iii. Patient referral and consultation

   iv. Treatments and prescriptive practices

c. Practice protocols to be used by the AG-ACNP, including a list of texts and references

d. Additional provisions as agreed to by the NP and the collaborating physician

e. Physician consultation:

   i. Coverage for emergency absences of either the NP or the collaborating physician

   ii. How and when the AG-ACNP will seek consultation from the physician

f. Process for documentation, including notes, prescriptive practice, and/or procedural information

g. A plan for resolution of disagreement(s) between the NP and the collaborating physician regarding diagnosis and treatment

h. Who can change or renew the agreement, and how

i. Signatures

Multiple sample or template practice agreements are available on the Internet offered by the SBON, schools of nursing, and legal sources.

Step 5: Apply for Federal DEA Registration Number

In order to prescribe ANY medications in your role as an AG-ACNP, you need to obtain a federal DEA registration number. Information for applying can be found on apps.deadiversion.usdoj.gov/webforms/jsp/regapps/common/newAppLogin.jsp.

You will need the following information on hand when you fill out the online form (form 224):

a. Personal information

b. Business information, including name of facility, address, phone number, email address, contact name, and number

   i. You do need to use your employer's address.

   ii. Be as specific as possible when documenting the address of the facility; specifically identify building and/or room numbers so the mail is delivered to the correct location in a timely manner.

      iii. DEA registration requires renewal every 3 years. Failure to renew can occur while the renewal document has circulated within the institution. An NP cannot practice with an expired license.

   c. Drug schedule information you are requesting

      i. You will request schedules II, III, IV, V, and VI.

      ii. Schedule I drugs are defined as drugs with no currently accepted medical use and a high potential for abuse, including heroin, lysergic acid diethylamide (LSD), and marijuana (cannabis).

   d. State licensure: The AG-ACNP must provide current state license and controlled-substance registration (if applicable). The DEA website warns the applicant: "Failure to provide VALID and ACTIVE state license will be cause to declare the application as defective and it will be withdrawn WITHOUT refund" (DEA, 2017).

   e. Personal background information on controlled substances

   f. Payment

      i. Application fees are not refundable.

      ii. The cost of the application as of the printing of this book is $731.00 for a 3-year registration.

New applications can take 4 to 6 weeks to process (DEA, 2018).

Step 6: Obtain State Controlled-Substance License (if Applicable)

Many states require additional prescriptive authority in order to obtain prescriptive privileges for medications and controlled substances in the state. This is different from and in addition to the DEA registration. Visit your state's website to determine state-specific requirements.

Information required for state prescriptive authority includes:

   a. Personal information

   b. Institutional information, including address, phone, and work email address

      i. Be as specific as possible on the address; include building name and room numbers so the interoffice mail is delivered to the correct location in a timely manner.

      ii. State controlled-substance registrations require renewal. Failure to renew can occur while the renewal document has circulated within the institution. An NP cannot practice with an expired license.

   c. Supervising or collaborating physician information may include:

      i. Name, address, specialty, license number, DEA controlled-substance registration and state controlled-substance registration

      ii. Copies of medical license, DEA number, and state controlled-substance licenses

   d. Drug schedules requested: Identify schedules of drugs you are requesting.

Step 7: Subscribe to the State Prescription Drug Monitoring Program

We highly recommend, if not required by states, that NPs subscribe to the state prescription drug monitoring program (PMDP) system. A PDMP is an online database that collects and makes information available on prescription drugs, including the identity of the prescriber, patient, and dispensing pharmacy (Soelberg, Brown, Du Vivier, Meyer, & Ramachandran, 2017). Most states have implemented a PDMP. Rules mandating and directing their use varies by state. Some states have also facilitated interstate sharing of prescription information to improve PDMPs' effectiveness to reduce opioid overdoses and overdose deaths. While not all states require PMDP use for inpatient prescribing, it is good practice to ensure the safest care is provided to your patients and families.

Step 8: Institutional Credentialing

Once you have completed the first seven steps, including passing the national board certification, and securing state licensure, DEA registration, and state controlled-substance registration (if applicable), you will need to submit copies of each of these documents to the credentialing department of your employing institution. Each institution is required to credential you prior to you beginning employment in the AG-ACNP role. The institution will perform primary verification of your education, training, licensure, and DEA and state controlled-substance registration. How long this process takes is dependent on how quickly it takes to submit documents and how long the institutional process takes. It can take as short as a month and upwards of 4 months. Typically, the larger the institution, the more complex the process and the longer it may take.

Documentation

Submit copies of your national board certification, state AG-ACNP license, and DEA and state controlled-substance registrations to the credentialing office. If the position requires basic life support (BLS), advanced cardiac life support (ACLS), and/or fundamentals of critical care support (FCCS) or other certifications, submit copies of these as well. Confirm with the credentialing office that all paperwork has been received and is complete. Always keep copies for yourself.

The Process

During the credentialing process, it's common to meet with the billing office to obtain an NPI number, if not already done, and to sign paperwork for them to obtain credentialing for each insurance company in order for you to bill for your services as an AG-ACNP. You should expect to receive annual mandatory training in billing and compliance. Befriending the billing person(s) is key to success as a new AG-ACNP, as they will answer many of your coding and billing questions and help keep your billing practices and documentation accurate. They can and will teach you well.

Your credentialing packet will likely require multiple signatures by the various layers of management, which can take time given people's busy schedules. The packet must then be reviewed by the institution's credentialing board, which commonly has specific and hard deadlines for submission to ensure time for the board members to review packets prior to their meetings.

Complete each of the steps in an efficient manner. Pay close attention to details of each step and document timely response to emails asking for additional information. Expect delays in the process.

When to Relinquish Your RN Position

The credentialing process realistically takes 3 to 4 months after passing the certification exam or receiving a job offer, whichever is the latter event. Use caution when deciding when to resign from your nursing position. Be fully transparent with your nurse manager, letting him/her know that you have accepted employment in the AG-ACNP role and that the start date may move, depending on the process. Once you have been given an idea of how long the process usually takes in your state and institution, then you can identify a target date to transition. It is expected that professionals provide 4 weeks of notice of resignation. Inquire with the manager about flexibility of the departure date, as your start date may get moved further out depending on how long the credentialing process takes. Be cautious with your transition date to avoid a gap in income or insurance coverage if the start date is delayed by the credentialing process.

Step 9: Begin Employment

We strongly recommend ensuring you are fully credentialed prior to caring for patients in the AG-ACNP role. Remember, you cannot legally practice as an NP until you are licensed by your respective state, nor can you bill. There is no such thing as retrospective billing, regardless of what some might tell you.

■ REFERENCES

American Association of Nurse Practitioners. (2018). *State practice environment.* Retrieved from https://www.aanp.org/legislation-regulation/state-legislation/state-practice-environment

Buppert, C. (2018). *Nurse practitioner's business practice and legal guide* (6th ed.). Boulder, CO: Jones & Bartlett.

Centers for Medicare and Medicaid Services. (2015). *National provider identifier standard.* Retrieved from https://www.cms.gov/Regulations-and-Guidance/Administrative-Simplification/NationalProvIdentStand/

Soelberg, C. D., Brown, R. E. Jr., Du Vivier, D., Meyer, J. E., & Ramachandran, B. K. (2017). The US opioid crisis: Current federal and state legal issues. *Anesthesia and Analgesia, 125*(5), 1675–1681. doi: 10.1213/ANE.0000000000002403

U.S. Drug Enforcement Agency. (2017). *Application for registration under Controlled Substances Act of 1970.* Retrieved from https://apps.deadiversion.usdoj.gov/webforms/

U.S. Drug Enforcement Agency. (2018). *Drug schedules.* Retrieved from https://www.dea.gov/druginfo/ds.shtml

30 Should You Fail the Certification Exam

DAWN CARPENTER

Should you fail, take a deep breath and try to relax. It is not the end of the world and you will get through this difficult time. For a variety of reasons, failing an exam can happen to the best of graduates, including being overly nervous, inadequately prepared, not feeling well, and being fatigued.

DEAL WITH EMOTIONS

You may feel a wide range of emotions, including bewilderment, deep sadness, anger, fear, and/or panic. These emotions are normal and will lessen over a few days. Give yourself permission to cry, to be angry, and to be simply miserable for a few days. It's okay to wallow in a bit of self-pity. Your family and close friends will be there for you; lean on them for support as they want to help you.

PRACTICE SELF-CARE

You will likely beat yourself up over the exam failure. You may think to yourself, "I could have … " or "I should have … ." STOP! Be kind to yourself. This is not the end of the world; it is a minor setback in the larger scheme of life. Take this time to care for yourself. Allow a period of time to disengage from studying. Give your mind a break, taking a few days to not look at materials. Focus on fun things you like to do: exercise, spend time with family or friends, do some gardening, go shopping or to lunch with a friend, visit family out of town. This will then allow you be more objective when you return to the task. Pick yourself up by your bootstraps, regroup, and devise a plan to retest.

REFLECT

The first step is to reflect on what did not go well. Consider:

Personal Factors

- Were you healthy when you took the exam?
- Were you overly nervous or anxious?
- Were there unforeseen circumstances that threw you off on the day of the exam?
- Did you get a good night's sleep the night before?
- Did you feel overly stressed?
- Did you feel confident going in? Did you feel confident when you submitted the exam?
- Were you distracted in the test setting?

Preparation

- Did you feel that you knew the material?
- Did you feel adequately prepared? How did you prepare?
- What resources and materials were used and how much time was allocated?

Exam Content

- Did you feel you had mastery of the content?
- What questions or content areas threw you off?
- Were there areas you were not prepared for (i.e., ethics, policy) or were there physiological content areas that you could not answer (i.e., heart failure, neurological topics)?

Time

- Did you have sufficient time to complete the exam?
- Did you use the time during the exam wisely?
- Did you rush through the questions?
- How was your pacing throughout?
- Did you take any breaks during the exam? If so, for how long?

Test-Taking Strategies

- Did you change any answers? If so, what were the reasons you changed the responses?
- Did you misread any questions?
- Did you read all the answer options?
- Could you recall information when attempting to answer questions?

Preparation

- Did you adequately prepare for the exam?

- Did you allocate adequate time to review for the exam?

- Did you follow the steps in Section I of this book explicitly? Did you skip or gloss over a section or specifics?

- Did anything derail your study time?

  - Were the children distracting you from studying?

  - Did you stop paying for extra babysitting now that school was over to save money?

  - Was your significant other asking for extra time and attention?

  - Did you pick up extra shifts at your nursing position to make up for lost wages during school?

Resources and Materials

- Did you have enough study materials?

- Did you use your textbooks and PowerPoint slides from school?

- Did you take a face-to-face review course or an online review course?

- Did you purchase any review books or materials?

- Were these tools helpful?

- Did you get through all your planned review materials?

- Did you have enough practice questions? Did you do all the practice questions?

- Did you review the material related to the questions you got wrong more than one time?

Exam Feedback

Examine the report that is provided by the certification body. This has valuable data and can help assess your performance on the exam. Both certification bodies offer diagnostic information on how you performed in each category of questions on the exam. You will receive a raw score and what the minimal passing score was for that particular exam.

The *American Association of Critical-Care Nurses* (AACN) provides feedback on the exam in seven categories, which record both physiological systems and physiologic content. Some are reported in individual systems, while others have multiple systems combined into one category. In addition, there are two nonclinical categories of the exam. The results for these sections are reported out as your percentage passing for each section:

- Cardiovascular, pulmonary, and multisystem are reported separately.

- Endocrine, hematology, gastrointestinal, renal, and integumentary are combined.

- Musculoskeletal, neurology, and psychosocial are combined.

- Advocacy, caring practices, response to diversity, and facilitation of learning are combined.

- Collaboration, systems thinking, and clinical inquiry are combined.

The *American Nurses Credentialing Center* (ANCC) provides feedback on the exam in four distinct categories, with a rating of high, moderate, or low performance in each area. It is important to note that physiological systems are integrated throughout each of these systems. The four categories of information that are reported are:

- Foundations of practice
- Professional role
- Independent practice
- Healthcare systems

Review the report. What jumps out at you? Where did you score high versus low? Does this information surprise you? Are these areas where you had expected to struggle?

Faculty Input

Faculty, program coordinators, and/or program directors can help you assess your specific situation. They have been through this before with other students and can be a resource to you. Reach out to them, as they know your abilities. Inquire if your faculty has time to meet and review your reflections. Ask them to assess the feedback from the exam, integrate his or her insights about you, and inquire if they have any strategies or recommendations for you as you plan to retest. Discuss whether to retake the same exam or take the other exam. The evaluation of this information will assist you to develop and prioritize a plan to move forward.

■ RETESTING OPTIONS

The next step is to decide upon which exam you plan to take or retake. There are still two options to become certified. You could decide to retake the exam you failed or elect to take the other exam. This is a very personal decision and is based on your specific situation. The most important tip is not to just automatically reapply to take the same exam. Take some time to evaluate the situation and then make an informed decision before you put down more money.

AACN: If you fail the exam, you may reapply to retest through AACN. A discounted retest fee is available to candidates who took the exam within their most recent 90-day window. Graduates are eligible to retest up to four times in a 12-month period. To reapply, please refer to the *Certification Exam Policy Handbook*.

ANCC: If you fail the certification exam, you may retest after 60 days from your exam date. Graduates are eligible to retest up to three times in a 12-month period. You must meet eligibility requirements when the retest application is submitted. To reapply, please refer to the website.

With both organizations, you will need to retake the entire exam, not just the areas where you did poorly. This needs to be taken into consideration when devising a new study plan.

▪ DEVISE A NEW STUDY PLAN

Once you have completed the evaluation of your specific circumstances and determined which exam to take or retake, devise a renewed plan for success. Refer back to and re-read Section I of this book, "Preparing for the Exam," in detail. Perform each of these steps once again with a slightly different focus. This time you will focus on the areas you need to improve upon as the priority, yet still build in time and materials to review content with which you are already comfortable to maintain this knowledge base.

- Plan out study time.
- Reprioritize material.
- Fit topics into the schedule.
- Mitigate circumstances that kept you from adhering to study plans.

Reprioritize Material

Reestablish priorities for content review based on your performance and diagnostic information from the exam results. Combine this information with the exam blueprint for the exam you will be taking and build your study calendar. Then re-rate the topic areas.

Consider adding more detail and specificity to the schedule topics to keep you focused and make the tasks easier to break down into manageable chunks. For example, if neurology was challenging, break it down into smaller components, such as:

- Neurological
- Encephalopathy, delirium, dementia
  - Intracerebral bleeding
  - Neuromuscular disorders
  - Intracranial hypertension
  - Seizure disorders
  - Spinal cord disorders
- Stroke

Tip: Write out tables comparing and contrasting the differences in some of these diagnoses and treatments. This can be a powerful learning tool. Adding drawings, symbols, or arrows indicating increase/decrease of a detail will add to visual recall of the material.

Reassess Study Materials

If necessary obtain additional resources, including books, references, or clinical practice guidelines. Look at the areas that challenged you and utilize the resources listed in this book as well as the reference list for the certification exam you will be taking.

Do Lots of Practice Questions

It is critical to do lots and lots of practice questions. Make sure you have fresh questions to answer, so that you are not just recalling details from previous questions. It is imperative to use new questions to process and reason through new materials. Oftentimes, even if you do not memorize questions, you have put information into your notes that create associations that tie closely to previous questions. Thus when you review those notes, it can make the reused questions less challenging.

Review All Topics

Plan to review all material to be included on the exam, as you will be retaking the entire exam. As such, all content must be fresh in your mind. Utilize the same strategies you used for your areas of strength, as they clearly worked. What tools worked to learn that material? Did you use flash cards? Did you make notes? Did you do a lot of practice questions? Replicate these strategies in the content areas of weakness.

Other Preparation Suggestions: If you have not done these items, consider:

- Taking an additional or different review course
- Purchasing audio recordings of a review course

Mitigate Circumstances That Kept You From Adhering to Study Plans

Consider ways to manage things that derailed your studying. Consider utilizing babysitters so you can study. Go to the library to focus and study. Reduce your work schedule to make more time to study. Managing these elements and others are critical so you can optimize study time.

Difficulty Studying/Anxiety

If anxiety is keeping you from staying focused and is hindering your studying, reconsider accessing professional help. Your confidence level has taken a hit and you may need to add additional strategies to help get you through this temporary situation.

Assess your anxiety level.

- Are you nervous when you sit down to study?
- Do you fidget?
- Are you jittery?
- Does your heart race?
- Do you get short of breath?
- Do you have difficulty retaining the information you are reading/reviewing?
- Are you able to concentrate during study sessions?
- Do you find yourself using negative self-talk that erodes your confidence?
- Are you unable to get past the catastrophizing of the failure?
- Do you find yourself panicking when you think of taking the exam again?

If the answer to these questions is yes, then you will want to address this anxiety. Failure to manage anxiety can and will affect you again during studying and during the exam. Take control of the situation. Implement stress management techniques. A balanced diet, regular exercise, hydration, plenty of sleep, mindfulness exercises, and abstaining from alcohol are advised. Consult your primary care provider, who can refer you to a counselor or therapist and decide if medication management is warranted.

31

Employment Search, Interview, and Negotiations

ANTHONY McGUIRE, DAWN CARPENTER,
ALEXANDER MENARD, AND NIKHIL RASWANT

Employment opportunities frequently emerge during your academic program, through both clinical rotations and work contacts. Other times, students undertake an employment search. This section of the book explores and guides the new graduate adult-gerontology acute care nurse practitioner (AG-ACNP) to choose the right position. It offers guidance on the employment process from application to interview including the negotiation of the details pertaining to the position.

NETWORKING

Network through your preceptors, clinical faculty, alumni list serves, and word of mouth. Preceptors have invested time and energy to facilitate your clinical learning and, assuming you have demonstrated your knowledge, skills, and aptitude for the role, they may want you as their next colleague. Clinical faculty, alumni list serves, and word of mouth can be equally important relationships to connect you to additional employment opportunities. Do not hesitate to reach out to your preceptors, clinical faculty, program coordinators, or director to forward your resume to colleagues and hiring managers. It can be quite difficult for the new graduate to get past the online human resource application process that frequently seeks prior experience. Your local and regional professional organizations may send out "job lists" or hold events where you can network with their members.

EMPLOYMENT OPTIONS

Seek employment options that align with your interests and education and that fall within the scope and practice of the adult-gerontology acute care population.

Settings

AG-ACNPs are employed in a variety of physical environments or settings caring for the sickest patients. Thus, physical location of the patient is less important;

rather, patient acuity, complexity of care, and risk for rapidly changing conditions are the primary focus of the AG-ACNP role (AACN, 2017).

Common settings where AG-ACNPs are utilized include inpatient hospital departments, where the AG-ACNP stays in a specific unit for the full shift; procedural areas and service-based teams, where AG-ACNPs cover multiple patient care areas and/or may see patients in a clinic setting prior to procedures; and posthospitalization, such as postoperative visits. Table 31.1 outlines appropriate employment settings, shows where overlap can occur with primary care NPs, and, finally, lists inappropriate employment options for AG-ACNPs. Table 31.2 highlights and expands on the overlap of roles between acute and primary care (PC) NPs in a hospital setting, which are discussed in Table 31.1.

Table 31.1 Roles for AG-ACNPs		
Appropriate	**Overlap With Primary Care NPs**	**Inappropriate**

• Hospitalist role
• Intensivist role
• Emergency department (caring for young adults, older adults, and geriatric populations only)
• Inpatient service-based lines
  ▪ Acute care surgery
  ▪ Cardiology
  ▪ ID
  ▪ Renal
  ▪ GI
• Procedural areas
  ▪ Cardiac catheterization lab
  ▪ Interventional radiology
	• Specialty service lines, such as:
	  ▪ Oncology
	  ▪ Orthopedics
	  ▪ Thoracic surgery
	  ▪ Cardiology
	  ▪ GI
	• Urgent care
		• Pediatric primary care
		• Pediatric acute care
		• Obstetrics
		• Dermatology
		• Cosmetic surgery

GI, gastrointenstinal; ID, infectious disease.

Permanent Versus Temporary Employment Options

There are two primary paths or routes to employment: being hired directly into a permanent position or being hired into a residency or fellowship.

Permanent Employment Options

The traditional and most familiar way of securing an AG-ACNP position is to be hired as a permanent staff member. Typically there is a defined orientation period, which gives you time to acclimate to the facility and your new role.

Temporary Employment Options

There are two types of temporary employment options available to AG-ACNPs, postgraduate residency or fellowship programs, and locum tenens positions.

Table 31.2 Example of Patient Acuity Driving That NP Is Best Qualified to Manage Patients	
PC NP or FNP In the Hospital	**AG-ACNP In Outpatient Settings**
A PC NP could manage inpatient orthopedic patients who have elective knee or hip surgeries. The PC NP could see them in the office preprocedure and follow the patient throughout the hospitalization. However, if the patient has a worsening condition, such as NSTEMI, or becomes septic from a wound infection, the PC NP is no longer qualified to manage the higher acuity and an AG-ACNP must take over the management of the patient.	An AG-ACNP could work in a cardiology clinic, seeing patients with heart failure. Heart failure patients can progress from a relatively healthy state to acutely/critically ill at a rapid pace. The AG-ACNP understands the scope and range of treatments available for patients with multiple and progressive exacerbations of heart failure, including inotropes, synchronized pacemakers, ventricular assist devices, and heart transplant.
An AG-PCNP working in thoracic surgery could manage an inpatient. He/she could see the patient preoperatively for lung cancer, follow the patient throughout the hospital stay, and continue to care for the patient in clinic postoperatively. Again, if the patient develops a worsening condition, such as RAF, acute respiratory failure, or a pulmonary embolism, the AG-ACNP would need to care for the patient.	The AG-ACNP could work in an outpatient oncology clinic, where most of oncology care is delivered, caring for patients undergoing chemotherapy, as these patients can develop rapidly changing conditions such as sepsis. Sepsis in an immunocompromised patient may present with very subtle signs due to their poor reserve, making early recognition and prompt intervention of this lethal diagnosis essential to their survival.

FNP, family nurse practitioner; NSTEMI, non-ST elevated myocardial infarction; RAF, rapid atrial fibrillation.

Postgraduate Residency or Fellowship

A postgraduate NP residency or fellowship is an option for new graduate AG-ACNPs who have minimal nursing experience or desire to specialize in a specific area that requires in-depth knowledge about a population. Common areas of specialization for AG-ACNPs include critical care, surgery/trauma, and orthopedics. These programs typically offer temporary employment for a predetermined amount of time, typically 6 to 12 months.

The residency/fellowship offers structured learning in classroom, clinical, and simulation areas that correlates with precepted clinical practice. The numbers of residency and fellowship programs have been increasing in recent years. It is important to note that not all programs guarantee employment at the completion of the training. Compensation is typically less than a direct hire and usually requires additional work hours as part of the training program. The benefit of such a pathway is in-depth training and orientation in a structured program and preparation for a permanent position. Characteristics of quality residencies or fellowship programs include inclusion of formal didactic lectures, high-fidelity simulation, clinical supervision, and regular feedback (Brown, Poppe, Kaminetzky, Wipf, & Woods, 2015).

Locum Tenens

Locum tenens is another form of temporary employment for AG-ACNPs, similar to being a travel nurse. Locum tenens providers fill in for other permanent providers on a temporary basis. Tenure can range from a few weeks to up to 6 months or more. When employers face temporary staffing shortages due to hard-to-fill vacancies, prolonged illness, maternity leave, or other reasons, they may choose to hire locum tenens providers. Locum tenens providers fill their vacancies and maintain adequate staffing levels to ensure quality patient care is maintained. In addition, some hospitals utilize these temporary employees while they perform a permanent search. Other facilities may hire them to pilot the need for a new position (Blumenthal, Olenski, Tsugawa, & Jena, 2017).

While this employment option exists, it is not recommended for a new graduate AG-ACNP. To capably fulfill this type of position, you really need a solid foundation in practice for a minimum of a year, and two is preferable. Typically in these positions, there is minimal orientation to the organization and institutional policies. The greatest success in a locum tenens position involves experienced AG-ACNPs working in the same specialty area where they have been working.

■ APPLICATION PROCESS

There are three important aspects of the application process that deserve your best efforts: the cover letter, your resume or curriculum vitae (CV), and the interview. A good initial impression may turn your application into an interview and then, ultimately, into a job offer. A professional portfolio can provide an edge over other candidates. The differences between resumes, CVs and portfolios are discussed later in this chapter.

Cover Letter

A well-written cover letter is critical to prompt the reader to examine your resume/CV. Write the letter formally; format it as a business letter with careful attention to grammar, punctuation, and white space. Make the letter brief and to the point; three well-written, succinct paragraphs are sufficient. A poorly written letter will prompt the reader to move on; a letter that is too verbose may lose the reader's interest.

The first paragraph states the purpose of the letter. Convince the reader of your enthusiasm for the position and the organization. Avoid beginning with, "Enclosed you will find … ." The reader can readily see you enclosed your resume. Instead, begin with, "This letter is in response to a position as … ."

Sell yourself in the second paragraph. Clearly and succinctly outline your knowledge and skills, along with how these skills can move the organization's mission and vision forward. Give specific examples of which skills link to the organizational mission and/or vision. Do not express how the organization can improve you; instead, articulate how you can improve the organization.

Conclude by requesting an interview for the position, providing contact information. Be sure to include or attach your resume or CV to the letter or email. Follow your letter up with a phone call to the appropriate person. Always remember to address the letter to an individual as opposed to "to whom it may concern."

Resume Versus CV

A resume is a concise, one- to two-page listing of one's education, work experiences, and certifications—complete with dates of service and key responsibilities bulleted within each section. A CV provides a more complete picture of a candidate's educational and experiential qualifications, and is required in many professional and academic arenas. A CV is expected of providers who seek academic roles as well as larger institutions and academic medical centers.

New graduate AG-ACNPs typically start an employment search with a resume. As you progress through practice, opportunities may or are likely to arise for the AG-ACNP to do presentations, publications, service and research, and so on. At this time, the AG-ACNP may begin to build a CV. Either way, keep your resume current.

Resume

A resume is the first and most important representation of you that an interviewer will see. The resume helps to sell you as the ideal candidate. Update your resume at graduation and list your school and work experiences. Include employment other than just your nursing experiences. Translate experience into employment skills for the AG-ACNP role: time management, communication skills, finance experience, and reliability. There is no need to describe the functions of being a nurse in every position you have held. Hiring managers understand the differences between nursing roles in various hospital departments. Highlight leadership and educational elements, such as precepting new graduates, being a charge nurse, and committee involvement.

List your education, employment, state licensure, certifications, and extracurricular activities in distinct sections. Examples are available online and in the appendices of this chapter. Keep the resume to one page, two at most. Do not list your actual license numbers or certification numbers on your resume and/or CV.

A basic resume template is found in Appendix A. Sample resumes for a traditional experienced nurse and a direct entry graduate are found in Appendices B and C.

Curriculum Vitae

A CV is a biography of your professional life. It contains a comprehensive listing of educational and employment history along with information related to licensure, certifications, honor and awards, professional memberships and committees, professional activities, scholarly works (presentations/publications), research, and teaching activities.

Take care to make the CV orderly (logical flow) with proper grammar and spelling. Add to the CV on an annual basis so it will be ready to send each time you participate in a professional activity after you start your advanced practice career. Appendix A contains a CV template that can be customized to your use. Not all sections are required on the CV as shown, especially as you start your career. Once you participate in the activity, add it to the appropriate section. Do not list a category or section on your CV and state "none"; it is best to leave out the sections where there is nothing to list.

Basic and advanced CV templates are found in Appendices D and E.

Professional Portfolio

A professional portfolio is a unique way to showcase your educational and professional experiences. Perhaps you started this in your graduate program. A portfolio is a purposeful collection of selected and/or specialized works that reflects employment or academic achievements. The portfolio can be used as a springboard for future development and advancement within APRN practice or to further your education. The portfolio grows over time, just as a CV grows as a career advances. Regularly update your portfolio as accomplishments occur to keep it current.

Developing a portfolio can be a creative, professional endeavor. The portfolio can be presented as a professional three-ring binder or as an electronic "e-portfolio." One option to create an e-portfolio is at www.wix.com or www.wix.com/html5webbuilder/400?utm_campaign=vir_wixad_live#

Content to be included in a portfolio includes:

- Cover/title page with name, credentials and a professional photo
- Copy of your resume or CV
- Copies of current licenses
- Copies of current certifications
- Copies of academic transcripts
- Documentation of clinical experiences (i.e., graphs from Typhon), including descriptors of the population, diagnoses seen, general skills, and invasive skills performed throughout your AG-ACNP program
- Scholarly writing sample(s)
- Copies of or links to any publications
- PowerPoint presentations and posters
- Awards and recognitions
- Documentation of community service/volunteer work

The final product for an e-portfolio is a web link to share with prospective employers via online application, email, and/or on your resume. The website can be password protected so that only people to whom you have given permission can access the information.

Regular portfolio updates should be undertaken during annual performance reviews. It is a natural time to reflect on accomplishments and define goals for the coming year.

■ REFERENCES

Ask faculty, clinical faculty, preceptors, nurse managers, and program coordinators and directors proactively for recommendations. Obtain contact information, including full name, credentials, title, address, phone number, and email address, for each reference. Keep your references updated as you apply for positions. References do not need to be listed on your resume but will be required upon a job offer, so have them typed up and ready for distribution. Always remember to contact the person prior to listing them as a reference, so they are aware they may receive correspondence from your potential hire.

■ INTERVIEW

Interviewing for an AG-ACNP position can be anxiety provoking; the institution is assessing your fit within their team and you are determining if the position is a good fit for you, your family, and your lifestyle.

Prepare for the interview. They can range from a one-on-one interview with a single hiring manager to a daylong series of interviews or panel interviews with multiple team members. You will likely be competing with several applicants for a single position, so be prepared to make the best impression possible.

■ PREPARE

Present yourself professionally. A suit is recommended and expected when interviewing for an advanced practice role. Overdress rather than underdress for an interview, even if you know the interviewers. Put your best self forward, smile, make eye contact, and offer a firm handshake.

Do your homework about the institution, the position, and individuals with whom you will be interviewing. Be prepared to ask thoughtful questions. Search the institution's website to understand its mission, vision, and values. Read articles written by the interviewers to demonstrate interest and generate discussion during the interview.

The interview is your time to convey your worth to the institution. Complete a self-assessment before your interview. Prepare and practice responses to standard interview questions, including:

- Strengths
- Opportunities for improvement
- Why you want the position
- Why you are the best fit for the position

Reply to these questions out loud to hear how your answers come across. Have a classmate or colleague practice with you so you will become comfortable with the questions and they can give you feedback on the answers. Interviewers may ask behavioral interviewing questions to get a better sense of your critical thinking and thought processes. Examples:

- Give an example of when you worked on a team where conflict developed and how you reacted to it.
- Tell us how you made a positive impact in your last job.
- If a patient became angry with you during a visit, how would you handle it?
- Have you ever had to report anyone for a compliance concern? If so, tell us about it. If not, how would you go about it?
- You come to work one day and the senior attending provider smells of alcohol and is acting inappropriately. What would you do?
- You have a patient with the following chief complaint (be prepared for the population of the practice). What would be your next step?
- Discuss your differential diagnosis process.
- What are your thoughts on the current opioid crisis?

In addition, interviewers may ask clinical scenarios about the population to understand your level of understanding. Lastly, be prepared to respond to questions about any lapses in your employment history.

A typical interview will also invite you to ask questions. Take this opportunity to ask thoughtful questions about the position, institution, role, team, and so on. DO NOT ask about money or benefits at this time. The opportunity to gather this data will come if/when you receive a job offer.

Interviews are a two-way assessment. This is your opportunity to assess the role, expectations, and fit of the position, and to identify congruence with your expectations and needs. Be sure you fully understand the role and employment expectations. Ask to shadow a provider or the team to see the role and teamwork firsthand. If this is not possible, ask to meet with any other NPs or other team members.

▪ SUGGESTED INTERVIEW QUESTIONS

Come prepared with questions for the interviewers. Have the questions written down, as you may be nervous in the interview and forget them. Focus on learning about the position. Suggested questions include:

- What is the scope of the position: inpatient, outpatient, or both?
- What is a typical day and week like?
- Tell me the hours expected of the role: 8, 10, or 12 hours per day? Number of days per week? Any on-call hours? Night shifts? Weekends? Holidays?
- What procedures are expected of the position? How will I get trained to do them?
- Tell me about the orientation: To the institution? The position? Any classes or lectures? Are there recommended resources? Books? Journals? Professional memberships?
- Why is the position open? How long has the position been vacant?
- Who are the other team members? What are they like? How do they get along?
- Will I be able to meet them? Can I shadow the team for a few hours or a day?
- Who is the supervisor of the position, administrator or physician?
- Who will do my evaluations? When will I be evaluated? Within the first 3 months? 6 months? Then annually?
- Will I be expected to bill directly for the services provided?
- Given the organization's mission (name whatever that is), how would this position work to facilitate growth?
- One of my strengths is networking; is there room on the team to use this skill to grow the practice?

  Do not be timid; exude confidence!

▪ RECEIVING A JOB OFFER

Typically a job offer will come through the human resources (HR) department, rather than the hiring provider. The offer will include information on the salary and benefit package. If the offer is provided verbally, ask for it in writing or via email. Take time to consider the offer. A few days to a week is reasonable.

You could request an extension if you have other interviews pending or offers you are expecting.

Negotiating an AG-ACNP position involves consideration of multiple elements.

Be Prepared

Be prepared to receive an offer. Identify the average starting salary for an AG-ACNP in an acute care setting for the respective region, size of the population (urban, suburban, rural) area, and size of the institution (large academic medical center, teaching hospital, or community hospital). Look up the most recent AANP National NP Compensation Survey report and the *Advance for NPs and PAs* current salary survey. In addition, evaluate information by specialty service, if available, which can add additional context to salary expectations.

The Package

Salary is only one part of the employment compensation package. Take into consideration:

- Health, vision, and dental insurance
- Retirement plan contributions
- Short- and long-term disability insurance
- Amount of vacation time, educational time, holiday time
- Malpractice coverage
- Financial support to attend a professional conference
- Cell phones and/or pagers
- Provision of lab coats and laundering
- Reimbursement for professional licenses, certification, and federal Drug Enforcement Agency (DEA) registration.
- Continuing education expenses

Attendance at one annual national conference, including registration, flights, and hotel, can add up to a couple thousand dollars. An institution may offer a "professional practice allowance" whereby a preset dollar amount is allocated to the NP which could include reimbursement for conferences, licenses, certification renewals, educational programs, annual membership dues to professional organizations, books, subscriptions to journals, and so on. The new AG-ACNP should consider the total compensation package, not just the salary offer (Buppert, 2014).

■ NEGOTIATING A CONTRACT

Think of contract negotiation as a conversation; approach negotiations in a collaborative manner. Be prepared and informed on the issue of compensation and benefits, making the process objective and less personal. Keep emotion out of the discussion by remaining calm and focused.

Once you receive the offer, do not feel pressured to immediately accept the offer. Request a day or two to think before responding. Use this time to evaluate the offer objectively and compare it to the research you have done. Try to understand from where the other side is coming. Although you may have many years of nursing experience and be at the top of the pay scale, you are a new graduate AG-ACNP.

The opportunity to negotiate comes once you have had time to consider the details of the offer. Have a conversation regarding your expectations for salary and benefits. Inquire if they have any wiggle room to increase the offer. Let them know what you were looking for and see if they can meet your request.

When making a final decision, in addition to the salary and benefits, consider whether the position lets you practice to the full extent of your education and capabilities, while also considering schedule factors that may impact your desired quality of life (Melnic, 2018).

■ MALPRACTICE INSURANCE

Be informed about the amount of liability insurance coverage offered by the hiring institution. It is a very personal decision whether or not to have your own liability insurance outside of the institutional coverage. Insurance that covers you for an event after you separate service until the statute of limitations expires is called "tail coverage," and is highly recommended that the AG-ACNP have or obtain this type of coverage.

Obtaining your own malpractice insurance policy is a very personal decision. Buppert (2018) strongly recommends AG-ACNPs obtain their own if they might practice outside their professional setting, such as providing volunteer work.

An AG-ACNP who strictly maintains employment in an institution that provides umbrella coverage may still choose to obtain malpractice insurance coverage. In this case, you will likely have "occurrence" coverage, which covers the AG-ACNP only when the insurance policy is in effect. If the AG-ACNP chooses to leave the institution, the AG-ACNP may choose to keep a "claims made" insurance policy active by adding tail coverage, which provides insurance coverage to the AG-ACNP past the time employment ends until the statute of limitations has expired. Buppert (2018) recommends choosing an insurance company that has more than 10 years of experience and is financially stable.

■ HEALTH CLEARANCES

Once you have finalized negotiations with details of the position and benefits, realize the offer is contingent upon further onboarding processes, including the preemployment physical examination. In addition, requests for national background checks, drug testing, and fingerprinting are becoming more prevalent.

■ REFERENCES

American Association of Critical-Care Nurses. (2017). *AACN scope and standards for acute care nurse practitioner practice 2017* (L. Bell Ed.). Aliso Viejo, CA: Author.

Blumenthal, D. M., Olenski, A. R., Tsugawa, Y., & Jena, A. B. (2017). Association between treatment by locum tenens internal medicine physicians and 30-day mortality among hospitalized medicare beneficiaries. *JAMA, 318*(21), 2119–2129. doi:10.1001/jama.2017.17925

Brown, K., Poppe, A., Kaminetzky, C., Wipf, J., & Woods, N. F. (2015). Recommendations for nurse practitioner residency programs. *Nurse Educator, 40*(3), 148–151. doi:10.1097/NNE.0000000000000117

Buppert, C. (2014, July 17–22). *Negotiating terms of employment.* Paper presented at the AANP 2014, Nashville, TN.

Buppert, C. (2018). *Nurse practitioner's business practice and legal guide* (6th ed.). Boulder, CO: Jones & Bartlett.

Melnic, J. (2018). *Know your worth: Contract negotiation for NPs.* Retrieved from https://www.melnic.com/job-seekers/learning-center/job-search-tools/interview-skills/contract-negotiation-for-nps/

APPENDIX A—RESUME TEMPLATE

Name & Credentials
Address, Phone, Email

Objective: Obtain employment as an Adult Gerontology Acute Care Nurse Practitioner in a critical care unit.

EDUCATION

Graduate Education   Year

MS or DNP, in Adult Gerontology Acute Care Nurse Practitioner

Nurse Practitioner Clinical Rotations:

- Hospital and service   # hours
- Hospital and service   # hours

Undergraduate Education   Year

Bachelor of Science Degree in Nursing

LICENSES & CERTIFICATIONS

APRN license

Registered Nurse license   Year

Advanced Cardiac Life Support (ACLS)

Basic Life Support (BLS)

WORK EXPERIENCE

Nursing work experience:

Hospital, City, State

Nursing department or type of unit   Year

- Types of patients
- Charge nurse responsibilities
- Precepting new graduates

Other professional work: (non-nursing):

HONORS & AWARDS

APPENDIX B—SAMPLE RESUME FOR A TRADITIONAL NURSE TO MASTER'S (MS OR MSN) DEGREE

Name & Credentials
Address, Phone, Email

Objective: Obtain employment as an Adult-Gerontology Acute Care Nurse Practitioner in a critical care unit.

EDUCATION

University of Massachusetts Medical School, Graduate School of Nursing

MS in Nursing, Adult- Gerontology Acute Care Nurse Practitioner	2017
Curry College	2003
Bachelor of Science Degree in Nursing	
Quincy College	2002
Associate Degree in Nursing	

LICENSES & CERTIFICATIONS

MA Registered Nurse license	2002–Present
Certified Critical Care Nurse (CCRN)	
Certified Emergency Nurse (CEN)	
Advance Trauma Care for Nurses	
Advanced Cardiac Life Support (ACLS)	
MA Emergency Medical Technician	1996
Basic Life Support (BLS)	

WORK EXPERIENCE

Massachusetts General Hospital, Boston, MA

Post Anesthesia Care Unit, Staff Nurse	2010–Present

- Work with a variety of patients who have undergone various surgical interventions and operations.
- Provide care for pre-operative patients.
- Precept new staff nurses.

(continued)

Appendix B *(continued)*

EDUCATION

Medical Intensive Care, Staff Nurse   2005–present

- Practice primary nursing care within a multidisciplinary team to provide care to critically ill medical, transplant, and surgical patients.
- Conduct research focused on the improvement of medical staff interpretation of central venous pressure and pulmonary artery wave forms.
- Function as unit resource nurse.
- Precept new staff nurses to the unit.
- Member of the Ebola response team/biocontainment unit

Respiratory Acute Care Unit Staff Nurse   2002–2005

- Provided a multidisciplinary approach to complex medical, transplant, and trauma ventilator-dependent patients
- Performed duties of resource nurse

International Medical Surgical Response Team, Deputy Commander   2006–present

- Work with Department of Health and Human Services to provide medical/ surgical care to people who have been affected by a disaster.
- Promoted to Deputy Team Commander on 4/2010

EDUCATIONAL EXPERIENCES

Nurse Practitioner Clinical Rotations:

- UMass Memorial Medical Center—Medical ICU   360 hours
- UMass Memorial Medical Center—Surgical ICU   360 hours

Interprofessional Education

- **Communication and Care of Decedents and Their Families in the ICU Setting**
  Worked on a project to focus on development of recommendations to enhance communication for families of ICU patients upon death, including autopsy consideration, provider/staff communication and support with the family, patient/family wishes for the deceased patient, and family bereavement needs

(continued)

Appendix B *(continued)*

EDUCATION

Fall 2015–Spring 2016

- **Clinical Interprofessional Professional Curriculum**
    - With third-year medical students
    - Developed effective teamwork and putting patient interests first
    - Improving advocacy for patients through culture of teamwork

HONORS & AWARDS

England Regional Giving Excellence Meaning (GEM) Volunteer and Service Award Sponsored by Johnson & Johnson   2014

Distinguished Member of the Year, NDMS Response Team   2014

Awarded in recognition of outstanding dedication and performance of duty as an NDMS team member

President's Volunteer Service Award   2012

Awarded for humanitarian mission response to Indonesia posttsunami

Presented at the White House

APPENDIX C—SAMPLE RESUME FOR A DIRECT ENTRY NURSE TO DOCTOR OF NURSING PRACTICE (DNP) DEGREE

Name & Credentials
Address, Phone, Email

Objective: Obtain employment as an Adult Gerontology Acute Care Nurse Practitioner in a critical care unit.

NURSING EDUCATION

University of Massachusetts Medical School, Graduate School of Nursing

Doctor of Nursing Practice   **2016**

- DNP project: Developed a Military and Veterans Health elective course for interprofessional education

Master of Science in Nursing   **2015**

                                                                             2012

- Adult-Gerontology Acute Care Nurse Practitioner track
- Specialty in Cardiovascular Care and Critical Care
- Graduate Education Pathway Certificate of Completion in Registered Nursing

   Nurse Practitioner Clinical Rotations:

   UMass Memorial Medical Center—Surgical ICU (360 hours)

   UMass Memorial Medical Center—Medical ICU (360 hours)

OTHER EDUCATION

The Fletcher School of Law and Diplomacy, Tufts University

Master of Arts in Law and Diplomacy   **2007**
- Fields of Study: International Information and Communications; International Security

University of Maryland

Bachelor of Arts in Government and Politics; Minor in Chinese   **2003**
Studies

Beijing Language and Culture University

Chinese Language Certificate   **May 2002–Aug. 2002**

(continued)

Appendix C *(continued)*

NURSING EDUCATION

United States Naval Academy

Academic Concentration: Political Science   **Jun. 1997–Feb. 2001**

LICENSES & CERTIFICATIONS

Massachusetts Registered Nurse   **Sep. 2012–Apr. 2016**

Fundamentals of Critical Care Support Certification   **Current–Nov. 2016**

Advanced Cardiovascular Life Support Certification   **Current–May 2014**

Basic Life Support Certification   **Current–Mar. 2015**

HEALTHCARE EXPERIENCE

UMass Memorial Medical Center   **Worcester, MA**

Registered Nurse   **Apr. 2013–Present**

- Responsible for the planning, delivery, and management of direct patient care for hospitalized patients in the acute care setting, primarily on the 7 East hematology/oncology floor and 6 East general medicine/telemetry floor

Veterans Inc.   **Worcester, MA**

Volunteer Staff Registered Nurse   **Nov. 2011–Jun. 2013**

- Provide homeless residents with advocacy and counseling, prescription medicine reconciliation, health literacy education, and triage assessment.

Brigham and Women's Hospital   **Boston, MA**

Volunteer Patient Care Assistant, Emergency Department   **Feb. 2008–Mar. 2011**

OTHER PROFESSIONAL EXPERIENCE

Operational Medicine Institute   **Boston, MA**

Unconventional Diplomacy Fellow   **May 2008–Mar. 2011**

- Coordinated public information and cultural awareness training programs
- Acted as public health officer and community liaison in collaboration with the Harvard Humanitarian Initiative at the Love a Child Disaster Recovery Center, Fond Parisien, Haiti, following the 2010 earthquake; created and implemented a public health monitoring, surveillance, and information program

(continued)

Appendix C *(continued)*

NURSING EDUCATION

United Nations High Commissioner for Refugees,   **Hong Kong SAR**
Sub-Office Hong Kong

Public Information Advisor   **May 2006–Aug. 2006**

- Developed and conducted public information campaigns and activities to disseminate information on UNHCR and raise public awareness of refugee issues
- Designed and implemented fundraising programs, bringing in over US$300,000 in cash and in-kind donations

U.S. Department of State, U.S. Embassy Baghdad   **Baghdad, Iraq**

Press and Information Officer, Public Affairs Section   **Jun. 2004–Dec. 2004**

- Coordinated and handled all U.S. Mission interviews and media events; advised embassy press officers on developing media plans, official guidance, and media inquiries
- Acted as liaison between Iraqi Interim Government Prime Minister's Office and U.S. Mission Iraq

U.S. Department of Defense, Coalition Provisional Authority   **Baghdad, Iraq**

Press Assistant to the Spokesman, Office of Strategic Communications   **Sep. 2003–Jun. 2004**

- Served as CPA administrator's advance staff press lead; advanced venues for press events, press conferences, briefings, and interviews

HONORS & AWARDS

- UMMS: Community Service Award 2013, HRSA Comprehensive Geriatric Education Traineeship, Sigma Theta Tau International Nursing Honor Society
- U.S. Department of Defense Joint Civilian Service Commendation Award, Coalition Provisional Authority Service Citation, Kingdom of Spain Ministry of Foreign Affairs and Cooperation Letter of Appreciation, U.S. Navy Meritorious Unit Commendation, U.S. Navy Marksmanship Medal

APPENDIX D—BASIC CURRICULUM VITAE TEMPLATE FOR ENTRY POSITIONS

Your contact information

Name

Address

Telephone

Cell Phone

Email

EMPLOYMENT HISTORY

List in chronological order, include position details and dates

Work History

Academic Positions

Research and Training

EDUCATION

Include dates, majors, and details of degrees, training, and certification

Postdoctoral Training

Graduate School

Undergraduate University

PROFESSIONAL QUALIFICATIONS

Certifications and Accreditations

AWARDS

PUBLICATIONS

BOOKS

PROFESSIONAL MEMBERSHIPS

INTERESTS

APPENDIX E—ADVANCED CURRICULUM VITAE TEMPLATE FOR ACADEMIC POSITIONS

First Name Last Name, Degrees
Department
University/Institution
Street Address
City, State Zip code
(Area code) phone number
email@address.com

Education

Postdoctoral Training

Academic Appointments

Major Leadership Positions

Other Positions and Employment

Honors and Awards

Educational Activities

Educational Leadership, Administration, and Service

Teaching Activities in Programs and Courses

Clinical Education

Research Education

External Educational Activities

Education for the Public/Community Education

Educational Development: Curricula and Educational Materials

Advising and Mentoring

Students

Residents

Postdoctoral Trainees

Faculty

Research

Leadership Positions

Grants

Current

Completed

(continued)

Appendix E *(continued)*

Education

Pending

Current Unfunded Projects

Healthcare Delivery

Leadership Positions

Certification and Licensure

Clinical Discipline

Clinical Activities

Clinical Innovations, Safety, and Quality Improvement Projects

Clinical Guidelines and Protocols

Scholarship

Peer-Reviewed publications

Books and Chapters

Preprints and Other Interim Research Products

Policy Statements, White Papers, Reports

Nonpeer-Reviewed publications

Nonprint/Online materials

Patents

Devices/Software Applications

Invited Presentations

International

National

Regional

Local

Other Presentations, Posters, and Abstracts

International

National

Regional

Local

Academic Service

Internal Administration and Service

Department

School

(continued)

Appendix E *(continued)*

Education

Health System

University

Professional Memberships and Activities

Editorial Responsibilities

External Professional Service

International

National

Regional

Professional Development

Adapted from: www.umassmed.edu/ofa/development/cv/

32

Progressing Into Practice

DAWN CARPENTER

RECERTIFICATION

Plan ahead to maintain your licenses and certifications. Track what expires when, and have a plan to renew well before the expiration dates. Nurse practitioners (NPs) have a professional responsibility to maintain all licenses, national board certifications, and federally and state-controlled licenses as well as any required certifications (e.g., basic life support [BLS], advanced cardiac life support [ACLS], fundamentals of critical care support [FCCS], advanced trauma life support [ATLS], etc.). You are responsible for tracking expiration dates and for timely renewals. At the advanced practice level, you should not expect a manager to send reminders to renew or submit paperwork. In addition, do not expect a grace period should anything expire. The onus of responsibility is on the professional.

Renew National Board Certification

National board certifications currently require renewal every 5 years; they can be completed through the American Association of Critical-Care Nurses (AACN) or American Nurses Credentialing Center (ANCC) websites. Check the websites and renewal handbooks for their respective processes and requirements. The organizations send out reminders of impending expiration and requirements for renewal in sufficient time to allow you to complete any that may remain. Start now to confirm what is needed and acceptable for successful renewal. Develop a plan to achieve these goals as you progress in your career.

Both organizations require continuing education hours in your practice area, including specific pharmacology hours. Other activities, such as precepting, teaching, publication, research, and volunteerism, can be considered if the specific requirements for each are met. Understanding these specific requirements now and combining that knowledge with a strategic plan will make recertification simple and stress free.

The renewal process is relatively easy once you have met the requirements. To be efficient, develop a system to track contact hours and pharmacology hours as you progress through the certification period. Maintain a paper trail, as the certification organizations and state boards of nursing (SBON) perform random audits to ensure compliance with requirements. Keep hard copies of contact-hour completion certificates in case you are selected for an audit. Keep all documents in one place and organize them by date, in either chronological or reverse chronological order.

Ask if your employer tracks participation in contact-hour–bearing activities, such as monthly educational conferences, grand rounds, morbidity and mortality conferences, and other educational activities that occur at the institution. If so, obtain an annual listing of these activities for your files.

Renew Federal Drug Enforcement Agency Registration

The federal Drug Enforcement Agency (DEA) registration requires renewal every 3 years. Remember, the recertification paperwork will arrive at your place of employment, not at your home. Its failure to arrive at your department will not excuse you for failing to renew in a timely fashion. Once your FDA registration expires, you will need to start a new application. There is no grace period for renewal.

Renew State Licensing and Controlled-Substance Registration

Renewal of NP state licensing and controlled-substance registration varies by state. In both cases, you are responsible for tracking expiration dates, knowing the renewal requirements, and completing the renewal processes in sufficient time to avoid lapses.

State regulations change year to year to stay current with society's needs. It is up to the adult-gerontology acute care nurse practitioner (AG-ACNP) to stay abreast of new and revised state requirements for continuing education. Many states continue to add training requirements, such as

a. Safe opioid-prescribing training

b. Interpersonal violence screening and recognition

c. Child abuse screening and recognition

d. Pharmacology education requirements

e. Addiction treatment and management training

Words of Advice

Loose documents can get lost or misplaced. Always keep copies of your documents. Keep notes on such key information as date of submission, payment method, and amount. Be sure to maintain a paper trail. Email the medical staff office copies or photos of your documents, and copy yourself on these emails—and save them—so you can provide evidence of compliance on short notice.

Set reminders in your calendars a month or two before each of these licenses and certifications expire to allow sufficient time for renewal.

Failure to maintain current state licensure, DEA registration, state controlled-substance registration, or national board certification will result in the AG-ACNP being removed from the work and prevented from providing care to patients. Both patient care and colleagues will be significantly impacted while you work to renew a document. Be aware that once a document has expired, it may not be possible to renew and you may be required to reapply. Furthermore, depending on the institution, you likely will not get paid during this time away from of work.

Tips to Avoid Lapses

- Enter expiration dates into your calendar for automatic reminders.
- Set the reminder approximately 8 weeks ahead of the expiration date to allow time for renewal.
- Keep the license and registration numbers, with expiration dates, in the notes section of your phone or other secure location for easy access.
- Do not carry cards or licenses in your wallet, thus preventing the possible theft of your professional identity in case your wallet is lost or stolen.

■ STARTING A NEW POSITION

There are three primary domains for the new AG-ACNP to learn when starting a new position. These domains are: (a) the patient population, (b) the institution, and (c) the staff.

Study the Patient Population

Recognize that your educational program has prepared you for "entry into practice"—that is, it has ensured you have met the minimum standard to safely care for adult and geriatric patients who are acutely and/or chronically ill or have acutely changing health statuses. There is a significant depth and breadth of information that must be mastered to effectively and efficiently care for a specific population in practice. The learning curve during the first year of practice is steep. Therefore, continue to read daily to increase your knowledge about the population for whom you will be caring. Join national organizations to receive information on current evidence as it is published.

Read

The AG-ACNP needs to gain greater insights regarding the

- Common and uncommon conditions for this population
- Range of the health/illness continuum
- Anticipated illness trajectory
- Expected recovery

The AG-ACNP should expect to

- Diagnose a range of complications.
- Prescribe a range of treatments.
- Perform possible procedures that are required.

Understanding the current standards of care, landmark studies, and current areas of research and future research is essential to become a proficient, experienced provider.

Ask for a list of recommended books, clinical practice guidelines, clinical trials, and other resources specific to this population. Get a jump-start on your orientation by reading while you wait for the credentialing process to be complete. As an AG-ACNP, you are expected to be self-directed in continuing your education, as lifelong learning is a tenet of quality healthcare.

A good orientation will provide a variety of learning opportunities. Formal and informal lectures, grand rounds, a journal club, morbidity and mortality conferences, and so forth are all ways to augment learning. Attend as many of these opportunities as possible, including coming in on your days off, as this is part of your professional development.

The professional AG-ACNP should also access resources, articles, and toolkits from national organizations in the area of specialty practice. There are great resources available on their websites that can enhance your preparation to care for the population.

Join Professional Organizations

As you enter the professional field, it is appropriate and expected that you will join the appropriate professional organizations. There are multiple such organizations. Depending on the area of subspecialty, AG-ACNPs working in critical care, for example, could join AACN, Society of Critical Care Medicine, American College of Chest Physicians, Neurocritical Care Society, American College of Surgeons, and American Thoracic Society, among others. Ask members of your team to recommend organizations to you. In addition, many organizations have regional chapter memberships that provide excellent networking opportunities.

Read the professional organizations' journals, listen to podcasts, and follow Twitter feeds or Facebook posts. Stay current with advancements to ensure you provide contemporary quality care. Be sure to attend local, regional, and national conferences.

Membership can lead to involvement in these organizations. Committee work, presentations at conferences, or participation in research at the local/regional level can grow into involvement at the national level. Be sure to record this involvement on your curriculum vitae as you progress in your career.

Learn the Institution

Some AG-ACNPs are hired for a position in the organization where they have practiced as an RN or student, thus this component of the learning curve may be less steep. In these cases, the AG-ACNP is likely to be familiar with the institutional policies and processes, computer systems, staff, and so forth. Review these policies and processes through the lens of the AG-ACNP and see how they affect you in your new role.

Conversely, if you are hired by an institution where you have never worked or done a clinical rotation, the learning curve is considerably steeper. The new AG-ACNP will need to master three major areas: (a) the fine details of the position and its job responsibilities, (b) computer systems, and (c) departmental nuances.

Job Responsibilities

It is impossible to relay all aspects and details of a position during a job interview. Take time early in the orientation to review the specifics of the position, including the work flow, who does what and when, and so forth. Pay particular attention to such areas as:

- How is a typical day organized—getting handoff, prerounding, formal rounds, and clinic schedule? Who returns calls to patients? Is there any cross coverage of each other's patients?

- How to obtain a consult:
  - Does it just get entered into the computer? Is a phone call required to complete the communication?
  - Remember to call consults early in the day, as many hospitals have policies requiring inpatient consults to be completed that same day. Consults called earlier in the day will lead to more efficient use of the consultant's time and better coordination of patient care.

- How to schedule tests: AG-ACNPs frequently aid in the scheduling of diagnostic testing or therapeutic procedures. Find out who is responsible for which ones, and how such scheduling is executed.

- Filling out screening forms:
  - What diagnostic testing requires screening forms (e.g., CT scans with contrast, MRI metal screen, MRI with contrast)?
  - Identify forms the AG-ACNP is responsible for completing. Be cognizant that delays in filling out forms can result in delays in patient care.

- Procedures:
  - What procedures are you expected to perform?
  - How and when will you be trained, and by whom?
  - How do you get these procedures added to your credentialing records?
  - How do you maintain proficiency with procedures?

- Obtaining informed consent:
  - What is the institutional policy on obtaining informed consent?
  - What needs informed consent at the institution? ICU admission? Transfusion of blood products? Arterial lines? Central venous catheters?
  - Identify who has highest legal authority to consent when a patient does not have capacity to consent; this varies by state.

Tips for Success

- Keep notes in a pocket notebook or in the notes section of your phone.
- Refer to notes regularly, sometimes daily at first.
- Keep a list of names and departmental phone numbers for quick reference when you need answers to questions.

Computer Systems

Identify and obtain access to computer programs essential to the work of a AG-ACNP. Healthcare systems vary: There may be one integrated electronic health record, or the AG-ACNP may need to access a variety of programs. Systems the AG-ANCP should have access to include, for example:

- Radiology imaging systems
- ECG
- Echocardiogram (ECHO)
- Microbiology

These may require additional training on how to access and manipulate images and data. Learning to navigate complicated computer systems can be a challenge, so take full advantage of all computer training classes. Reading and interpreting x-rays and CT and ECHO scans can be a challenge, so ask to use some of your orientation time with a designated radiologist and/or cardiologist to hone those skills.

Billing

The AG-ACNP needs to have been hired by the group practice to be able to bill. AG-ACNPs hired by a hospital cannot bill for services. Coding and billing is frequently challenging for the new AG-ACNP. Institutions are required to provide billing and compliance training at the time of hire and regularly thereafter. New AG-ACNPs need to review the specifics of coding and billing a few times to fully grasp the concepts and accurately apply them to the notes and the care provided. Coding and billing is best learned by applying it to patient care.

Tips for Success

- Get to know your billing people. They are a valuable source for help in ensuring your documentation meets regulatory requirements and other billing standards.
- Review the documentation and discuss billing codes and time requirements with your preceptor or collaborating physician for every patient on a daily basis, until you become comfortable with the billing requirements.

Policies/Procedures

Whether you are new to the institution or not, review where institutional policies and processes are maintained and how to access them. View the policies through the lens of the AG-ACNP. For example, review incident reporting and determine if the AG-ACNP is expected to file reports, how to report, and what needs to be reported (e.g., unplanned events, such as extubations, or complications of procedures).

Departmental Nuances

Get to know how various departments operate. Departments that are critical for new AG-ACNPs to understand include pharmacy, respiratory therapy, nutrition, rehabilitation services (physical therapy, occupational therapy, and speech language pathology), social work, and case management. Learn how to access the staff and get to know their routines and hours of coverage. Learn how to order consults, specific diagnostic testing, and/or treatments. Pharmacy is a department worth particular mention because it contains significant components—specifically, the formulary, medication stewardship, and national drug shortages—that can impact the new AG-ACNP's ability to be efficient in the early months of a new career.

Pharmacy

Understand the institution's formulary, resource stewardship, and cost-containment strategies. As a new graduate AG-ACNP, you will still be refining your prescribing knowledge, including appropriate drug choices, alternatives, rationales for route of administration, and appropriate dosing for elderly patients and/or those with renal or hepatic impairments.

Formulary

Most institutions and patient prescription plans have contracts with pharmacy distributors, which have defined medications on their formulary. For example, an institution may have famotidine (Pepcid) as the preferred H2 blocker on formulary. Thus, if the AG-ACNP orders ranitidine (Zantac), there may be an automatic substitution policy that would convert the order to famotidine. Be aware if this process occurs and what to do if a patient has an explicit reason not to be prescribed famotidine. Alternatively, for outpatient prescriptions that are out of the patient's insurance prescription plan formulary, the additional cost of the nonformulary medication will be extended to the patient to pay out of pocket.

Stewardship

Resistance to antibiotics has created a focus on antibiotic stewardship. Thus, be aware of institutional automatic stop policies and/or restrictions on ordering specific antibiotics. For example, it is common for Automatic Stop Orders (ASOs) to be in place for perioperative antibiotics not to exceed 24 hours postop, or an order of antibiotic treatment to end after 7 days of treatment. Be aware of these policies; in the event that a treatment needs to exceed 7 days, the AG-ACNP may need to reorder the antibiotic to avoid a lapse in coverage that could cause detrimental effects to the patient.

In addition, as hospitals struggle with containing costs, it is common for institutions to have policies restricting who can order specific medications or how long the drug can be used. Many antibiotics are restricted for use so that they maintain efficacy when they are truly needed. Other medications, such as dexmedetomidine (Precedex), can be quite expensive and its use may be restricted to shorter durations to minimize costs.

Drug Shortages

Medication, electrolyte, and intravenous fluid shortages are a common and multifactorial problem that can stem from national disasters, how drugs are manufactured in cycles, medication recalls, and so forth. Learn how these shortages and their resolution are communicated within the institution. If a medication or electrolyte is ordered but is not available, how is it handled? Will the pharmacy call the provider to change or rewrite the order, or is there an automatic substitution policy?

Get to Know the Staff

The third domain for the new AG-ACNP to learn when starting a new position is to become familiar with the skill and competency of the staff you will be working with, including physician colleagues, NP or physician assistant (PA) colleagues, staff nurses, respiratory therapists, and the multitude of other departmental staff. Gain an understanding of the team's knowledge, skills, and preferences as they also learn your knowledge, skills, and critical thinking.

Assessing the Staff

Getting to know the staff is more than simply learning their names and roles; be sure to assess their knowledge and skills. Longevity does not always translate into proficiency, a solid knowledge base, or sound decision making. Identify who your resources are.

Nursing units with newer staff are more likely to need greater attention, with additional teaching and coaching to achieve the best patient outcomes. Conversely, a highly seasoned and experienced staff member may be on the verge of burnout. Ask for background and history from a well-respected peer or collaborating provider, but be sure to perform your own assessment of each staff member.

Identify the formal and informal leaders who can provide information on processes and procedures. Get to know the unit secretaries and patient care technicians (PCTs), who possess a wealth of knowledge and expertise. They know how to get things done and where things are kept. Do not undervalue or underappreciate them.

Expect to Be Challenged

The staff will also assess your knowledge, skills, and decision making. Expect to be questioned or challenged as they determine your ability to explain and articulate rationales for your decisions. To build staff's confidence in your knowledge and skill, share your thought process and reasoning. Take the time to explain why you are requesting specific interventions, define the expected or desired outcomes, and specify those details of which you want to be informed.

Provider Specific Preferences

Learning the preferences and nuances of colleagues and collaborating providers takes time. Keep in mind that there are multiple ways to achieve the same great outcomes for patient care. Healthcare is as much an art as it is a science. Evidence-based care includes individual experiences as well as the best evidence. For this reason, there is variability in practice patterns and preferences despite widely utilized clinical practice guidelines. It is helpful to inquire if collaborating providers and colleagues have specific preferences or nuances in their approach to care.

Tips for Success

- Ask the collaborating providers about their preferences and items to which they pay particular attention.
- Ask your preceptor and colleagues for insights so you can be prepared.
- Write these preferences in a notebook and refer to them before each shift.
- Update your notes regularly.

■ GET ESTABLISHED

As you proceed into practice and become established, realize it may take you a year in your new role to feel confident. The learning curve is steep in the first year, so be patient with yourself. Ask for feedback on your performance and how you can improve. As you become established in your practice, be sure to track practice hours and procedures. Lastly, once you have a year or two of experience, consider precepting a student AG-ACNP.

Get Feedback

Obtaining feedback on how you are doing is key to continued professional growth. You may need to ask for this feedback from experienced colleagues and physician staff. Ask specific questions:

- How are my patient presentations? Are they organized and coherent?
- How are my treatment plans? Are they thorough and complete?
- In what areas should I do more reading?
- How am I perceived by the staff?
- How was my management of this specific patient situation? Is there anything I could have done differently? Any suggestions for me for the next time I encounter this situation?

Obtain feedback from a variety of people on a regular basis. Many times this information is not offered, especially in situations where formal orientation evaluation processes are not fully developed.

Ask for feedback on your documentation and billing. Ask to meet with a documentation specialist or coder to assess the completeness and accuracy of your documentation. Review your billing data on a regular basis and ask how you compare to the group. Are you underbilling or overbilling for services?

After you perform a procedure, take a few minutes to debrief the person who trained you or supervised the procedure. Specifically, ask what you did well and what you should or could do differently next time.

Practice-Hour Documentation

Documentation of clinical practice hours is exceptionally important to retain and maintain as you progress through your career. It is impossible to predict where life will take you. You may end up moving from a collaborative practice state to a state that has independent practice. Thus, possessing documentation of previous supervised practice hours is imperative for licensure in the state with independent practice.

Keeping clinical logs, such as Typhon, or other electronic or written records of clinical hours in an educational program is also essential. As you progress through your career, obtain written documentation to support the supervised clinical hours that includes dates, number of hours, and by whom they were supervised, as they will be required when applying for independent practice in another state. It is not uncommon for collaborating providers to retire andmove away, becoming unreachable when this documentation is needed years later. By keeping meticulous records throughout your career, you will have what you need when the time comes.

Track Procedures

For the same reason previously mentioned, track the procedures you perform. Should you happen to change employers and need to demonstrate proficiency or that you meet the criteria to be credentialed, you will require documentation. Some organizations have a computer system to log procedures and others do not. In the latter case, you will need to create your own tracking system in a Word document or Excel spreadsheet.

Give Back

As this book comes to a close, take a moment to reflect on the wonderful opportunities that were provided you to get you where you are right now. Consider how you can help the next generation of AG-ACNPs. Your time and expertise can support the next cohort of learners become successful in their new field.

Once you have a year or two of experience, reach out to your faculty or program coordinator/director to offer to precept an AG-ACNP student or lecture to the current class. NPs are frequently tasked with precepting medical students or PA students. My challenge to you is to reach out to your faculty or closest AG-ACNP program to request to precept an AG-ACNP student.

Alternatively, financial donations to your school can support educational tools or scholarships. Consider a donation to your alma mater.

Index